INTRODUCTION TO RADIOGRAPHY AND PATIENT CARE

INTRODUCTION TO RADIOGRAPHY AND PATIENT CARE

Second Edition

ARLENE M. ADLER, MEd, RT(R), FAERS

Professor and Director
Radiologic Sciences Programs
Indiana University Northwest
Gary, Indiana

RICHARD R. CARLTON, MS, RT(R)(CV), FAERS

Assistant Professor of Radiologic Sciences
Arkansas State University
State University, Arkansas

DTF

W.B. SAUNDERS COMPANY
A Division of Harcourt Brace & Company
Philadelphia London Toronto Montreal Sydney Tokyo

W.B. SAUNDERS COMPANY
A Division of Harcourt Brace & Company

The Curtis Center
Independence Square West
Philadelphia, Pennsylvania 19106

Library of Congress Cataloging-in-Publication Data

Introduction to radiography and patient care / [edited by] Arlene M. Adler, Richard R. Carlton.—2nd ed.

p.   cm.

Includes bibliographical references and index.

ISBN 0–7216–7662–6

1. Radiology, Medical.   2. Radiologic technologists.   I. Adler, Arlene McKenna.   II. Carlton, Richard R.   [DNLM: 1. Radiography.
2. Professional—Patient Relations.   WN200 I6155 1999]

R898.I55   1999   616.07′572′—dc21

DNLM/DLC   98–25697

INTRODUCTION TO RADIOGRAPHY AND PATIENT CARE   ISBN 0–7216–7662–6

Printed in the United States of America.

Last digit is the print number: 9   8   7   6   5   4   3   2   1

NWST
ALE0374

To

Don, Meredith, and Katie Adler

and to

D. Raleigh and Hazel Carlton

Contributors

Arlene M. Adler, MEd, RT(R), FAERS
Professor and Director, Radiologic
   Sciences Programs, Indiana
   University Northwest, Gary, Indiana
Introduction to Radiologic Technology;
   Professional Organizations; History
   Taking

Janice L. Akin, MS
Manager, Educational Services, St.
   Margaret Mercy Healthcare Centers,
   Hammond and Dyer, Indiana
Educational Survival Skills

Jane A. Auger, MD
Resident in Diagnostic Imaging, Brown
   University/Rhode Island Hospital,
   Providence, Rhode Island
Radiographic Imaging

Judith Baron, MS, RT(R)
Professor Emerita, Medical Imaging
   and Biology, College of Lake County,
   Grayslake, Illinois
Contrast Media

Jan Bruckner, PhD, PT
Director of Research, Department of
   Physical Therapy, Thomas Jefferson
   University, Philadelphia, Pennsylvania
Transfer Techniques

Robert A. Buerki, PhD
Professor, Division of Pharmacy
   Practice and Administration, The
   Ohio State University College of
   Pharmacy, Columbus, Ohio
Professional Ethics

Nadia A. Bugg, PhD, RT(R)
Professor/Graduate Coordinator,
   Radiologic Sciences, Midwestern
   State University, Wichita Falls, Texas
Pharmacology

Richard R. Carlton, MS, RT(R)(CV), FAERS
Assistant Professor of Radiologic
   Sciences, Arkansas State University,
   State University, Arkansas
Introduction to Radiologic Technology;
   Professional Organizations; Patient
   Interactions; History Taking

Steven B. Dowd, EdD, RT(R), (QM), (MR)(M)
Associate Professor, Division of Medical
   Imaging and Therapy, University of
   Alabama at Birmingham,
   Birmingham, Alabama
Aseptic Techniques; Nonaseptic Techniques

Jody L. Ellis, MPA, RT(R)
Program Director, Radiologic
   Technology Program, South
   Suburban College, South Holland,
   Illinois
Infection Control

Joanne S. Greathouse, EdS, RT(R)
Associate Director, Joint Review
   Committee on Education in
   Radiologic Technology, Chicago,
   Illinois
Medical Emergencies

Scott T. Gregory, MS, RT(R)
Chairperson Emeritus and Associate
   Professor Emeritus, Department of
   Radiologic Sciences, Medical College
   of Georgia, Augusta, Georgia
Radiographic and Fluoroscopic Equipment

Karen Jefferies, BS, RT(R)
Assistant Professor, Program in
   Radiography, Wright College,
   Chicago, Illinois
Basic Radiation Protection and Radiobiology

Marlene E. Ledbetter, MEd, RT(R)
Associate Professor, Radiologic Sciences, and Clinical Coordinator, Radiography, Indiana University Northwest, Gary, Indiana
Introduction to Clinical Education

Denise E. Moore, BS, RT(R)
Professor and Chairperson, Radiologic Technology Program, Sinclair Community College, Dayton, Ohio
Vital Signs and Oxygen

C. William Mulkey, EdD, RT(R), FASRT, FAERS
Program Director, Radiologic Sciences, Midlands Technical College, Columbia, South Carolina
Patient Interactions

Gail A. Nielsen, BSHCA, RT(R), FAHRA
Manager, Managed Care, Health Information Analysis and Business Development, Allen Memorial Hospital, Waterloo, Iowa
Radiologic Services Administration

Ann Obergfell, JD, RT(R)
Associate Professor, Radiologic Technology Program, University of Louisville, Louisville, Kentucky
Medical Law

Cheryl Oprisko, JD, RRT
Assistant Professor and Director of Respiratory Therapy Program, Indiana University Northwest, Gary, Indiana
Vital Signs and Oxygen

Margaret A. Skurka, MS, RRA, CCS
Professor, Health Information Management, Allied Health Sciences Division, Indiana University Northwest, Gary, Indiana
Health Records and Health Information Management

Dennis Spragg, MS Ed, RT(R)
Chairman/Associate Professor of Medical Imaging, Lima Technical College, Lima, Ohio
Immobilization Techniques

Louis D. Vottero, MS
Professor Emeritus, Department of Pharmacy and Health Care Administration, Ohio Northern University, Ada, Ohio
Professional Ethics

Foreword to First Edition

Introduction to Radiography and Patient Care provides an exceptional overview of the radiologic sciences profession and its patient care aspects, which will make the discovery process about them one of the high points in a student's educational career. In 1965, after graduating from high school, I began working an an electrocardiography technician. Through that experience, which I continued for three years, I knew I wanted a career in a health care profession but was unsure about which one. Working in a hospital gave me the unusual opportunity to begin observing various professionals in their everyday work. I found radiologic technology interesting but didn't known where to turn to find out more about it. This book would have been the missing resource I needed.

Individual readers will find different sections rewarding. In Units I and II, the student is provided information about the vast number of opportunities available to the radiologic technologist and about the vital role of radiologic technologists in the health care team. Those who are willing to use the skills they will learn by reading this book will have many avenues open to them. This knowledge and the learned skills will enable them to continue to move toward a rewarding future no matter what direction they would like that future to be.

I have had the pleasure to speak with many radiologic technologists from across the country and have found it amazing how few have a grasp of the function and need for our professional organizations. This text provides information that should be invaluable in encouraging individuals to involve themselves in the growth of the profession through the only mechanism available—their professional organizations.

As I read through each page, several things came to mind. First, I recognized the purpose of the book and the important aspect it will play in the educational process. I saw it not only as a publication to enlighten students about the radiologic sciences professions but also as a resource for technologists, such as myself, who have been in the field for a while. It delves into areas not covered in my radiologic technology education. In addition, I was impressed with the quality of the writing. It made me wish I had been involved in writing it as well.

The technical nature of the radiologic technologist's work is vast, and most educational experiences deal with this technical aspect. However, with the dynamic changes occurring in health care, much more emphasis is being placed, and rightfully so, on the nontechnical aspect of our profession: *service*. This book will help expand the student's knowledge base in these areas. Patients have no concept of film quality because they rarely see that outcome. Thus, they can rely only on the appearance, attitude, and other patient care observances of the technologist to assure them that quality procedures are being performed.

Unit III does an excellent job of enhancing the educational experience of the students in the vital patient care aspects of their profession. It covers both the affective aspects of patient care, such as communication and good history-taking, as well as the more technical sides, such as infection control and aseptic techniques. Unit IV provides a good introduction to the medical legal and ethical issues of the profession.

The list of contributing authors is impressive. I am pleased to say that not only are these individuals highly talented and knowledgeable, but I consider myself fortunate enough to be able to refer to many of them as "friends." Reading this book has deepened my professional respect for these individuals. Their desire to provide this high-quality educational tool in such an excellent format should be highly commended by all radiologic technologists.

It is with great pride that I recommend this book to all educators for use and incorporation into their programs. Technologists who have been practicing in the profession should also find it rewarding. I learned a great deal by reading the book and am confident that others will have the same positive experience. We all need to continually grow and expand our knowledge.

John F. Kennedy frequently defined happiness as "the full use of your powers along the lines of excellence." The authors of *Introduction to Radiography and Patient Care* should be most pleased with the outcome of their efforts. Each reader will be enriched by the experience. We all strive toward the goal of excellence, and I believe this book will help our future technologists achieve that goal.

BARBARA A. BURNHAM, RT(R), FASRT, FAHRA

Preface

The enthusiasm with which the first edition of *Introduction to Radiography and Patient Care* has been received over the past five years has justified the efforts of our group of authors from both the radiologic sciences and the other health professions. In speaking with the original team of writers as well as the new faces we've recruited for this second edition, we are most proud of the fact that we have become the starting point for the professional careers of so many radiographers. It's a sacred professional trust that we take very seriously, and we hope you will agree that this is evident in the numerous updates, clarifications, expanded coverage, and new topics we've added as a result of the commentary we've received from students and faculty. To continue to keep students and faculty current and up-to-date, we have developed a web site for the text at **www.clt.astate.edu/rcarlton/Intro.htm.**

We remain committed to providing a reasonably priced but comprehensive introduction to our profession. We continue to strive to provide the breadth necessary to permit well-informed and properly oriented students their first real clinical practice. We attempt to pry open the doors to technical areas sufficiently that students will respect not only what they know but how much they *don't* know as well. We have found that the most dangerous person in a school may well be the first year student who has had an introduction to psychology but has not yet glimpsed the vast depth of knowledge in this field. The danger, of course, is not in what the student knows, but in the failure to appreciate what they *don't* know. We hope we have avoided setting anyone up for this error by treating our readers as serious new professionals perfectly capable of deducing the potential dangers of the clinical environment while at the same time beginning to learn how to function competently in a manner that begins to make a contribution to our field.

The major changes in this edition include:

- expanded and current standard (universal) precautions
- a new section on chest tubes and lines
- updated and expanded information on radiation protection for pregnant students
- expanded information on drug interactions with water-soluble iodine contrast media
- significant revisions and an additional case study in professional ethics
- updated materials on the security of health information
- an expanded patient history-taking guide
- a complete update of state licensing agencies in Appendix C
- addition of the ASRT radiography practice standards in Appendix A

We continue to assume full responsibility for any errors, including those that may be construed as having arisen from quoting others out of context. We have made every effort to ensure the accuracy of the information. We ask that you remember that it is the responsibility of every practitioner to evaluate the appropriateness of a particular procedure in the context of an actual clinical situation. Consequently, neither the authors nor the publisher takes responsibility or accepts any liability for the actions of persons applying the information contained herein in an unprofessional manner.

We highly value your point of view. We have learned that the most precious commodity for an author is criticism. As the reader, your perceptions are very important to us, and we always appreciate your communications regarding any aspect of the book you like, dislike, or would like to see changed. As in all our books, we point out that a book such as this is never finished, but merely abandoned until the next edition.

ARLENE M. ADLER, MED, RT(R), FAERS
aadler@iunhaw1.iun.indiana.edu

RICHARD R. CARLTON, MS, RT(R)(CV), FAERS
rcarlton@crow.astate.edu

> For additional up-to-date information, contact our web site at
>
> www.clt.astate.edu/rcarlton/Intro.htm

Acknowledgments

Students are always the best teachers, and I've had some of the very greatest at Lima Technical College in Lima, Ohio; City College of San Francisco; Mills-Peninsula School of Radiologic Technology, Burlingame, California; Memphis' Methodist School of Radiologic Technology; and at Arkansas State University. I thank you all for listening and valuing what I have tried to teach you. Without the constant and solid support of Lyn Hubbard and Jeannean Gray, the RadSci faculty at Arkansas State, I doubt this edition would have been finished. It was a pleasure working with Jeannean and our new model, her daughter Taylor, for which I thank you both. Our appreciation is extended to Curtis Steele, the Art Department Chair at Arkansas State, for the great job updating our photographs. Finally, and nowhere near last, I must confess to Ray Winters and our Dean, Dr. Susan Hanrahan, that I am at a loss to express my thanks for bringing me to Arkansas State and giving me a role in the new wave of radiologic sciences education.

RICHARD R. CARLTON, MS, RT(R)(CV), FAERS

Preface to First Edition

This textbook was designed to meet the needs of programs requiring an introductory text for the profession of radiologic technology while also encompassing the concepts of basic patient care skills. In speaking to educators across the country, we found that many programs provide introductory concepts within their patient care course, but students had to purchase two or more textbooks for this one course. We have tried to combine this material into one comprehensive text.

The text is divided into four units for a total of 22 chapters. The first unit, entitled The Profession of Radiologic Technology, contains three chapters on an introduction to radiologic technology, professional organizations, and educational survival skills. The second unit, Introduction to the Clinical Environment, contains five chapters on an introduction to clinical education, radiologic services administration, radiographic imaging, radiographic and fluoroscopic equipment, and basic radiation protection and radiobiology. The third unit details Patient Care and contains eleven chapters on such content as patient interactions, history taking, transfer techniques, immobilization techniques, vital signs and oxygen, infection control, aseptic techniques, nonaseptic techniques, medical emergencies, pharmacology, and contrast media. The last unit outlines Ethical and Legal Issues and contains three chapters on professional ethics, medical records and health information, and medical law.

Throughout our travels as radiography educators we have come in contact with many wonderful professionals who have contributed, each in his or her own way, to enhancing our profession. We decided to call on the talents of many of these educators and practitioners when we began planning this text. A wealth of talent has been gathered together to produce this book. While most of this talent belongs to radiologic technologists, we did call on certain allied health specialists to assist us as well. For example, the chapter on transfer techniques was written by a physical therapy educator; the chapter on vital signs and oxygen was written by two respiratory therapy educators; and the chapter on medical records and health information was written by a health information technology educator. In addition, a radiographer/lawyer wrote the chapter on medical law.

Although we assume full responsibility for any errors, including those that may be construed as having arisen from quoting others out of context, we have made every effort to ensure the accuracy of the information. It is important to remember that it is the responsibility of every practitioner to evaluate the appropriateness of a particular procedure in the context of an actual clinical situation. Consequently, neither the authors nor the publishers take responsibility or accept any liability for the actions of persons applying the information contained herein in an unprofessional manner. This information is designed to enhance and supplement the instructional methodologies of educators in accredited programs in radiography, radiation therapy technology, nuclear medicine technology, and sonography and should not be applied, especially to human subjects, without this essential background.

As the reader, your perceptions are very important to us. We would very much appreciate communicating with you regarding any aspect of the book you like, dislike, or would like to see changed. We especially appreciate constructive comments and notice of errors. Your comments will be welcomed and valued. A book such as this is never finished, but merely abandoned for the time being.

ARLENE M. ADLER, MEd, RT(R)

RICHARD R. CARLTON, MS, RT(R)(CV)

Acknowledgments for the First Edition

The professional assistance provided by the following persons proved invaluable as we developed the chapters: Marlene E. Ledbetter, M.Ed., R.T. (R); Carol Collins, R.T.; Steven Crawford, B.S., R.T. (R); Jody L. Ellis, B.A., R.T. (R); Barb Hanna, R.T. (R); Robin Jones, B.S., R.T. (R); Carla Mock, B.S., R.T. (R); Traci O'Donnell, A.S., R.T. (R); Sandy Piehl, M.P.A., R.T. (T) (R); LaVerne Ramaeker, Ed.D., R.T. (R); Laura Richards, R.T. (R); Marie Ross, A.S., R.T. (R); Deb Sobota, A.S., R.T. (R); Sue Wilson, A.S., R.T. (R); and Sue Woods, A.S., R.T. (R), all with the Radiologic Sciences Programs at Indiana University Northwest; Dennis Spragg, M.S.Ed., R.T. (R); Andy Shappell, B.S., R.T. (R); Mike Wurst, R.N., E.M.T–P., Chairman Emergency Medical Technician Program; Chris McDonald, R.P.T., Chairman, Physical Therapist Assistant Program; Sandy Kinkle, R.N.; Bob Casto, M.S., R.R.T.; and Tish Hatfield, B.S., R.R.T., all of Lima Technical College; and Susan Robinson at Riley Children's Hospital, Indiana University Medical Center, Indianapolis.

Bill Mulkey wishes to acknowledge his wife, Paula, for her unselfishness and for being the radiographer this book teaches us all to be.

Steve Dowd wishes to acknowledge the support of Mark Harbaugh, Ph.D., Joan Lewis, M.S.N., and the Radiography Program Class of 1992, all of Lincoln Land Community College; Mike Drafke, M.S., R.T. (R), for providing critical review; and Bettye Wilson, M.A.Ed., R.T. (R), of the University of Alabama Radiography Program, for providing radiographs and securing some of the items used in the photos.

Judy Baron's chapter was due in part to efforts by Mark Gajewski, Margaret Goodwin, Shane Harvey, Nancy Kolb, Dr. Richard Mintzer, Dr. Bernard Sakowicz, David Skarbek, Pamela Thurow, and Margaret Weaver in providing radiographs and contrast media package inserts and for reviewing, typing, and retyping the manuscript.

Most of the photographs were made possible through the courtesy and cooperation of the Radiology Department at St. Rita's Medical Center in Lima, Ohio. Special thanks are owed Edyta Postolowicz, Dennis Stryker, Brian Nye, John Jacobs, Jill Steinbrenner, and Sally Singer. Without Judy Piehl, radiology nurse at St. Rita's, we would never have been able to acquire all the props for our photo sessions. Appreciation is also extended to our photographers, Jenny Torbett from the Biomedical Communications Department at the Ohio State University, and George D. Greathouse of Richmond, Virginia. Many of our photographs were great because of the spectacular performance of the best pediatric model ever, Meredith Adler.

ARLENE M. ADLER, MED, RT(R), FAERS
RICHARD R. CARLTON, MS, RT(R)(CV), FAERS

Contents

UNIT III

Patient Care

UNIT IV

Ethical and Legal Issues

UNIT

1

The Profession of Radiologic Technology

CHAPTER 1

INTRODUCTION TO RADIOLOGIC TECHNOLOGY

Arlene M. Adler, MEd, RT(R), FAERS
Richard R. Carlton, MS, RT(R) (CV), FAERS

During World War I the demand for x-ray technicians in military hospitals was so great that a shortage of technical workers became acute at home. The value of the well-trained technician was emphasized, and the radiologist was no longer satisfied with someone who knew only how to throw the switch and develop films.

MARGARET HOING, THE FIRST LADY OF RADIOLOGIC TECHNOLOGY
A HISTORY OF THE AMERICAN SOCIETY OF X-RAY TECHNICIANS, 1952

OBJECTIVES

On completion of this chapter, the student will be able to:

1 Explain the use of radiation in medicine.
2 Describe the discovery of x-rays.
3 Define terms related to radiologic technology.
4 Explain the career opportunities within the profession of radiologic technology.
5 Identify the various specialties within a radiology department.
6 Describe the typical responsibilities of the members of the radiology team.
7 Explain the career ladder opportunities within a radiology department.
8 Discuss the roles of other members of the health care team.

GLOSSARY

Cardiovascular Interventional Technology (CIT): radiologic procedures for the diagnosis and treatment of diseases of the cardiovascular system

Computed Tomography (CT): recording of a predetermined plane in the body by use of an x-ray beam that is measured by a scintillation counter, recorded on a magnetic disk, and then processed by a computer for display on a cathode ray tube

Diagnostic Medical Sonography: visualization of deep structures of the body by recording the reflections of pulses of ultrasonic waves directed into the tissue

Energy: capacity to operate or work

Ionization: any process by which a neutral atom gains or loses an electron, thus acquiring a net charge

Magnetic Resonance Imaging (MRI): process of using a magnetic field and radio frequencies to create sectional images of the body

Mammography: radiography of the breast

Nuclear Medicine Technology: branch of radiology that involves the introduction of radioactive substances into the body for both diagnostic and therapeutic purposes

Radiation: energy transmitted by waves through space or through a medium

Radiation Therapy: branch of radiology involved in the treatment of disease by means of x-rays or radioactive substances

Radiography: making of film records (radiographs) of internal structures of the body by passage of x-rays or gamma rays through the body to act on specially sensitized film

Radiologic Technologist: general term applied to an individual who performs radiography, radiation therapy, or nuclear medicine technology

Radiologist: physician who specializes in the use of roentgen rays and other forms of radiation in the diagnosis and treatment of disease

Radiology: branch of the health sciences dealing with radioactive substances and radiant energy and with the diagnosis and treatment of disease by means of both ionizing (eg, roentgen rays) and non-ionizing (eg, ultrasound) radiation

Roentgen Ray: synonym for x-ray

X-ray: electromagnetic vibrations of short wavelength that are produced when electrons moving at high velocity impinge on various substances, especially the heavy metals

Synonym for x-ray

Medical Radiation Sciences

When the term *radiation* is used, it generally evokes concern and a sense of danger. This is unfortunate because not only is radiation helpful, it is essential to life. **Radiation** is energy that is transmitted by waves through space or through a medium (matter). It has permeated the universe since the beginning of time. Radiation is a natural part of all of our lives. For example, the sun radiates light energy and a stove radiates heat energy.

Energy is the capacity to operate or work. There are many different forms of energy, including mechanical, electrical, heat, nuclear, and electromagnetic. Many forms of energy are used in medicine to create images of anatomic structures or physiologic actions. These images are essential for the proper diagnosis of disease and treatment of the patient. All of these energy forms can be described as radiation because they can be, and in many instances must be, transmitted through matter.

Some higher-energy forms, including x-rays, have the ability to ionize atoms in matter. **Ion-**

ization is any process by which a neutral atom gains or loses an electron, thus acquiring a net charge. This process has the ability to disrupt the composition of the matter and, as a result, is capable of disrupting life processes. Special protection should be provided to prevent excessive exposure to ionizing radiation.

Sound is a form of mechanical energy. It is transmitted through matter, and images can be created of the returning sound waves. Diagnostic medical sonography is the field of study that creates anatomic images from sound waves that have passed through the body. Sound waves are a form of non-ionizing radiation.

Electrocardiography and electroencephalography are methods of imaging the electrical activities of the heart and of the brain, respectively. The graphs they produce provide useful information about the physiologic activities of these organs.

The body's naturally emitted heat energy can produce images for diagnostic purposes as well. These images are called *thermograms*, and they can be useful in demonstrating such conditions as changes in the body's circulation.

Nuclear energy is emitted by the nucleus of an atom. Nuclear medicine technology uses this type of energy to create images of both anatomic structures and physiologic actions. It involves the introduction of a radioactive substance into the body for diagnostic and therapeutic purposes. These substances emit gamma radiation from their nuclei. Gamma radiation is a form of electromagnetic energy that has the ability to ionize atoms. As a result, proper radiation protection is important in the nuclear medicine department.

There are many forms of electromagnetic energy (Fig. 1–1). Many of these are used in medicine to deliver high-quality patient care. For example, light is an essential energy form in many of the scopes physicians use to view inside the body. In addition, x-rays are a man-made form of electromagnetic energy. They are created when electrons moving at high speed are suddenly stopped. X-rays, also called **roentgen rays** after their discoverer, Röntgen, allow physicians to visualize many of the anatomic structures that were once visible only at surgery.

Radiography is the making of film records, known as *radiographs*, of internal structures of the body by passage of x-rays or gamma rays through the body to act on specially sensitized film. In the diagnostic radiography department, images are created using x-rays that pass through the body (Fig. 1–2). In addition, very high energy x-rays are used in the radiation therapy department for the treatment of many forms of cancer. In both of these departments, proper radiation protection is essential.

Radio waves are another form of electromagnetic radiation. They are a non-ionizing form of radiation and are important in the creation of magnetic resonance images (Fig. 1–3).

Medical radiation science involves the study of the use of radiation throughout medicine. It should be apparent that many forms of radiation are used in all branches of medicine.

The History of Radiologic Technology

—compare to anode.

The field of radiologic technology was born on November 8, 1895. On that day, Wilhelm Conrad Röntgen, a German physicist, was working in his laboratory at the University of Wurzburg. Röntgen had been experimenting with cathode rays and was exploring their properties outside glass tubes. He had covered the glass tube to prevent any visible light from escaping. During this work, Röntgen observed that a screen that had been painted with barium platinocyanide was emitting light (*fluorescing*). This effect had to be caused by invisible rays being emitted from the tube. During the next several weeks, Röntgen investigated these invisible rays. It was during his investigation that he saw the very first radiographic image, his own skeleton. Röntgen became the first radiographer when he produced a series of photographs of radiographic images, most notably the image of his wife's hand (Fig. 1–4). He termed these invisible rays x-rays because x was the mathematical symbol for an unknown variable.

Wilhelm Conrad Röntgen was born in Lennep, Germany, on March 27, 1845. In 1872, he married Anna Bertha Ludwig (1839–1919), and they had one adopted daughter. In 1888, he began working at the University of Wurzburg in the physics department. During the 1870s and 1880s, many physics departments were experimenting with cathode rays, electrons emanating from the negative (cathode) terminal of a tube. The tube that Röntgen was working with during his discovery was a Crookes tube. Sir William Crookes (1832–1919) used a large, partially evacuated glass tube that encompassed a cathode and an anode attached to an electrical supply. His tube was the early version of the

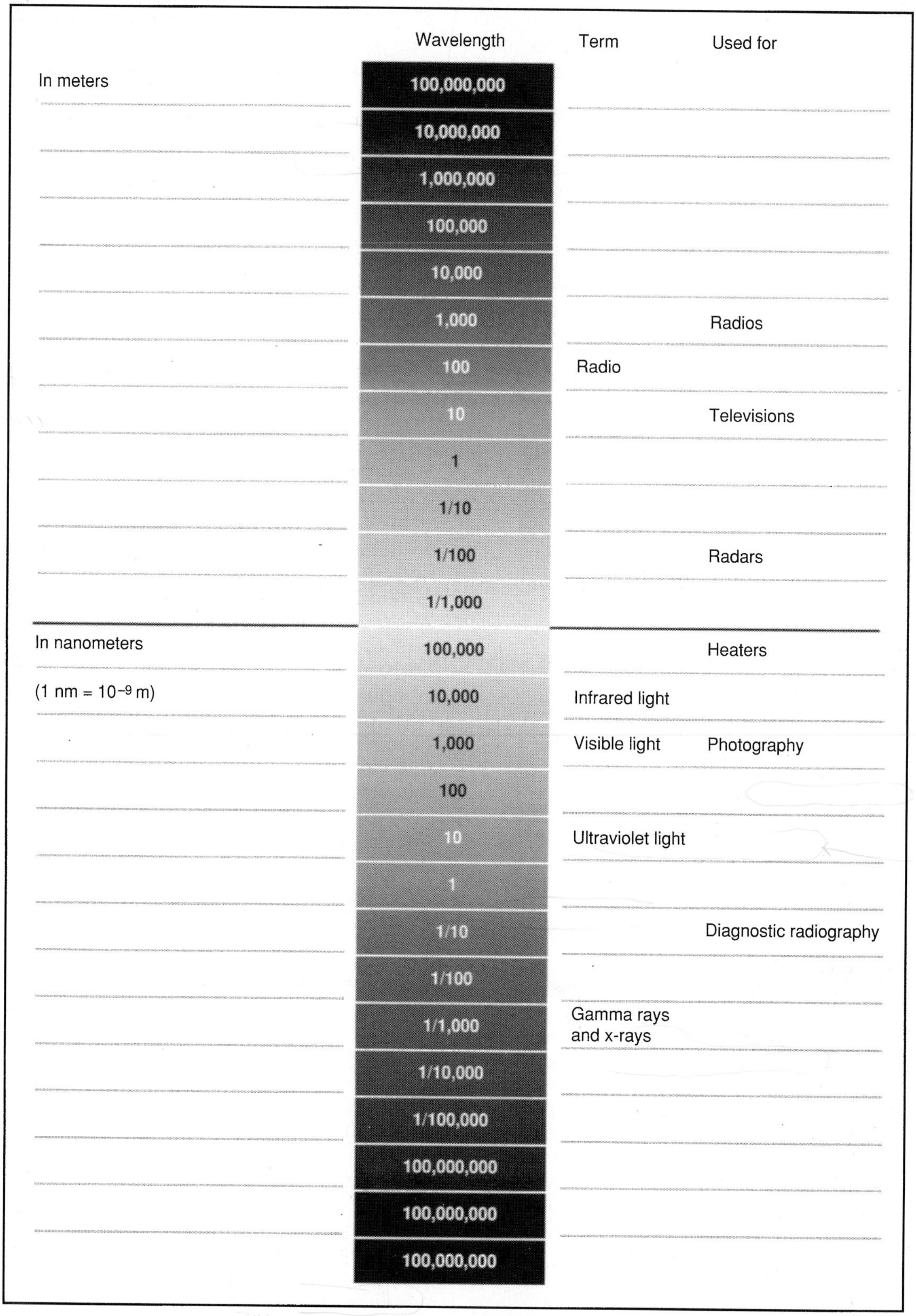

	Wavelength	Term	Used for
In meters	100,000,000		
	10,000,000		
	1,000,000		
	100,000		
	10,000		
	1,000		Radios
	100	Radio	
	10		Televisions
	1		
	1/10		
	1/100		Radars
	1/1,000		
In nanometers	100,000		Heaters
(1 nm = 10^{-9} m)	10,000	Infrared light	
	1,000	Visible light	Photography
	100		
	10	Ultraviolet light	
	1		
	1/10		Diagnostic radiography
	1/100		
	1/1,000	Gamma rays and x-rays	
	1/10,000		
	1/100,000		
	100,000,000		
	100,000,000		
	100,000,000		

FIGURE 1–1. The electromagnetic spectrum.

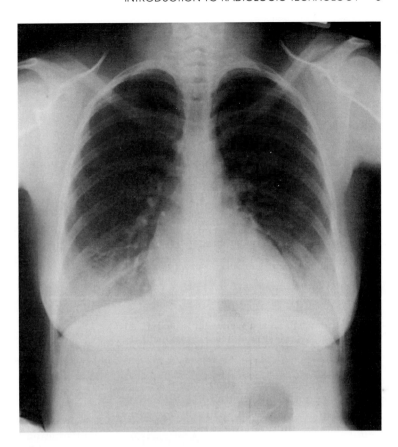

FIGURE 1–2. Radiograph of the chest. (Courtesy of Robin Jones, B.S., R.T.(R.), Methodist Hospital Southlake Campus, Merrillville, Indiana.

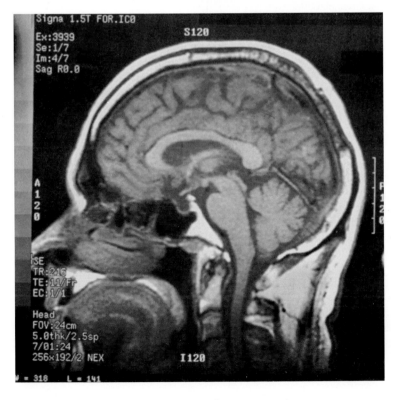

FIGURE 1–3. Sagittal image of the brain created using magnetic resonance imaging. (Courtesy of Robin Jones, B.S., R.T.(R.), Methodist Hospital Southlake Campus, Merrillville, Indiana.)

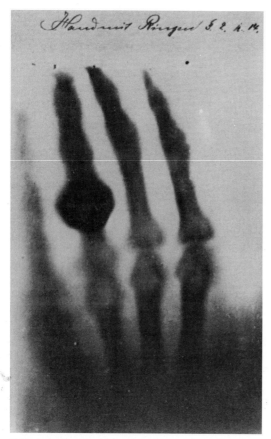

FIGURE 1–4. The first radiograph was an image of Wilhelm Röntgen's wife's hand.

modern fluorescent light. Crookes actually produced x-rays during his experimentation in the 1870s but failed to grasp the significance of his finding. He often found that photographic plates stored near his work table were fogged. He even returned fogged photographic plates to the manufacturer, claiming they were defective. Many physicists created x-rays during the course of their work with cathode rays, but Röntgen was the first to appreciate the significance of the penetrating rays.

The actual day that the significance of Röntgen's finding became clear to him is the subject of much debate; however, Friday, November 8, 1895, is believed by historians to be the day that Röntgen created the famous image of his wife's hand (see Fig. 1–4). On Saturday, December 28, 1895, Röntgen submitted his first report, titled "On a New Kind of Rays," to the Wurzburg Physico-Medical Society. Through his investigative methods, Röntgen identified

the properties of x-rays. His methods were so thorough that no significant additions have been made to his work.

For his efforts, W.C. Röntgen was honored, in 1901, with the first Nobel Prize in physics. He refused to patent any part of his discovery and rejected many commercial company offers. As a result, he saw little financial reward for his work. He died on February 10, 1923, of colon cancer.

Opportunities in Radiologic Technology

Radiologic technology is the technical science that deals with the use of x-rays or radioactive substances for diagnostic or therapeutic purposes in medicine. **Radiologic technologist** is a general term applied to individuals qualified to use x-rays (radiography) or radioactive substances (nuclear medicine) to produce images of the internal parts of the body for interpretation by a physician known as a **radiologist**. Radiologic technology also involves the use of x-rays or radioactive substances in the treatment of disease (radiation therapy).

In addition to the use of x-rays and radioactive substances, radiologic technologists have become involved in using high-frequency sound waves (diagnostic medical sonography) and magnetic fields and radio waves (magnetic resonance imaging) to create images of the internal anatomy of the body.

RADIOGRAPHY

A radiologic technologist specializing in the use of x-rays to create images of the body is known as a *radiographer* (Fig. 1–5). Radiographers perform a wide variety of diagnostic x-ray procedures, including examinations of the skeletal system, the chest, and the abdomen. They administer contrast media to visualize the gastrointestinal tract and the genitourinary system. They also assist the radiologist during more specialized contrast media procedures, such as those used to visualize the spinal cord (myelography) and the joint spaces (arthrography).

To become a registered radiographer, an individual must complete an accredited radiography

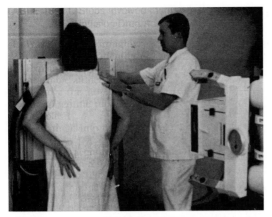

FIGURE 1–5. A radiographer positions a patient for a radiographic examination.

program. Programs are most commonly sponsored by hospitals, community colleges, and universities. Upon successful completion of an accredited program, individuals are awarded a certificate, an associate degree, or a baccalaureate degree and are eligible to take the national examination in radiography offered by the American Registry of Radiologic Technologists (ARRT). A registered radiographer uses the initials RT(R) after his or her name. This abbreviation means *registered technologist (radiography)*.

Appendix A contains Clinical Practice Standards for Radiography along with position descriptions for the staff radiographer, nuclear medicine technologist, radiation therapist, and diagnostic medical sonographer developed by the American Society of Radiologic Technologists (ASRT).

Cardiovascular Interventional Technology

Radiographers can specialize in performing radiologic examinations of the cardiovascular system, a discipline called **cardiovascular interventional technology.** These procedures involve the injection of iodinated contrast media for diagnosing diseases of the heart and blood vessels. *Angiography* is the radiologic examination of the blood vessels after injection of a contrast medium. Most often, the contrast material is injected through a catheter. The catheter can be directed to a variety of major arteries for visualization of these structures. By way of a catheter, it is relatively easy to inject contrast media into such structures as the carotid arteries

leading to the brain, the renal arteries leading to the kidneys, the femoral artery of the leg, and many other sites.

Placing a catheter into one of the chambers of the heart is termed *cardiac catheterization.* This catheter can then be directed into one or both of the two main arteries that supply blood to the heart itself. These arteries are called the *coronary arteries.*

Coronary arteriography is an extremely valuable tool in diagnosing atherosclerosis, which can block the coronary arteries and cause a heart attack (myocardial infarction). By way of a special catheter with a balloon tip, effective treatment of atherosclerosis is possible. This treatment of a blocked blood vessel is termed *angioplasty.* Angioplasty is used to treat patients without the need for invasive open heart surgery.

Cardiovascular interventional technology involves the use of highly specialized equipment and complex procedures. This specialization of equipment and supplies has resulted in a need for radiographers to be specially trained in this advanced technology. Most of this advanced education and training occurs through continuing education classes and on-the-job training. In 1991, the ARRT began offering an advanced-level certification examination in cardiovascular interventional technology. To qualify to take the examination, individuals must be ARRT-certified in radiography for at least 1 year and meet clinical requirements.

Mammography

Radiographers can specialize in performing radiologic examination of the breast, a procedure called **mammography.** Mammography is a valuable diagnostic tool for the early detection of breast disease, especially breast cancer. Current statistics indicate that 1 of every 10 females will develop breast cancer. Males are not excluded from this disease; about 1% of breast cancers are found in men. Early detection of breast cancer is important to successful treatment and cure. As a result, the American Cancer Society has recommended regular mammography screening for all women over 40 years of age.

This emphasis on screening mammography has resulted in an increase in the number of mammographic examinations being performed across the country. Special breast imaging centers have been built to accommodate the demand for these procedures. Equipment and supplies, such as film and screens, have been specially designed to create high-quality breast images. This specialization of equipment and supplies has resulted in a need for radiographers to be specially trained in this advanced technology. Most of this advanced education and training occurs through continuing education classes and on-the-job training. In 1992, the ARRT began offering an advanced-level certification examination in mammography. To qualify to take the examination, individuals need to be ARRT-certified in radiography and meet clinical requirements.

Computed Tomography

Computed tomography (CT) is the recording of a predetermined plane in the body by use of an x-ray beam that is measured by a scintillation counter, recorded on a magnetic disk, and then processed by a computer for display on a cathode ray tube. This technology has allowed physicians to visualize patient anatomy from various sectional planes.

Computed tomography involves the use of highly specialized equipment and complex procedures. This specialization of equipment and supplies has resulted in a need for radiographers to be specially trained in this advanced technology. Most of this advanced education and training occurs through continuing education

courses and on-the-job training. In 1995, the ARRT began offering an advanced-level certification examination in CT. To qualify to take the examination, individuals need to be ARRT-certified in radiography or radiation therapy technology and meet clinical requirements.

NUCLEAR MEDICINE

The branch of radiologic technology that involves procedures that require the use of radioactive materials for diagnostic or therapeutic purposes is **nuclear medicine technology** (Fig. 1–6). Nuclear medicine procedures usually involve the imaging of a patient's organs—such as the liver, heart, or brain—after the introduction of a radioactive material known as a *radiopharmaceutical*. Radiopharmaceuticals are usually administered intravenously but can be administered orally or by inhalation. Procedures can also be performed on specimens such as blood or urine. Samples from a patient can be combined with a radioactive substance to measure various constituents in the sample.

To become a registered nuclear medicine technologist, it is necessary to complete an accredited nuclear medicine technology program. There are more than 100 such programs in the United States. Most commonly sponsored by hospitals, community colleges, or universities, these programs vary in length from 1 year to a 4-year baccalaureate program. One-year pro-

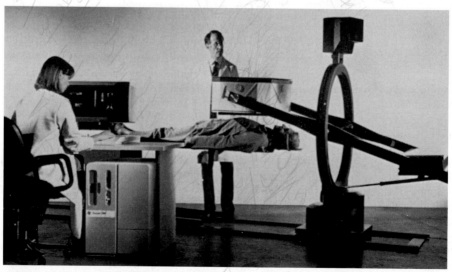

FIGURE 1–6. A nuclear medicine technologist performs procedures requiring the use of radioactive substances. (Courtesy of General Electric Medical Systems, Waukesha, Wisconsin.)

grams are usually designed for individuals who already hold credentials in radiography, medical technology, or nursing, or who possess a bachelor's degree in one of the basic sciences. Graduates of an accredited program are eligible to take the national examination in nuclear medicine technology offered by either the ARRT or the Nuclear Medicine Technology Certification Board (NMTCB). Successful completion of one of these two examinations is usually required for employment. An ARRT-certified individual uses the initials RT(N) after his or her name, meaning *registered technologist (nuclear medicine technology)*. An NMTCB-certified individual uses the initials CNMT after his or her name, signifying *certified nuclear medicine technologist*.

RADIATION THERAPY

A **radiation therapy** technologist, or *radiation therapist*, is an individual who administers radiation treatments to patients according to the prescription and instructions of a physician known as a *radiation oncologist* (Fig. 1–7). Radiation oncology involves the use of high-energy ionizing radiation to treat primarily malignant tumors (cancer). Therapists are responsible for administering a planned course of prescribed radiation treatments using high-technology therapeutic equipment and accessories. They provide specialized patient care and observe the clinical progress of their patients.

To become a registered radiation therapy technologist, it is necessary to complete an accredited radiation therapy technology program, of which there are more than 100 in the United States. Programs are most commonly sponsored by hospitals, community colleges, or universities and vary in length from 1 year to 4-year baccalaureate programs. One-year programs are usually designed for individuals who already have credentials in radiography or who can demonstrate competence in the areas identified in the essentials for a radiation therapy technology program. Graduates of an accredited program are eligible to take the national examination in radiation therapy technology offered by the ARRT. An ARRT-certified individual uses the initials RT(T) after his or her name. This abbreviation means *registered technologist (radiation therapy technology)*.

new book. See p. 14 (adds bone densitometry and CT.

DIAGNOSTIC MEDICAL SONOGRAPHY

Diagnostic medical sonography is the visualization of structures of the body by recording the reflections of pulses of high-frequency sound (ultrasound) waves directed into the tissue. An individual who specializes in this field is known as a *diagnostic medical sonographer* (Fig.

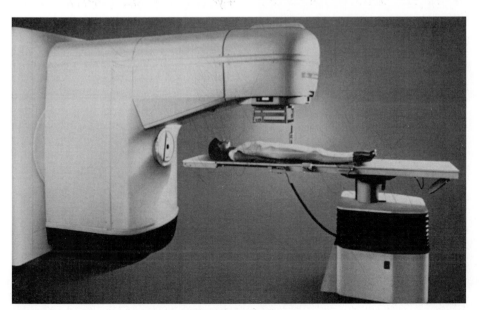

FIGURE 1–7. A radiation therapist administers radiation treatments, primarily to cancer patients. (Courtesy of General Electric Medical Systems, Waukesha, Wisconsin.)

1–8). Sonographers often have previous experience as radiographers, but this is not required.

To become a sonographer, individuals may complete an accredited diagnostic medical sonography program or may be trained on the job. On-the-job training is typically provided only to individuals who have previous experience in another allied health specialty such as radiography. Graduates of accredited programs or experienced sonographers are eligible to take a national examination offered by the American Registry of Diagnostic Medical Sonographers (ARDMS). A *registered diagnostic medical sonographer* uses the initials RDMS after his or her name.

MAGNETIC RESONANCE IMAGING

Magnetic resonance imaging (MRI) uses a strong magnetic field and radio waves along with a computer to generate sectional images of patient anatomy. Like CT, this advanced technology uses highly specialized equipment and requires specialized education and training. Most of this education and training occurs through continuing education courses and on-the-job training, although a few formal educational programs do exist. For the most part,

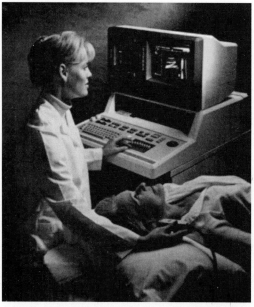

FIGURE 1–8. A diagnostic medical sonographer uses high-frequency sound waves to create images. (Courtesy of General Electric Medical Systems, Waukesha, Wisconsin.)

MRI technologists have credentials in radiography. Many of these individuals are also experienced CT technologists. In 1995, the ARRT began offering an advanced-level certification examination in MRI. To qualify to take the examination, individuals need to be ARRT-certified in radiography, nuclear medicine technology, or radiation therapy technology and meet clinical requirements.

ADDITIONAL OPPORTUNITIES

Regardless of the area in which one chooses to specialize within the profession of radiologic technology, additional opportunities exist in education, management, and commercial firms.

Education

Individuals who have an interest in teaching in any of the specific disciplines can find opportunities in hospitals, colleges, and universities. Careers include clinical instructor, didactic faculty member, clinical coordinator, and program director.

A clinical instructor teaches students primarily on a one-on-one basis in the clinical setting. A didactic faculty member teaches students typically through classroom lectures and laboratory activities. A clinical coordinator has teaching responsibilities along with administrative duties in overseeing clinical education, most often in programs using many clinical education centers. A program director has teaching responsibilities as well as overall administrative responsibility for the entire educational program. Advanced coursework in education is desirable for these positions. Program directors are required to have a baccalaureate degree.

Administration

Individuals who have an interest in the management of the radiology services in a given facility can specialize for a wide spectrum of supervisory and administrative positions. Many departments have supervisory positions in areas such as CT, MRI, cardiovascular interventional technology, sonography, and quality management. In 1997, the ARRT began offering an advanced-level certification examination in quality management. To be eligible to take the examination, individuals need to be ARRT-certified in radiography, nuclear medicine technology, or radiation therapy technology and meet clinical requirements. In addition, depending on the department size, there are upper-management positions such as a chief technologist and radiology manager or administrator. Along with experience, advanced coursework in management is desirable for these positions.

Commercial Firms

Opportunities for radiologic technologists and sonographers exist in a variety of areas within commercial companies involved in the selling of x-ray equipment, film, processing chemicals, and related x-ray supplies. These companies need sales representatives with technical knowledge of the radiologic procedures and equipment as well as the ability to sell. In addition, companies hire technical specialists who are not directly involved in sales but who are involved with the education and training of the staff at the sites where the equipment is installed. Sales representatives and technical specialists generally have some travel requirements as a part of their responsibilities.

The Health Care Team

A wide array of specialists make up the health care team. More than 200 different health careers have been identified. Most of these careers have been grouped into the large category known as allied health. *Allied health* is a term that includes all of the health-related disciplines with the exception of nursing and the MODVOPP careers. *MODVOPP* is an acronym that stands for *m*edicine, *o*steopathy, *d*entistry, *v*eterinary medicine, *o*ptometry, *p*harmacy, and *p*odiatry.

Although not all of the various disciplines can be detailed here, some of the health care services that a radiologic technologist encounters on regular basis are highlighted. These services include medicine and osteopathy, nursing, and the allied health careers that encompass many of the diagnostic services, therapeutic services, and health information services. Individuals employed in health care find opportunities in all kinds of environments such as hospitals, clinics, doctors' offices, long-term care facilities, schools, and industry.

Many of the health care workers share the titles of technologist, technician, and therapist.

Technologist is a general term that applies to an individual skilled in a practical art. This health care provider applies knowledge to practical and theoretical problems in the field. *Technician* is a term that applies to an individual who performs procedures that require attention to technical detail. Technicians work under the direction of another health care provider. Often the terms *technologist* and *technician* are used interchangeably. This can create problems in disciplines in which the terms are used to denote differing levels of education. In the clinical laboratory sciences, a medical technologist (MT) possesses a 4-year degree, and a medical laboratory technician (MLT) has completed a 2-year program. In general, technologists are involved in higher-level problem-solving skills and have more extensive educational preparation than do technicians. Technologists and technicians work throughout all areas of health care. Many provide direct patient care, and others serve in support roles.

Therapists specialize in carrying out treatments designed to correct or improve the function of a particular body part or system. Therapists possess varied levels of educational experiences. Most therapists have either a 2-year or a 4-year college degree.

MEDICINE AND OSTEOPATHY

Physicians are primary care providers who promote the optimal health of their patients and who provide for patients' care during an illness. Two principal types of physicians are the medical doctor (MD) and the doctor of osteopathy (DO). Medical doctors generally complete a baccalaureate degree program with a science major such as biology or chemistry and then complete 4 years of medical school. Doctors of osteopathy have educations similar to those of medical doctors. The philosophy of osteopathic medicine is different from the philosophy of traditional medicine. In addition to learning the important concepts of medicine, doctors of osteopathy are trained to do manipulations of muscles and bones as a part of the healing process. Both medical doctors and doctors of osteopathy must be state-licensed to practice.

After medical school, most medical doctors and doctors of osteopathy complete additional training, known as a residency, in an area of specialization. Residencies are usually 3 or 4 years long. They may include the following branches of medicine:

Anesthesiology—the study of the use of medication to cause loss of sensation during surgery

Cardiology—the study of diseases of the cardiovascular system

Family Practice—the study of diseases in patients of all ages

Geriatrics—the study of diseases of the aged

Gynecology—the study of diseases of the female reproductive system

Internal Medicine—the study of diseases of the internal organs of the chest and abdomen

Neurology—the study of diseases of the brain and nervous system

Obstetrics—the study of pregnancy and childbirth

Oncology—the study of the treatment of tumors

Orthopedics—the study of diseases of muscles and bones

Pediatrics—the study of diseases in children

Radiology—the study of the use of x-rays and radioactive substances to diagnose and treat diseases

Surgery—the study of the use of operative procedures to treat diseases

Urology—the study of diseases of the urinary system

In addition, many physicians subspecialize, such as a pediatric cardiovascular surgeon whose primary duties include performing surgery on the heart and blood vessels of children.

NURSING

A nurse provides direct patient care, typically under the direction of physicians. Nurses are classified as nursing assistants, licensed practical nurses (LPN), or registered nurses (RN). Registered nurses have a variety of duties depending on their area of expertise. Nurses often choose to work exclusively in one specialty area, such as pediatrics, orthopedics, intensive care, or the emergency department. To become a registered nurse, an individual must pass a state licensing examination after completion of a 2-, 3-, or 4-year program of study.

Advanced education for the nurse can lead to work as a nurse practitioner, a nurse midwife, or a nurse anesthetist. A nurse practitioner performs physical examinations, orders and inter-

prets some tests, and in some states may prescribe medications. A nurse midwife provides perinatal care and can deliver babies under the supervision of an obstetrician. A nurse anesthetist provides anesthesia under the supervision of an anesthesiologist.

Nursing assistants and licensed practical nurses generally work under the direction of a registered nurse or a physician to provide basic care to patients. Nursing assistants generally have limited training, most of which is done on the job. Licensed practical nurses complete a 1-year program and may legally administer drugs except by the intravenous route. *Not allowed*

DIAGNOSTIC SERVICES

Health care workers in diagnostic service areas perform tests or evaluations that aid the physician in determining the presence or absence of a disease or condition. Many health care specialists perform diagnostic procedures. Electrocardiographic technicians operate equipment that records the electrical impulses of the heart. Electroencephalographic technologists operate equipment to record the electrical impulses of the brain.

The clinical laboratory sciences involve a wide variety of careers in health care. A medical technologist (MT) works in the laboratory performing tests and analyzing results. Several areas of specialization exist in the laboratory, including hematology, microbiology, clinical chemistry, immunology, and blood banking. Medical laboratory technicians (MLT) generally work under the supervision of a medical technologist or physician to perform basic laboratory tests in all the various departments of the laboratory. Other laboratory personnel include the cytotechnologist, who specializes in the preparation and screening of cells, and the histologic technologist, who specializes in the preparation of tissues.

Radiology is predominantly a diagnostic service. These careers have already been detailed.

Educational requirements for careers in the diagnostic services vary considerably across the disciplines, but most require 2 to 4 years of education beyond high school.

THERAPEUTIC SERVICES

Therapists provide services designed to help patients overcome some form of physical or psychological disability. Examples include occupational therapists, who teach useful skills to patients with physical or emotional illnesses; physical therapists, who help restore muscle strength and coordination through exercise and the use of special devices such as braces or crutches; radiation therapists, who treat patients with cancer using high-energy x-rays and gamma rays; and respiratory therapists, who help treat patients with breathing difficulties. Educational requirements vary considerably across the disciplines, but most require 2 to 4 years of education beyond high school.

HEALTH INFORMATION SERVICES

Health information services involve careers that are responsible for the management of health information such as that contained in the patient's health record. These careers do not involve direct patient contact but are essential to the efficient operation of any health care facility. For example, health information technologists are involved in the coding of patient conditions, and these codes are used to determine the amount of money a facility is reimbursed for providing care to a patient.

Educational requirements for careers in health information management vary considerably across disciplines, but most require 2 to 4 years of education beyond high school.

OTHER HEALTH SERVICES

A vast number of other careers exist within the health care environment. Other health services include such disciplines as dental health, dietetics, psychosocial health care, and emergency care.

Summary

Radiation is energy transmitted by waves through space or through a medium (matter). It is both helpful and essential for life. Energy is the capacity to operate or work. One form of energy is electromagnetic energy, which includes radio waves, light, and x-rays. Many forms of energy are used in medicine to help diagnose and treat patients. Some higher-energy forms, such as x-rays, are capable of causing ionization. This process is capable of causing biologic damage, and caution should be exercised to prevent unnecessary exposure to ionizing radiation.

X-rays were discovered by Wilhelm Conrad Röntgen on November 8, 1895. For his discovery, Röntgen was awarded the first Nobel Prize in Physics in 1901.

Radiologic technology is the technical science that deals with the use of x-rays or radioactive substances for diagnostic or therapeutic purposes in medicine. *Radiologic technologist* is a general term applied to an individual qualified to use x-rays (radiography) or radioactive substances (nuclear medicine) to produce images of the internal parts of the body for interpretation by a physician known as a *radiologist*. Radiologic technologists also use x-rays or radioactive substances in the treatment of disease (radiation therapy).

In addition to using x-rays and radioactive substances, radiologic technologists have become involved in using high-frequency sound waves (diagnostic medical sonography) and magnetic fields and radio waves (magnetic resonance imaging) to create images of the internal anatomy of the body. Additional opportunities also exist for radiologic technologists in education, management, and commercial firms.

The health care team comprises a wide array of specialists. More than 200 different health careers have been identified, most of which have been grouped into the large category known as allied health. *Allied health* is a term that includes all of the health-related disciplines with the exception of nursing and the MODVOPP careers. *MODVOPP* is an acronym standing for *m*edicine, *o*steopathy, *d*entistry, *v*eterinary medicine, *o*ptometry, *p*harmacy, and *p*odiatry.

Radiologic technologists work as a part of the health care team and interact with many of the other health care members on a regular basis. These other members are employed in such health services as medicine and osteopathy, nursing, and the allied health careers that encompass many of the diagnostic services, therapeutic services, and health information services.

Individuals employed in health care find opportunities in all kinds of environments, such as hospitals, clinics, doctors' offices, long-term care facilities, schools, and industry.

◀R REVIEW QUESTIONS

1 The term used to describe energy transmitted through matter is:

a) ionization
b) physiology
c) radiation
d) therapy

2 Special protection should be taken to prevent excessive exposure to:
a) energy
b) electromagnetic energy
c) ionizing radiation
d) radio waves

3 Which of the following specialties uses a non-ionizing form of radiation?
a) nuclear medicine technology
b) radiation therapy
c) radiography
d) sonography

4 The discovery of x-rays occurred in:
a) 1858
b) 1876
c) 1895
d) 1898

5 An individual specializing in the use of x-rays to create images of the body is known as a:
a) diagnostic medical sonographer
b) nuclear medicine technologist
c) radiographer
d) radiation therapist

6 An effective treatment of atherosclerosis that uses a special catheter with a balloon tip is termed:
a) angiography
b) angioplasty
c) arteriography
d) cardiac catheterization

7 A discipline that visualizes sectional anatomy by the recording of a predetermined plane in the body is:
a) computed tomography
b) cardiovascular interventional technology

c) nuclear medicine technology
d) radiation therapy

8 Radiography of the breast is termed:
a) angiography
b) cytotechnology
c) histology
d) mammography

9 The study of diseases of muscles and bones is termed:
a) neurology
b) orthopedics
c) oncology
d) urology

10 An individual who specializes in carrying out treatments designed to correct or improve the function of a particular body part or system is known as a:
a) diagnostician
b) histologist
c) technologist
d) therapist

BIBLIOGRAPHY

American Medical Association: Allied Health Education Directory. 25th ed. Chicago, American Medical Association, 1997.

Carlton R, Adler AM: Principles of Radiographic Imaging: An Art and a Science. 2nd ed. Albany, NY, Delmar Publishers, 1997.

Curry TS, Dowdey JE, Murry RC: Christensen's Physics of Diagnostic Radiology. 4th ed. Philadelphia, Lea & Febiger, 1990.

Eisenberg RL: Radiology: An Illustrated History. St. Louis, Mosby–Year Book, 1992.

Gerdin JA: Health Careers Today. St. Louis, Mosby–Year Book, 1991.

Grigg ERN: The Trail of the Invisible Light. Springfield, IL, Charles C Thomas, 1965.

Gurley LT, Calloway WJ: Introduction to Radiologic Technology. 4th ed. St. Louis, Mosby–Year Book, 1996.

Papp J: Quality Management in the Imaging Sciences. St. Louis, Mosby–Year Book, 1998.

Röntgen WC: On a new kind of rays. Nature 53:1369, 1896.

Simmers L: Diversified Health Occupations. 2nd ed. Albany, NY, Delmar Publishers, 1988.

CHAPTER 2

PROFESSIONAL ORGANIZATIONS

Richard R. Carlton, MS, RT(R) (CV), FAERS
Arlene M. Adler, MEd, RT(R), FAERS

Be active in your local, state and national organizations; never be satisfied until the highest goal has been attained.

PROFESSOR ED. C. JERMAN, THE FATHER OF RADIOLOGIC TECHNOLOGY, CIRCA 1920

Accreditation of Schools
Joint Review Committee on Education in Diagnostic Medical Sonography
Joint Review Committee on Education in Nuclear Medicine Technology
Joint Review Committee on Education in Radiologic Technology

Certification of Individuals
American Registry of Diagnostic Medical Sonographers
American Registry of Radiologic Technologists
Nuclear Medicine Technology Certification Board
State Licensing Agencies

Professional Societies
American Healthcare Radiology Administrators
American Society of Radiologic Technologists
Association of Educators in Radiological Sciences
Association of Vascular and Interventional Radiographers
International Society of Radiographers and Radiologic Technologists

Society of Diagnostic Medical Sonographers
Society of Magnetic Resonance in Medicine/Society for Magnetic Resonance Imaging
Society of Nuclear Medicine—Technologist Section
State and Local Radiologic Technology Societies

Radiologist and Physicist Organizations
American Association of Physicists in Medicine
American Board of Radiology
American College of Radiology
American Institute of Ultrasound in Medicine
American Medical Association
American Roentgen Ray Society
American Society for Therapeutic Radiology and Oncology
Radiological Society of North America
Society of Nuclear Medicine

Summary

OBJECTIVES

On completion of this chapter, the student will be able to:

1 Differentiate accreditation, certification, and representation functions of various professional organizations.
2 Describe the organizations that carry out the professional aspects of a specific radiologic technology area of specialization.

3 Describe the relationship of various radiologist and physicist organizations with radiologic technology.

GLOSSARY

Accreditation: voluntary peer process through which an agency grants recognition to an institution for a program of study that meets specified criteria

Certification: voluntary process through which an agency grants recognition to an individual upon demonstration, usually by examination, of specialized professional skills.

"Essentials": document specifying the minimum quality standards for the accreditation of programs as approved by the appropriate joint review committee sponsors

Joint Review Committee: group of persons appointed by sponsoring organizations to oversee the accreditation process

Licensure: process by which a governmental agency (usually a state) grants permission to individuals to practice their profession

Registry: listing of individuals holding certification in a particular profession

Sponsoring Organization: professional organization that appoints members to a joint review committee board

"Standards": document specifying the requirements for accreditation of an educational program by a joint review committee.

Accreditation of Schools

Accreditation of schools sets the conditions under which new members may qualify for entry into the profession. Accredited programs have satisfactorily demonstrated compliance with educational standards developed by and for the profession. These standards are set by the organizations that sponsor the accrediting agency. Each **sponsoring organization** appoints one or more members to the board of directors known as a **joint review committee.** This board is the governing body of the organization, and its members make recommendations on the accreditation status of schools. The sponsoring organizations of the JRCs approve a document formerly known as the **"Essentials"** and now known as the **"Standards"** which details exactly how an accredited program must

operate. These documents typically require a program to demonstrate its purposes, resources, effectiveness of its outcomes, and other elements deemed important by the sponsoring organizations.

The process of accreditation begins with an application from the program. On approval of the application, a comprehensive document known as a *self-study* must be compiled by the program according to guidelines set by the accrediting agency. On submission of this document, a team of site visitors is sent to verify the information provided in the self-study. Site visitors are volunteers from the profession who serve without pay, although their expenses are paid by the program being visited. The site-visiting team submits a report to the accrediting agency, and this report is reviewed by the agency staff and presented to the board for a vote on recommended accreditation status. Typical accreditation award classifications include provisional, probationary, and up to 8–year status. Fees are collected for the application and the site-visit expenses, as is an annual fee from the sponsor of the program and from each clinical education site.

Accreditation is a voluntary peer-review process. Although accreditation is voluntary, few programs choose not to undergo the accreditation process. Nearly all schools value their accreditation status highly and work hard to maintain standards that meet all the accreditation recommendations. A list of accrediting agencies, certification agencies, and professional societies with addresses and telephone numbers is supplied in Appendix B.

JOINT REVIEW COMMITTEE ON EDUCATION IN DIAGNOSTIC MEDICAL SONOGRAPHY

The Joint Review Committee on Education in Diagnostic Medical Sonography (JRCDMS) was established in 1979 and is currently sponsored by seven organizations: the American College of Cardiology, the American College of Radiology, the American Institute of Ultrasound in Medicine, the American Medical

Association (AMA), the American Society of Echocardiography, the American Society of Radiologic Technologists, and the Society of Diagnostic Medical Sonographers. The JRCDMS accredits about 75 diagnostic medical sonography programs.

JOINT REVIEW COMMITTEE ON EDUCATION IN NUCLEAR MEDICINE TECHNOLOGY

The Joint Review Committee on Education in Nuclear Medicine Technology (JRCNMT) was established in 1970 and is currently sponsored by six organizations: the American College of Radiology, the American Society for Medical Technology, the American Society of Clinical Pathologists, the American Society of Radiologic Technologists, the Society of Nuclear Medicine, and the Society of Nuclear Medicine—Technologist Section. The JRCNMT accredits about 100 nuclear medicine technology programs.

JOINT REVIEW COMMITTEE ON EDUCATION IN RADIOLOGIC TECHNOLOGY

Radiography is considered by many to be the fifth oldest allied health profession because the first "Essentials" was established in 1944, after occupational therapy, medical technology, physical therapy, and medical records administration. It was not until 1969 that the Joint Review Committee on Education in Radiologic Technology (JRCERT) was established. The JRCERT is currently sponsored by the American College of Radiology, the American Society of Radiologic Technologists, and the Association of Educators in Radiological Sciences. The JRCERT accredits some 625 radiography programs (more than any other allied health profession) as well as about 100 radiation therapy technology programs.

Certification of Individuals

Professional **certification** is a process through which an agency grants recognition to an individual upon demonstration, usually by examination, of specialized professional skills. It is a voluntary process and is the responsibility of the person, not of the person's school or employer. Each certification organization sets requirements for the recognition of professionals through registration, certification, or other recognition of skills by examination. Fees are charged for these services. Especially important are the annual fees for continued recognition. Failure to pay these fees or meet other requirements, such as verification of continuing education activities, results in the removal of an individual from the registration lists of the profession. Reinstatement usually does not involve retaking an examination, but there is often a special fee.

Actually, a **registry** is simply a listing of individuals holding a particular certification. It is common for the term *registry* to be applied to the agency that carries out the certification function and maintains the registry list. Each registry is sponsored by appropriate professional organizations. The sponsoring organizations appoint the members of the board, and this board then determines the standards for the registry, such as eligibility requirements, examination questions, fees, and ethical standards.

Nearly all hospitals in the United States require appropriate professional certification as a condition of employment. Physicians who desire quality imaging also insist on appropriate professional certification for the technologists who perform radiography, ultrasonography, and mammography in their offices and clinics.

AMERICAN REGISTRY OF DIAGNOSTIC MEDICAL SONOGRAPHERS

The American Registry of Diagnostic Medical Sonographers (ARDMS) offers voluntary certification through examination to eligible sonographers and vascular technologists. Since its inception in 1975, the ARDMS has certified some 30,000 individuals. The ARDMS offers three credentials: Registered Diagnostic Medical Sonographer (RDMS), Registered Diagnostic Cardiac Sonographer (RDCS), and Registered Vascular Technologist (RVT).

AMERICAN REGISTRY OF RADIOLOGIC TECHNOLOGISTS

The American Registry of Radiologic Technologists (ARRT) was founded in 1922 by the Radiological Society of North America (RSNA), with the support of the American Roentgen Ray Society and the cooperation of the Canadian Association of Radiologists and the American Society of X-Ray Technicians (now known as the ASRT). In 1936 the ARRT was incorporated, and in 1944 the American College of Radiology and the ASRT became cosponsors of the ARRT. Currently, the ASRT appoints five members to the ARRT board and the ACR appoints four members.

The purposes of the ARRT include encouraging the study and elevating the standards of radiologic technology, examining and certifying eligible candidates, and periodically publishing a listing of registrants. This is accomplished through voluntary certification by examination. Once an individual has passed the appropriate examination, he or she is listed in the registry and granted the right to use an appropriate professional title. These designations are Registered Technologist (RT), with a specialty designation for Radiographer (R), Radiation Therapy (T), Nuclear Medicine (N), Cardiovascular Interventional Technology (CV), Mammography (M), Computed Tomography (CT), Magnetic Resonance Imaging (MR), or Quality Management (QM). For example, a registered radiographer is designated as RT(R) (ARRT). This designation is a registered trademark and its use by non-ARRT-registered individuals is illegal.

Individuals must pay an annual fee to maintain active status with the ARRT and must adhere to the ARRT code of ethics. Members of the profession who violate the code of ethics, usually through criminal activity, may have their registration revoked. For example, former registered technologists who have been convicted of stealing from their employers often have their registration revoked. ARRT registrants must also certify that they have attended 24 hours of continuing education during the previous 2 years to maintain their registration status. Continuing education became mandatory for ARRT registrants in 1995.

The ARRT began offering registration in nuclear medicine technology and radiation therapy in 1962 and started advanced-level examinations in 1991. By 1997, the ARRT listed more than 220,000 registered technologists, thousands of whom were certified in more than one professional specialty. Registered technologists hold more than 10,000 certifications in radiation therapy, more than 10,000 in nuclear medicine, more than 2500 in cardiovascular intervention, more than 35,000 in mammography, more than

7500 in computed tomography, and more than 5000 in magnetic resonance imaging.

NUCLEAR MEDICINE TECHNOLOGY CERTIFICATION BOARD

The Nuclear Medicine Technology Certification Board (NMTCB) was founded in 1977. Current sponsors include the Society of Nuclear Medicine, the Society of Nuclear Medicine—Technologist Section, the American Society of Clinical Pathologists, the College of Physicists, the American Society of Medical Technology, and the Association of Physicists in Medicine. The NMTCB consists of 15 persons plus an advisory council, whose chair also sits on the board.

The purposes of the NMTCB include examining and certifying eligible candidates and periodically publishing a listing of registrants. This is accomplished through voluntary certification by examination. Once an individual has passed the appropriate examination, he or she becomes registered and is granted the right to use the title CNMT. The NMTCB has about 15,000 registrants.

STATE LICENSING AGENCIES

Requirements to practice the radiologic professions vary from state to state. About half the states and territories require a license, which can usually be obtained on providing proof of certification from the appropriate national certification organization (a process known as **licensure**). The laws in effect vary tremendously from one state to another and may vary from year to year within a state as a result of new legislation. Most radiologic professionals do not experience difficulty in moving employment from one state to another since proper licensing is usually a matter of submitting the appropriate paperwork and fees. It is important to verify current licensing requirements before practicing in a new state because penalties may be prescribed by law for practicing without a license. A list of state licensing bodies and their addresses and phone numbers is supplied in Appendix C.

Professional Societies

Professional societies represent the interests of various groups to the public and to governmental bodies. The radiologic sciences have many such organizations, with new ones forming and others combining or ceasing operations from time to time. These organizations usually publish professional journals, conduct educational meetings, and represent their members to governmental bodies. They also often provide continuing education verification, scholarships, special reports, information networking, recruitment and promotional materials, malpractice insurance, and other services for their members. Some of the more important professional societies are described here. Contact information, including Internet web sites, can be found in Appendix B.

AMERICAN HEALTHCARE RADIOLOGY ADMINISTRATORS

The American Healthcare Radiology Administrators (AHRA) was organized to promote management practice in the administration of imaging services. Membership is open to professionals engaged in the practice of radiology administration in both hospital and nonhospital settings, as well as to others in service or education who have limited management responsibilities.

The AHRA provides a broad range of services for its members, including the journal *Radiology Management*, a newsletter, and monographs. The association holds regular educational meetings and an annual conference. The AHRA has strong cooperative ties with other professional associations and has spearheaded the Summit on Manpower, a consortium of radiology and health care organizations concerned with labor shortages in radiology.

AMERICAN SOCIETY OF RADIOLOGIC TECHNOLOGISTS

The American Society of Radiologic Technologists (ASRT) was founded in 1920. As the most prominent national professional voice for radiologic technologists, the ASRT represents individual practitioners, educators, managers and administrators, and students in radiography, radiation therapy, and nuclear medicine, as well as the many specialties within each modality. The ASRT has about 65,000 members (about 30% of the registered technologists in the United States).

The goals of the ASRT are to advance the professions of radiologic technology and imaging specialties, to maintain high standards of education, to enhance the quality of patient care, and to further the welfare and socioeconomics of radiologic technologists. The ASRT publishes a peer-reviewed, refereed journal, *Radiologic Technology*; conducts regional and national conferences; and produces educational programs of all types.

ASSOCIATION OF EDUCATORS IN RADIOLOGICAL SCIENCES

The Association of Educators in Radiological Sciences (AERS) was founded in 1967. Its primary purposes are to encourage the exchange of teaching concepts, to help establish minimum standards for teaching radiologic technologies, and to advance radiologic education by encouraging educational research and technical writing by its members. The AERS is a national association of educators. The association holds meetings and publishes *Radiologic Science and Education AERS Quarterly* and other educational data.

ASSOCIATION OF VASCULAR AND INTERVENTIONAL RADIOGRAPHERS

The Association of Vascular and Interventional Radiographers (AVIR) was organized to represent radiographers and allied health care professionals specializing in cardiovascular and interventional radiology. AVIR offers members a quarterly newsletter and a national conference in conjunction with the Society of Cardiovascular and Interventional Radiology and the American Radiological Nurses Association.

INTERNATIONAL SOCIETY OF RADIOGRAPHERS AND RADIOLOGIC TECHNOLOGISTS

The International Society of Radiographers and Radiologic Technologists (ISRRT) was founded in 1959 as an organization of national societies of radiologic technologists. The ISRRT is an international, nongovernmental organization with official relations with the World Health Organization.

The primary objectives of the ISRRT are to facilitate communication among radiologic technologists worldwide, to advance the science and practice of radiologic technology, and to identify and help meet the needs of radiologic technologists in developing nations.

The ISRRT sponsors three types of international meetings: world congresses, regional meetings, and teachers' seminars. These meetings are held on a 4-year cycle, with one type of meeting scheduled each year and the fourth year off. Three regions hold meetings: Europe and Africa, Asia and Australasia, and the Americas. The world congresses and the teachers' seminars rotate among the regions of the world. The ISRRT publishes a semiannual newsletter, proceedings of meetings, and translations of various documents of interest to the profession.

Over 50 member countries are represented by the ISRRT. Each member country appoints a representative to the ISRRT World Council, which serves as the governing body. The Secretary-General of the organization serves as the liasion for the council as well as the office. The ISRRT offers associate membership to individuals wishing to support the organization.

SOCIETY OF DIAGNOSTIC MEDICAL SONOGRAPHERS

The Society of Diagnostic Medical Sonographers (SDMS) is the largest professional society for sonographers, representing every specialty and level of expertise. The SDMS was founded in 1970 to answer the needs of nonphysicians who were performing diagnostic sonographic procedures. Its goals are to promote, advance, and educate its members and the medical community in the science of diagnostic medical sonography and thereby to contribute to the enhancement of patient care. This is accomplished through educational programs, scientific and professional publications, and representation and collaboration with other organizations.

SOCIETY OF MAGNETIC RESONANCE IN MEDICINE/SOCIETY FOR MAGNETIC RESONANCE IMAGING

The Society of Magnetic Resonance in Medicine (SMRM) was founded in 1981 and now has more than 2500 members. Its major purpose is to further the development and application of magnetic resonance techniques in medicine and biology by promoting communications, re-

search development applications, and the availability of information in the fields of magnetic resonance imaging and spectroscopy. To accomplish this purpose, the society holds meetings and workshops, publishes journals and other documents, provides information and advice on those aspects of public policy concerned with magnetic resonance in medicine, and otherwise performs charitable, scientific, and educational functions with respect to magnetic resonance in medicine and biology. SMRM's periodicals include a newsletter, *Resonance*, and a journal, *Magnetic Resonance in Medicine*.

The Society of Magnetic Resonance in Medicine and the Society for Magnetic Resonance Imaging (SMRI) also support a joint Section for Magnetic Resonance Technologists (SMRT). SMRI publishes a journal, *Magnetic Resonance Imaging Technology*.

SOCIETY OF NUCLEAR MEDICINE— TECHNOLOGIST SECTION

The Society of Nuclear Medicine (SNM) is a multidisciplinary organization of physicians, physicists, chemists, radiopharmacists, technologists, and others interested in the diagnostic, therapeutic, and investigational use of radiopharmaceuticals. Founded in Seattle in 1954, it is the largest scientific organization dedicated to nuclear medicine.

The Technologist Section of SNM was formed in 1970 to meet the needs of the nuclear medicine technologist. It is a scientific organization formed with, but operating autonomously from, the SNM to promote the continued development and improvement of the art and science of nuclear medicine technology. Its ongoing objectives are to enhance the development of nuclear medicine technology, to stimulate continuing education activities, and to develop a forum for the exchange of ideas and information. The Technologist Section provides nuclear medicine technologists with a mechanism to deal directly with issues that concern them, such as continuing education, academic affairs, and socioeconomic issues. The organization publishes a journal called *JNMT.*

STATE AND LOCAL RADIOLOGIC TECHNOLOGY SOCIETIES

Nearly all states and many cities and regions have local professional societies that carry out many of the functions of the larger national organizations for their states or regions. In many instances, these organizations serve as chapters or affiliates of the larger groups, although these connections may be formal or simply loose affiliations. State and local societies often make special efforts to cater to the needs of students and new members of professions with opportunities to begin a career through scholarships, student competitions, publishing, exhibits, and committee work, as well as through positions as board members.

Radiologist and Physicist Organizations

AMERICAN ASSOCIATION OF PHYSICISTS IN MEDICINE

The American Association of Physicists in Medicine (AAPM) is the most prominent organization of radiation physicists. Its annual meeting is held in conjunction with the RSNA meeting each year in Chicago.

AMERICAN BOARD OF RADIOLOGY

The American Board of Radiology (ABR) was established in 1934 to conduct the certification of radiologists. There are three certification divisions: radiology, diagnostic radiology, and therapeutic radiology. The basic requirement for eligibility for these examinations is an MD degree plus 4 years of residency training. A written examination must be passed before a candidate is eligible for the oral examination. The ABR also offers certification for radiologic physicists and a special competence examination in nuclear medicine.

AMERICAN COLLEGE OF RADIOLOGY

With more than 28,000 members, the American College of Radiology (ACR) is the principal organization of physicians trained in radiology and medical radiation physics in the United States. The ACR is a professional society whose primary purposes are to advance the science of radiology, to improve service to the patient, to study the socioeconomic aspects of the practice of radiology, and to encourage continuing edu-

cation for radiologists and persons practicing in allied professional fields.

AMERICAN INSTITUTE OF ULTRASOUND IN MEDICINE

Physicians, engineers, scientists, sonographers, and other professionals involved with diagnostic medical sonography make up the American Institute of Ultrasound in Medicine (AIUM). The AIUM promotes the application of ultrasound in clinical medicine, diagnostically, and in research; promotes the study of its effects on tissue; recommends standards for its applications; and promotes education in the use of ultrasonics for medical purposes.

AMERICAN MEDICAL ASSOCIATION

The AMA was founded in Philadelphia in 1847 and is considered to be the largest and most active medical organization in the world. More than 250,000 American physicians (about 70% of those practicing) belong to the AMA. The activities of the AMA include promotion and regulation of all aspects of medicine in the United States, including the allied health professions. The AMA publishes the most widely distributed medical journal in the world, *The Journal of the American Medical Association*, also known as *JAMA*, which is published weekly.

AMERICAN ROENTGEN RAY SOCIETY

The American Roentgen Ray Society (ARRS) is the oldest American radiologic society. Founded in 1900 in St. Louis, the society had about 7000 members by the early 1990s. Its primary objectives are educational, which are met through meetings and publication of the *American Journal of Roentgenology*.

AMERICAN SOCIETY FOR THERAPEUTIC RADIOLOGY AND ONCOLOGY

The purpose of the American Society for Therapeutic Radiology and Oncology (ASTRO) is to extend the benefits of radiation therapy to patients with cancer or other disorders, to advance its scientific basis, and to provide for the education and professional fellowship of its members.

The society was formally incorporated in 1958 as an organization of physicians who believed that radiation, formerly used only as a diagnostic tool, had potential value as an interventional modality in the treatment of malignant disease. Today, ASTRO has over 4000 members and is the leading organization for radiation oncology, biology, and physics. ASTRO publishes a newsletter and an annual membership directory. The organization also makes a major commitment to education and research through awards, fellowships, travel grants, and contributions to accredited technology programs.

RADIOLOGICAL SOCIETY OF NORTH AMERICA

The Western Roentgen Society was founded in Chicago in 1915 in response to a need for a national radiology organization because the American Roentgen Ray Society had become an eastern organization. In 1920, it was renamed the Radiological Society of North America (RSNA) to reflect the nature of its membership. Since 1918, the RSNA has published the most influential journal in American radiology, which is known simply as *Radiology* and often referred to as "the gray journal" because of its traditional color representing the shades of gray that make up the radiologic image. In 1981, a second journal, *RadioGraphics*, was added. The RSNA had 25,000 members by 1990, and it conducts the world's largest radiology meeting, with more than 50,000 registrants, each November.

SOCIETY OF NUCLEAR MEDICINE

See the section on the Society of Nuclear Medicine—Technologist Section.

Summary

A major part of the fabric of a profession is its organizations, especially the accrediting agencies for educational programs, the certification bodies for individuals, and the professional societies that represent the interests of the profession to the public and government.

Radiologic technology accreditation is carried out through the various joint review committees. The joint review committees are the Joint Review Committee on Education in Diagnostic Medical Sonography, the Joint Review Committee on Education in Nuclear Medicine, and the Joint Review Committee on Education in Radiologic Technology (which performs both radiography and radiation therapy accreditation).

Individuals are certified by the various registries and by state and territorial licensing agencies. The national registries are the American Registry of Diagnostic Medical Sonographers (ARDMS), the American Registry of Radiologic Technologists (ARRT), and the Nuclear Medicine Technology Certification Board (NMTCB). The ARRT offers registration in radiography, nuclear medicine, radiation therapy, cardiovascular interventional technology, mammography, computed tomography, magnetic resonance imaging, dosimetry, and quality management.

Radiologic technologists are represented by numerous professional societies at the international, national, state, and local levels. Among the most prominent of these organizations are the American Healthcare Radiology Administrators, the American Society of Radiologic Technologists, the Association of Educators in Radiological Sciences, the Association of Vascular and Interventional Radiographers, the International Society of Radiographers and Radiologic Technologists, the Society of Diagnostic Medical Sonographers, the Society of Magnetic Resonance in Medicine, the Society for Magnetic Resonance Imaging, and the Society of Nuclear Medicine—Technologist Section.

Radiologists and physicists are also represented by numerous organizations. Among those with the strongest ties to radiologic technology are the American Association of Physicists in Medicine, the American College of Radiology, the American Institute of Ultrasound in Medicine, the American Medical Association, the American Roentgen Ray Society, the American Society for Therapeutic Radiology and Oncology, the Radiological Society of North America, and the Society of Nuclear Medicine.

Together, these organizations constitute the full strength of the radiologic sciences profession by their activities in accreditation, certification, and representation.

◀R REVIEW QUESTIONS

1 Which of the following is a voluntary process through which an agency grants

recognition to an individual upon demonstration, usually by examination, of specialized professional skills?
a) accreditation
b) certification
c) licensure
d) registration

2 Which of the following is a listing of individuals holding certification in a particular profession?
a) accreditation
b) certification
c) licensure
d) registry

3 What organization certifies individuals in radiography?
a) American Society of Radiologic Technologists
b) American Registry of Radiologic Technologists
c) Joint Review Committee on Education in Radiologic Technology
d) Radiological Society of North America

4 Which of the following organizations represents the interests of radiologic technologists to the public and federal government?
a) American Registry of Radiologic Technologists
b) American Society of Radiologic Technologists
c) International Society of Radiographers and Radiologic Technologists
d) American Roentgen Ray Society

5 What purpose is served by the "Standards" document for a profession?
a) It sets the legal and ethical standards for a profession.
b) It determines the minimum standards for an individual to become certified by a registry organization.
c) It establishes the sponsorship of a joint review committee.
d) It specifies the requirements for accreditation of an educational program by a joint review committee.

6 Which of the following is the process by which a governmental agency (usually at the state level) grants permission to individuals to practice their profession?
a) accreditation
b) certification
c) licensure
d) registration

7 Which title is granted to a radiographer after successful completion of the American Registry of Radiologic Technologist's examination in radiography?
a) Radiologic Technologist
b) Radiologic Technologist, Radiographer
c) Registered Technologist
d) Registered Technologist, Radiographer

8 Which of the following organizations is a sponsor of the Joint Review Committee on Education in Radiologic Technology and the American Registry of Radiologic Technologists?
a) Society of Nuclear Medicine
b) American Society of Radiologic Technologists
c) American Healthcare Radiology Administrators
d) Radiological Society of North America

9 Which of the following is a voluntary peer process through which an agency grants recognition to an institution for a program of study that meets specified criteria?
a) accreditation
b) certification
c) licensure
d) registration

10 Approximately how many individuals are registered by the American Registry of Radiologic Technologists?
a) 1000
b) 10,000
c) 20,000
d) 200,000

BIBLIOGRAPHY

American Medical Association: Allied Health Education Directory. 25th ed. Chicago, American Medical Association, 1997.
Eisenberg RL: Radiology: An Illustrated History. St. Louis, Mosby–Year Book, 1992.

CHAPTER 3

EDUCATIONAL SURVIVAL SKILLS

Janice L. Akin, MS

The real voyage of discovery consists not in seeking new landscapes but in having new eyes.

MARCEL PROUST

OBJECTIVES

On completion of this chapter, the student will be able to:

1 Discuss the causes and symptoms of stress.
2 Explain behaviors and thoughts that increase the fight-or-flight response.
3 Analyze interventions that can be used to reduce or buffer stressors.
4 Describe several survival techniques to reduce stress.
5 Enumerate steps to manage time through organization, setting limits, and self-evaluation.
6 Explain the benefit of uplifts in relation to hassles.
7 Identify foods that can be eaten to supply the body nutritionally with additional vitamin C, B complex, and magnesium.
8 Adapt study techniques to enhance retention and building of information into complex concepts.
9 List steps for successful test taking.

GLOSSARY

Buffers: activities that decrease the negative effects of stress but do not change the stressors

Fight-or-Flight Response: physiologic response resulting from anger and fear and triggered by a real or imagined threat

Hassles: unexpected negative changes or events

In-Control Language: statements that reflect an attitude of choice and evoke positive feelings

Out-of-Control Language: words or phrases that express a lack of control over a situation

Stress: demand on time, energy, and resources with an element of threat

Stressors: events, both real and imagined, that increase feeling of anxiety

Time Management: practice of self-management related to how time is consumed

Uplifts: planned positive activities to balance hassles

Worry: time and energy spent concerned for things over which we have little or no control

What Is Stress?

The busy world of the student is filled with new ideas, concepts, and changing focus. Little thought is given to managing the stressors associated with so much change. The attention given to life in general as a student is to *survive* in almost any way possible. The hope is to survive midterms and finals; to survive the changing demands of clinical instructors; and to survive working, family responsibilities, and school demands. The feeling associated with this survival effort may leave the student anxious, tired, humorless, irritable, uncreative, but on rare occasions thrilled. The path through all of these emotions provides the background for finally saying, "I'm stressed out!" The focus of this chapter is on possible interventions to manage or control stressors, including time management, study habits and test-taking strategies, and other self-care interventions.

Stress is produced by events that are perceived as demands on time, energy, or resources with the threat that there will not be enough energy, time, or resources to fulfill an obligation. It is difficult to study for a big examination when there is a feeling that there will not be enough time to complete the task. The pressure is on, and the result can be overwhelming anxiety. In fact, if the threat is real enough to the individual, the heart rate increases, breathing becomes shallow and rapid, and there may be a surge of energy that seems better handled while pacing the floor. The body is ready for a big event and does not distinguish between readiness for a 100-yard dash and readiness for a paper and pencil test. The chemistry of the body responds to the brain's message and prepares for physical activity. When the response of the body is to stay and continue studying, the chemicals of the body have to dissipate on their own.

Usually, we deal with more than one event at a time—home and family responsibilities, school, and work. In combination, these events produce a compounding effect. Finally we say, "I'm stressed out!" It's the plea for help when the limits of tolerance for juggling many responsibilities have been reached.

FIGHT-OR-FLIGHT RESPONSE

The **fight-or-flight response** is the physiologic response to a real or imagined threat arising from emotions of both fear and anger. It is the body's way of preparing for change that is perceived as threatening. This response served our species well many years ago when there were threats to our survival. It provided a way to battle the elements. The physiologic responses include the release of hormones to increase metabolism, increases in fats and sugars for energy, and increases in heart rate and respiration. Blood flows at a greater than normal rate to the long muscles of the extremities, and the central nervous system is stimulated. This is the preparation for battle or escape.

An example of triggering of the fight-or-flight response is when the phone rings at 2 AM, waking one from a deep sleep. All systems are "go" as soon as the ring is heard in anticipation of bad news; the body is ready for the "battle." It turns out to be a wrong number. The outcome presented no emotional or physical injury, but the body readied itself automatically for a physical response. For several minutes after the event, a person is under the influence of the body's chemical response to the potential threat. Until the body readjusts to the nonthreatening environment, neither sleep nor relaxation will return. This same response occurs in the face of threats such as missed deadlines, loss of self-esteem, poor test results, loss of friendship, overcommitment, and inability to set limits for oneself. Living in a state of constant alert over time can result in serious physical or emotional illness.

It is important to recognize that attitudes about oneself and the environment play a role in our ability to counter or cause a stress response. What is in our mind is in our body. If self-defeating, negative thoughts are predominant, both consciously and subconsciously, the body responds with an excessive release of chemicals; over time it succumbs to the wear and tear on organs, resulting in serious illness. Positive thoughts and an optimistic viewpoint can actually decrease the potential for ill health and reduce the metabolism that chemically triggers the fight-or-flight response. Positive thoughts also serve as a self-fulfilling prophecy: attitudes that accurately predict gloom or happiness dictate whether we manage daily stressors positively or negatively.

CAUSES AND EFFECTS

The compounding effect of stress over several weeks to months can contribute to poor emotional and physical health. Examples include repeated colds, ulcers, muscle stiffness, elevated cholesterol, excessive sleeping, irritability, and headaches. Stress-related symptoms are often discounted and not considered serious, but these problems are early warnings and can have an impact on individuals physically and emotionally.

Stress can be caused by such things as traffic, meeting a deadline, expecting all A's, family problems, overcommitment, new boyfriend or girlfriend, financial problems, and car trouble. These are **stressors.** What may be stressful to one person may not affect someone else because of perspectives, life experiences, and personal circumstances. Stress is individual, and interventions used to reduce or buffer stress can only be effective when individually identified. What is helpful for one person may not be helpful to another. The important point is to recognize your stressors, to develop interventions, and to recognize the need for taking responsibility for yourself.

Interventions

CHANGE

For most people, major life events are very stressful and in some cases overwhelming. Most people have observed others experience and cope with major changes such as divorce, death of a family member or friend, marriage, job loss, or career change. By observing these major events, the observer makes decisions about how he or she would handle a similar situation if confronted. What has not been learned is how to handle minor changes, or **hassles.** In a busy life, these minor changes have great impact. Examples are an unexpected detour in the normal travel route to work or school, a last-minute change in examination time, a family argument, and car trouble. These unexpected events create

great stress, and the body responds in the fight-or-flight mode. Once again, the body produces a chemical response, and these chemicals dissipate slowly through increased respiration, increased heart rate, muscle tension, and occasionally digestive upset. Responding to these stressors may occur frequently enough that the body does not have time enough to get back to a homeostatic condition. In other words, the body can be constantly on alert as a result of the back-to-back changing conditions that are so much a part of a busy, responsible existence.

There are ways to counter minor changes by balancing unexpected change with planned positive activity. The minor changes often elicit negative responses in the form of anger, depression, poor self-concept, frustration, or defeat. Planned positive activities provide opportunities to experience joy, happiness positive self-concept, optimism, and a sense of well-being. These activities, or **uplifts,** often are simple and easy to carry out. Examples include complimenting someone, watching a favorite television program, taking a walk, being efficient and organized, relaxing, having fun, hugging, and laughing.

In your chosen field of study, new concepts will be introduced, the language of the art will have to be mastered, and deadlines will need to be met both for the welfare of the patient and for the efficiency of the department. As goals are accomplished, great relief and joy are experienced, but reaching these goals without some planned positive activities will take an emotional and physical toll.

SURVIVAL TECHNIQUE FOR CHANGE. Plan positive activities, called *uplifts,* to balance unexpected negative change, or *hassles.*

LANGUAGE

Stress tends to be contagious. When someone is in a period of great stress, such as around the time of final examinations, their words often clearly express the fear and frustration felt as a result of the concern that there will not be enough time, energy, or resources to get everything accomplished. The expression of this may alarm others as well as augment the individual's feeling of frustration.

Many things influence how we feel about events occurring around us every day. Internal events (fight or flight) happen even as a result of the **out-of-control language** we use. The use of words or phrases that express a lack of control promotes this feeling of being out of control, which is apparent in such statements as "I *have* to study for a test" and "I *never* get to do what I want to do." Words used to express a feeling of not having any control include such statements as "I have to," "I must," "I never," "it's awful," and "it's unfair."

Not only are these examples of language that express loss of control, but much emotion is tied to each. It is virtually impossible to say "never," "must," "have to," "awful," and "unfair" without some strong emotion associated with each. Just saying each awakens feelings of anger, frustration, or despair in the speaker.

If out-of-control words can evoke negative feelings, it is also true that **in-control language** will produce positive feelings. Substitute terminology producing feelings of more control and less fight-or-flight response include such statements as "I decided," "I choose," "I want to," "I like," and "I can." It is difficult to have strong negative feelings when saying things like "I have decided to study this evening for my test" and "I choose to use this method to complete this procedure." Each statement reflects an attitude of choice and evokes positive feelings. These statements produce the expectation of reaching an attainable goal as well as feelings of determination, self-control, and pleasure.

Often, terms that maximize stress responses are used when in fact personal choices have been made, but we express them negatively: "I have to go to class." It is hoped that the unsaid portion is, "I choose this field of study, and I have to go to class to reach my goal." Not only are we expressing these choices negatively, but we often lose sight of the goal. It is the vision of who or what we will become that drives our choices; with practice, our language can reflect these decisions positively.

SURVIVAL TECHNIQUE FOR LANGUAGE. Practice language that reflects choice and expresses control over a situation. In-control language reduces the flight-or-fight response.

WORRY

During high stress times, everyone tends to be overly concerned about outcomes and to engage in a mental activity of "What will I do if. . . ." This is **worry.** "What will I do if I fail this exam?" "What if I don't complete all my clinical competencies in time?" "What if my family feels neglected?" "What if my car won't last until I graduate?" "What if I lose my job? How will I pay for tuition?" Each is a real possibility for many students, but until it is a reality, it represents unnecessary energy being expended through borrowing trouble. Worry robs energy! Less than 5% of what we worry about actually happens. Part of worry is time and energy spent being concerned about things over which we have no control. We often have little control over the mechanical functioning of our car, especially when preventive maintenance is practiced. We worry about situations that may not be ours to worry about, such as a classmate's passing an examination. We worry about possibilities that could be removed from our thoughts by taking some action. Not to take action is procrastination. If we could stop putting off an unpleasant or overly challenging activity because of laziness, poor management of time, or the fear of not being perfect, a significant part of worry would be eliminated. The big problem with procrastination is that a constant feeling of guilt goes with putting off unpleasant tasks. The best news about procrastination and the worry that accompanies it is that we have full control over it. Do something to reduce the anxiety! Doing something wrong may be better than doing nothing at all!

Consider worry this way. Most of what we worry about never happens or turns out better than we thought it would. A small portion of what worries us is the result of procrastination that can be eliminated by taking action. A minor part of worry is concern over matters that are not ours to be concerned about and that may involve the worries that other people have. Less than 5% of what we worry about actually happens.

SURVIVAL TECHNIQUE FOR WORRY. When worrying, use this checklist to anticipate the degree of control one has over the situation:

- Probably won't happen
- Will turn out better than expected
- Can change outcome by taking action
- Not my concern
- No control over the outcome
- Am I making a mountain out of a molehill?

MANAGING TIME

An important part of managing stress is learning to manage time. Most commonly, it is felt that there is not enough time to accomplish all that needs to be done or all that we want to do. Since there is no control over the amount of time available, it is then necessary to practice **time management,** which is self-management related to how time is consumed.

Many external interruptions are thieves of time. These include phone calls, mistakes and incomplete information about assignments or jobs, and outside activities. These items can be controlled by setting limits on length of phone calls if you choose to receive calls, getting a full understanding of assignments by taking a few minutes longer to clarify, and limiting outside activities temporarily.

Failure to set parameters on available time is also important. Often, too many tasks are attempted at once. This happens to the student who has responsibilities that include not only school assignments but also home and family responsibilities. Besides attempting too much at once, other compounding issues include setting unrealistic deadlines, not saying no, procrastinating, and a general lack of organization.

The biggest thief of time is indecision. The fear of making a mistake or not being perfect prompts indecision. With much to be done in a limited time, loss of energy through worry and indecision is destructive and wasteful. If indecision is the product of fearing a mistake, consider thinking of a mistake as an opportunity to learn and improve on future activities and decisions.

Setting deadlines can provide opportunities to schedule time for study, to make and take phone calls, to assist family members, and to socialize. Scheduling activities gives some assurance of being able to meet obligations without slighting anyone. A potential problem associated with scheduling activities is that of being trapped by the schedule. Deadlines can give rise to feelings of desperation and helplessness, especially when there has been an overestimation of the number of activities that can be accomplished within the allotted time frame, for example, allowing 3 hours to study for a test along with some other minor activities in an evening only to discover that the 3-hour time frame was not enough. One is then trapped into having to meet the other obligations and yet still find time to complete the studying.

Although it is wise to schedule activities, realistic time frames must be set. Unrealistic estimates of the time needed to complete a paper, study for an examination, or travel to class can give rise to feelings of panic. This panic can

trigger the fight-or-flight response, which then defeats the purpose of time management. The best way to combat the result of underestimating time needed is to build in contingency plans. If a paper takes longer to write than expected, what alternatives do I have? Is there another route to school if the street repair ties up traffic? Providing a way out reduces feelings of panic and the negative effects of the fight-or-flight response.

The best way to manage time is to practice self-management. This involves four steps:

1 *Know yourself.* Evaluate your personal style and recognize the times you are in peaks and valleys of effectiveness. Capitalize on your peak times and plan to do those activities that are most demanding. Ask yourself if you are a morning person or a night owl. When do you think most clearly and how much time can you concentrate on one activity? Generally, the best results come from studying for 50 to 60 minutes in one block of time, then breaking for 10 minutes. Repeating this cycle reduces fatigue and allows for more productive use of time.

2 *Prioritize responsibilities.* Identify all the roles you have that involve responsibility—that is, student, employee, housekeeper. Prioritize all of these roles from greatest to least priority. Evaluate time available after classes and after personal needs and obligations are met. Careful evaluation of activities and responsibilities should be done to determine which can be realistically continued and which need to be delegated to someone else.

3 *Prioritize activities.* Set priorities according to goals and the length of time that will be needed to complete an activity. It may be helpful to set a plan for a full week, month, or term and to schedule study, research, and social activities during those blocks of time. By looking at a long-term plan, rushing at the last minute can be avoided and social obligations can be met. Goals such as graduating, completing a semester, or getting a B in a course must be set so that activities will be driven by the goal.

4 *Plan for self-care.* Because we all have a need for relaxation, which includes exercise, games, rest, and socializing, this time should be anticipated and planned. For some people, planning for self-care is necessary because they learned the work-

before-play work ethic. Chances are, all the work will never be done and, consequently, little attention is given to social activities, leading to a negative view of life in general. For others, the opposite may be the norm. The lack of discipline to complete work may lead to disappointing results educationally. A balance is required between work and play so that the goals can be met successfully and with enthusiasm.

SURVIVAL TECHNIQUE FOR MANAGING TIME. Plan your time and set goals by:

- knowing when you are most effective
- prioritizing and delegating responsibility where additional resources exist
- planning and scheduling activities as far in advance as possible to avoid last-minute rushing
- scheduling time for relaxation and fun

Buffering Stressors

Even with all the positive steps to reduce stress, it cannot be eliminated. Because much of the stress experienced day to day cannot be changed, the next best intervention is to buffer the effects of stress. Just as a mute muffles the harsh notes of a brass instrument, **buffers** are necessary to reduce the harmful effects of the fight-or-flight response.

EXERCISE

The fight-or-flight response readies the body for action. Circulation increases in the long muscles, and the heart rate and respiration rate increase to supply more oxygen to the muscles. Sugars and fats are dumped into the system to supply the needed energy for physical activity. If you are berated in front of your peers, anger, rage, fear, and indignation boil in your system and can be felt immediately. A chemical, norepinephrine, is released into the body when preparing for action. This chemical heightens the emotional response caused by the stress. If irritation by someone or something is the cause, the response is anger, which is often out of proportion to the magnitude of the event. If threatened, the result may be unreasonable fear. This accounts for the extreme reactions often elicited in the form of irritability and loss of sense of humor when someone has been under stress for prolonged periods without proper interventions.

Participation in regular aerobic activity—continuous, rhythmic activity that involves large muscles—is necessary to dissipate the undesirable chemicals in the system due to stress. *Aerobic* means with air to perform the activity. Examples are running, walking, biking, and other noncompetitive exercise. Because of the desire to win, exercise during a competitive event may work to increase tension rather than to decrease it.

Exercise not only is necessary to dissipate undesirable chemicals produced by the body but also can be a means to prevent negative physical and emotional responses. A minimum of 30 minutes of aerobic exercise three to five times a week can have some very positive health benefits. Some physical benefits are reduced risk of heart disease, decreased blood cholesterol levels, and reduced muscle tension.

Many of our efforts in society are directed at getting and keeping the competitive edge. Ego-involved activities almost never result in feelings of reduced stress. In fact, they may have the reverse effect. The noncompetitive forms of exercise are the most beneficial mentally. Exercising is done because it feels right. There is a sense of well-being as a result of the activity. This sense of well-being after exercising is a result not only of reducing harmful chemicals produced under stress but also of the release of "happy" chemicals in the brain that produce a sense of pleasure, the most notable of which are the endorphins. Endorphins released in the brain during physical activity have a relaxing effect on the body and provide a sense of well-being. This contributes to what is commonly called the "runner's high." Those who exercise regularly look forward to the relaxing benefits of the aerobic activity. This usually promotes better sleep patterns, more energy, increased stress tolerance, and suppressed appetite.

If possible, find a friend to participate with you. You will become encouragement for each other. Time spent with a friend walking provides some social time as well. Sharing a mutual interest is a rewarding and satisfying experience.

SURVIVAL TECHNIQUE FOR BUFFERING STRESS. Exercise aerobically three to five times per week for a minimum of 30 minutes as a buffer to the chemicals produced in the body as a result of the fight-or-flight response.

NUTRITION

It seems that when we are most busy we are least able to provide good nutrition for ourselves. Stress can be buffered by eating three well-balanced meals each day. When our body undergoes the fight-or-flight response on any regular basis, three vitamins and minerals that are important to us both physically and mentally—vitamin C, B complex, and magnesium—are greatly reduced.

Vitamin C has been shown to be especially important in supporting the immune system to help protect from colds, sore throats, and other infections. Frequently, when someone experiences a stressor such as getting through final examinations, he or she may develop a cold and sore throat at that time. As vitamin C is depleted, our resistance is decreased. One way to replace the depleted vitamin C is to start a diet that includes dark green leafy vegetables, fruits, broccoli, brussels sprouts, potatoes, and tomatoes.

The complex of B vitamins seems to support and provide necessary energy to sustain us from day to day. When under a great deal of stress, we may oversleep or feel groggy much of the time. Lost B complex can be replaced by eating bananas, green leafy vegetables, lean meat, poultry, milk, eggs, and whole grains.

Magnesium supports the immune system also. Replacement of magnesium comes from eating bananas, fish, nuts, and whole grains.

A diet rich in carbohydrates (such as white bread) and simple sugars tends to cause sudden rises and falls in blood sugar levels. This fluctuation can cause sleepiness, sluggishness, and mental lethargy. Also, because of the response of insulin to the introduction of sugar into the digestive tract, blood sugar levels fall sharply. This rapid decrease in blood sugar levels provides the physiologic conditions that can lead to misinterpreting information or making mountains out of molehills. Vending machine foods and fast foods are often major sources of carbohydrates and need to be avoided or at least carefully selected.

Good nutrition includes a diet that provides proper, appropriate servings from all food groups (Fig. 3–1 and Table 3–1). The servings recommended on the pyramid represent an intake of approximately 2200 calories per day. For an active young adult, the appropriate daily calorie intake may need to be adjusted to 2200 to 2800. Maintaining a good nutritional balance will not change your stressors, but it will place

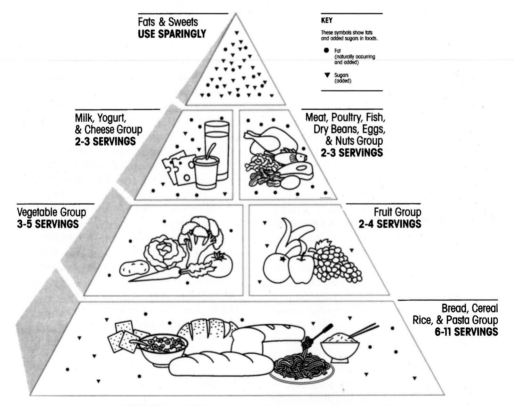

FIGURE 3–1. US Department of Agriculture's food pyramid.

TABLE 3–1. Serving Sizes for the Basic Food Groups

Food Group*	One Serving
Bread and cereals	1 slice bread *or* ½ cup cooked cereal *or* 1 oz ready-to-eat cereal
Vegetables	1 cup raw, leafy *or* ½ cup cooked or chopped raw *or* ¾ cup vegetable juice
Fruits	1 apple, banana, or orange *or* ⅓ cup cooked or canned fruit *or* ¾ cup fruit juice
Milk and cheese	1 cup milk or yogurt *or* 1½ oz natural or 2 oz processed cheese
Meat, poultry, and fish	2–3 oz meat, poultry, or fish *or* ½ cup dry beans *or* 1 egg *or* 2 tablespoons peanut butter

*Fats and sugars should be consumed sparingly.

you at an advantage for staying both physically and mentally healthy during stressful events.

VISUALIZATION AND MEDITATION

Other buffers to stress include visualization and meditation. Through visualization one can take a minivacation by mentally revisiting a pleasant experience for 10 or 15 seconds. Maybe you recall the peace of sitting on a beach and hearing the waves lap the shore. It could be the silence and coolness of getting up early and witnessing a sunrise. Maybe it is the remembrance of a camp fire, including the smells of wood burning, the sound of wood snapping, the feel of the heat from the flames, and the joy of sharing the experience with friends. Each of these mental events actually provides an opportunity to escape and relax by reliving the events momentarily. It also reduces the feeling of stress and the fight-or-flight response, thus providing a brief but real opportunity to get in touch with feelings of relaxation. This helps to buffer day-to-day stresses.

Meditation also provides a mechanism to escape stress by emptying the mind of all thoughts and focusing on only one word or one statement. In Christian meditation, it may be the process of sharing the weight of responsibility or the blessing of support through God's love and acceptance.

Other buffers to stress include progressive relaxation, deep muscle relaxation (usually guided by audio tape), biofeedback, and guided imagery.

SURVIVAL TECHNIQUE FOR BUFFERING STRESS. Eat three nutritionally balanced meals each day to replace lost vitamins and minerals adversely affected by stress. Regularly practice visualization or some form of meditation.

Study Skills and Test Taking

STUDY SKILL TECHNIQUES

During the next few years of college and advanced-level study, you will be required to learn technical information that is tested during each term. Additionally, you will have to recall pieces of learned information much later and add them to new, more advanced concepts. Because of the building of information into complex concepts, it is imperative that higher-level learning, not just a brief regurgitation of facts, occurs. An excellent way to increase the effectiveness of study time is to apply the concept of time management to develop good study skills. This involves five techniques:

1 *Review the material soon after it is introduced.* Most information introduced in class is forgotten within 24 hours unless steps are taken to reinforce it (Fig. 3–2). Students often do not begin to study for a test before the week of the test. Usually, a great deal of time has elapsed and much material has been forgotten. A common theme expressed during last-minute study is, "The instructor didn't explain very well," or "She never told us that!" If the material were reviewed immediately or within a short time after class, the information could be reinforced and remembered for a longer period. It would also help identify questionable areas where understanding is lacking.

2 *Use as many senses as possible.* In review of information, writing key elements or words has been shown to be beneficial. This visual stimulation through writing imprints additional and longer-lasting information in the brain, which enhances recall later. Besides writing the information, recite the material aloud. Saying the words helps formulate another dimension of the concept

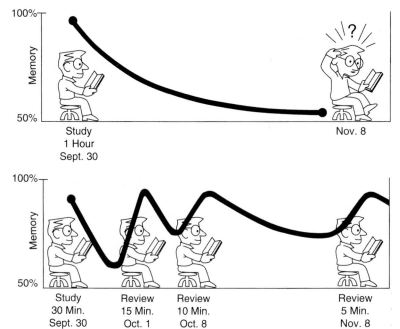

FIGURE 3–2. *Top,* "Massed" study. *Bottom,* Spaced reviews. (Reprinted with permission from Staton TF: How to Study. 6th ed. Nashville, How To Study, 1977, p 47.)

and allows practice at saying unfamiliar terms. The combination of seeing, saying, and hearing—using several senses—has been shown to provide opportunities for greater retention of information and recall.

3 *Plan a regular schedule of study.* Waiting until the last minute to study increases anxiety to a point that it may actually interfere with the ability to learn and recall information. Frustration sets in as the time ticks away. Studying or cramming for a test at the last minute may lead to confusion about details. Cramming provides only short-term recall. Plan regular review and study of all subjects from the time the material is first introduced. This may be as simple as planning to reread notes every other day for a short time. Studies have shown that short, regular periods of study and review result in greater recall than a long period of study followed by a long period of no exposure to the information. Studying for 1 hour per week before a test with no review in between can result in a 50% loss of recall.

4 *Study in a group.* Studying in small groups of no more than five helps to test your understanding of the material. The variety of perceptions offers opportunities to conceptualize the information from more than one viewpoint. If a large amount of material has to be covered, divide it among the group, each person preparing an area that may be within the individual's interest and expertise. Working in a group provides an opportunity to feel supported and encouraged, thus enhancing a personal expectation of success. The study group needs to focus on a goal with mutual agreement on purpose of meeting and task to be accomplished. This is necessary to avoid the temptation to use the time for socializing rather than study. Once the business of study is completed, it is important and appropriate to relax and enjoy the company of the group.

5 *Attitude helps remembering.* If you have a positive attitude about the reason for studying, it enhances your ability to learn and remember. You have set a goal for your professional future. Approach it with enthusiasm and a "can do" attitude. Become part of the self-fulfilling prophecy that says you are in control of your successes and failures. A feeling of control in turn reduces the stress response and enhances your chances for a healthy period of learning.

SURVIVAL TECHNIQUE FOR STUDY SKILLS

- Review new material soon after introduction.

- Use as many senses as possible—seeing, saying, and writing.
- Plan a regular study schedule.
- Study with a group occasionally.
- Develop a postitive, "can do" attitude.

TEST-TAKING TIPS

In addition to possessing good study skills, it is also helpful to follow a few *test-taking strategies.* Here are some useful tips for test-taking success:

1 Take the day off from study before the test to relax and prepare yourself. Last-minute cramming adds to anxiety and the possibility of "freezing" on the test.
2 Wear bright-colored clothes for the test. Color has great effect on moods and alertness. It also reflects feelings about oneself. Bright colors promote positive and optimistic feelings about oneself.
3 Avoid a diet full of carbohydrates the day before and the day of the test. "Carbo loading" may be helpful in a runner preparing for a long-distance race but not for a person sitting and taking a paper and pencil test. The carbohydrates convert to sugar, providing the runner with extra energy as he or she runs. Carbohydrates and sugars leave the nonrunner sluggish and sleepy because of the need to metabolize all the sugar without exerting much energy. A well-balanced diet that includes proteins and carbohydrates provides better mental alertness necessary when taking a test.
4 Get a good night's sleep before the examination. Rest allows for clearer thinking and better interpretation.
5 Get to the test early to allow yourself time to relax before beginning. Rushing at the last minute increases anxiety, which can decrease your mental effectiveness.
6 Scan the test and answer all the questions you are sure you know. Don't waste time initially on those that are problematic for you. Go back and repeat the procedure, allowing yourself a little more time to answer. Leave questions that are difficult to recall until the last. This way, if it is a time-limited examination, most questions will be answered even if you are caught short of time.
7 Review your test when done and make cor-rections as needed. Do not be afraid to change answers. Some recall may have occurred during the test as some questions provide a key to answers for other questions. Make certain you have answered all the questions. If you are answering on an answer sheet that requires blackening circles or boxes, be certain that the number of the question corresponds with the number on the answer sheet.
8 When the test is over, put it behind you. Use the results as an opportunity to enhance your knowledge in the future. And now, begin the study process all over again. Think positively!

Summary

Stress is a demand on time, energy, and resources with some fear of not being able to meet goals or obligations. Change is a large component of stress, and managing an ever-changing environment is the way to survival. The language we use can increase or decrease feelings of control. The issues we worry about need to be evaluated to determine whether our worries are within our control. Are these mountains created from molehills or can I convert my worry energy to action to diminish the problem? Much of the stress experience can be altered by practicing better time management, including prioritizing by setting limits, making decisions, establishing goals, and managing self-care.

Buffering of stress occurs when the effects of the fight-or-flight response can be offset through other activities. Most of our stressors will not go away, but we can exercise regularly, eat well-balanced diets, and use some form of meditation or visualization to temporarily reduce the physical and emotional effects of stress. These activities will not change our stressors, but they can offer an opportunity to balance some of the negative.

For students, a great deal of stress is the result of the physical and emotional effort of preparing for classroom and clinical tests. Successful test taking depends on good time management and appropriate study skills as well as on good nutrition and rest. Developing individualized study skills involves managing time to allow for regular review, periodic study in groups, and practicing methods to enhance learning and remembering. Letting as many senses as possible reinforce information assists in imprinting information on the brain. This is especially important as concepts are "built" from course to course. A systematic approach to taking the test prevents you from running out of time before all questions have been considered. Complete all the easiest questions first and return to more difficult questions later. This helps you relax and build confidence, and it helps trigger recall, since questions are often interrelated.

Most of all, maintain a positive, "can do" attitude. Attitude becomes a self-fulfilling prophecy. If you believe you can achieve your goals, you will. Associate with others who think positively. A positive attitude is contagious and needs to be fostered by you and by those around you.

◀R REVIEW QUESTIONS

1 Stress is defined as:
   a) a feeling of anxiety and fear
   b) not having enough time to complete commitments
   c) a breaking point
   d) demand on time, energy, and resources with some threat included

2 Causes of stress include:
   a) individual perception of wants
   b) poor physical health
   c) lack of time management
   d) all of the above

3 The best ways to reduce stress are by:
   a) managing finances better and saving money
   b) controlling time, thinking positively, and buffering stressors
   c) choosing a nonmedical profession and vacationing often
   d) not worrying and relaxing

4 When taking a test always:
   a) cram the night before
   b) arrive early and review notes just prior to test
   c) answer all questions you know first, then go back and repeat, leaving the most difficult questions for last
   d) review your test but do not change answers

5 In-control language:
   a) is used when driving to class
   b) is positive and expresses choice
   c) identifies where others are wrong
   d) is critical and powerful

6 The biggest thief of time is:
   a) indecision
   b) worry
   c) traffic
   d) mistakes

7 When managing time, practice self-management, which includes:
   a) setting your alarm and limiting phone calls
   b) doing only the important tasks
   c) prioritizing, setting limits, and providing for self-care
   d) stopping worrying

8 Good study habits include:
   a) reading out loud and writing down important facts
   b) planned group activity
   c) a regular plan for study and review
   d) all of the above

9 Stress buffers include:
   a) exercise and good nutrition
   b) taking a personal day off work
   c) not studying the night before a test
   d) not worrying

10 Vitamins and minerals depleted as a result of stress are:
   a) iron, B_{12}, and C
   b) B complex, C, and magnesium
   c) magnesium, E, and B complex
   d) A, E, and C

BIBLIOGRAPHY

Appelbaum SH, Rohrs WF: Time Management for Healthcare Professionals. Rockville, MD, Aspen Publications, 1981.

Bragstad BJ, Stumpf SM: A Guidebook for Teaching Study Skills and Motivation. Newton, MA, Allyn & Bacon, 1982.

Crea J: On nutrition. Chicago Tribune, May 28, 1992.

Ellis D: Becoming a Master Student. 5th ed. Rapid City, SD, College Survival, 1985.

Fuchs NK: The Nutrition Detective. New York, St. Martin's Press, 1985.

Girdano DA: Controlling Stress and Tension: A Holistic Approach. 2nd ed. Englewood Cliffs, NJ, Prentice-Hall, 1986.

Hubbard R: Stress and Burnout in Health Care Professionals. Notre Dame, IN, University of Notre Dame, Administrative Development Program, 1987.

Kirtbawski PA: Test-taking skills: Giving yourself an edge. Nursing '90 20:6, 1990.

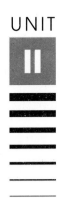

UNIT II

Introduction to the Clinical Environment

CHAPTER 4

INTRODUCTION TO CLINICAL EDUCATION

Marlene E. Ledbetter, MEd, RT(R)

Perfect health, like perfect beauty, is a rare thing, and so, it seems, is perfect disease.

PETER LATHAM
GENERAL REMARKS ON THE PRACTICE OF MEDICINE

OBJECTIVES

On completion of this chapter, the student will be able to:

1 Explain the purpose of the clinical education component.
2 Define terms that relate to the clinical education component of the radiography curriculum.
3 Describe the physical and human resources necessary for effective clinical education.
4 Explain the importance of adhering to major clinical education policies.
5 Discuss the methods used in effectively teaching clinical course content.
6 Describe methods of assessment that may be used to measure cognitive, psychomotor, and affective aspects of clinical education.
7 Summarize the clinical education process.

GLOSSARY

Affective: one of the three major categories or domains of learning, which includes behaviors guided by feelings and emotions that are influenced by one's interests, attitudes, values, and beliefs

Clinical: describes procedures and activities that occur in the clinic or hospital setting

Cognitive: one of the three major categories or domains of learning, which includes various levels of thought such as knowledge, understanding, reason, and judgment

Competency: demonstrable, successful achievement of a performance objective

Didactic: describes informational and instructional activities that may occur in formal or informal settings

Objective: concise description of an observable behavior to be achieved

Psychomotor: one of the three major categories or domains of learning, which includes behaviors involving physical actions, neuromuscular manipulations, and coordination

Overview of Clinical Education

Planned and structured learning experiences and activities in various clinical settings are necessary for an effective educational program for radiographers. For the student to fully appreciate the actual health care setting, and to allow for the observation, assistance, and performance requirements for the completion of diagnostic medical imaging procedures, learning in a clinical setting must occur. This is achieved by hospital-sponsored programs or through clinical affiliations between medical facilities and educational institutions.

GENERAL DESCRIPTION OF CLINICAL EDUCATION

Purpose of Clinical Education

The process of developing and refining the skills required to become a competent radiographer cannot be completed without hours spent in a setting that provides a variety of medical imaging procedures. Hospitals, clinics, and surgical centers are just a few of the locations that fulfill this need.

According to the "Standards for an Accredited Educational Program in Radiologic Sciences," an objective of the clinical curriculum is to provide competency-based educational experiences that promote synthesis of theory, use of current technology, competent clinical practice, and professional values. Areas of competence may include head and neck, abdominal, gastrointestinal, genitourinary, musculoskeletal, chest and breast, trauma, and bedside and surgical procedures. It is appropriate that all policies and procedures related to clinical education be published and provided to students, faculty, and clinical staff.

The clinical education centers are expected to conform to appropriate standards for accreditation by appropriate agencies.

Terminology

The **clinical** component of the radiography curriculum is those procedures and activities that occur in the clinic or hospital setting. Clinical experiences include one-on-one direct patient contact as opposed to theoretical or laboratory experiences. Interactions occur with inpatients, outpatients, and emergency and specialty patients of all ages.

Informational and instructional activities related to radiography make up the **didactic** portion of the curriculum. These activities may occur in settings such as the classroom, laboratory, instructional media viewing area, or learning resource center. The instructional activity should be well planned, with documented goals, objectives, and learning activities provided for the students.

In the early phases of the educational program, more time is spent in didactic instruction. Students then progress to an increasing amount of time in the clinical setting. The laboratory setting serves as a bridge to connect classroom with clinical activities (Fig. 4–1).

Most educational researchers agree that learning can be organized into three major categories or domains. The **cognitive** domain includes behaviors requiring various levels of thought: knowledge, understanding, reason, and judgment. The **psychomotor** domain includes behaviors involving physical actions, neuromuscular manipulations, and coordination. The **affective** domain includes behaviors guided by feelings and emotions that are influenced by one's interests, attitudes, values, and beliefs.

One element of the major categories or domains of learning is the performance **objective.** An objective is a description of an observable student behavior. Objectives must be concise, measurable, and achievable. They describe what behavior the student is to display, how well the student is to perform the behavior, and under what circumstances the behavior is to be achieved. Closely related to performance objectives is **competency,** the observable, successful achievement of the performance objectives.

The new student's eyes are open to anything and everything that goes on in the hospital or clinic as the clinical education segment of the program begins. This is the *observation* phase of the educational experience. This phase is extensive during the early portion of the program, tapering off as the new student gains confidence and can effectively integrate the appropriate cognitive, psychomotor, and affective behaviors. Still, throughout the length of the program there will be clinical situations that are totally new to the student. After gaining knowledge of the various procedures in a didactic setting and practicing the performance of the procedures in the laboratory setting, the student is ready to watch and give critical attention to all that is occurring in the clinical setting, noting the role of the various participating health professionals. As radiographers perform various diagnostic procedures, they serve as role models for the new student. The inquisitive student makes mental notes of how the procedure is being accomplished and begins to model or imitate the actions seen, whether correct or incorrect.

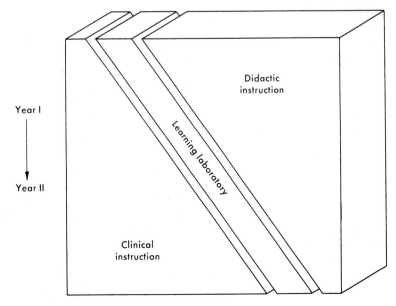

FIGURE 4–1. The articulation of didactic, laboratory, and clinical instruction. (Reprinted with permission from Ford C [ed]: Clinical Education for the Allied Health Professions. St. Louis, CV Mosby, 1978, p 121.)

Year I

Year II

Didactic instruction

Learning laboratory

Clinical instruction

When the student feels confident, it is time to proceed to *assistance*, the next phase of the educational program. In this phase, the student should begin aiding and supporting the radiographer in the performance of the diagnostic procedure. The student is now gaining hands-on experience, literally placing a hand on the patient to assist in movement to the examining table or helping the patient assume a specific position for the diagnostic procedure. If a number of manipulations of the patient is required, the student should feel free to discuss with the radiographer a desire to become more actively involved in the performance of the procedure. The radiographer will then be able to determine the appropriate extent of student assistance based on an assessment of the patient's needs.

After assisting the radiographer with various aspects of the diagnostic procedure, the student will eventually feel confident and will be ready to proceed toward the *performance* of the entire procedure without assistance from the radiographer, clinical instructor, or clinical supervisor. During the performance of the procedure, the student should accurately demonstrate all tasks included in the entire procedure at the level of skill determined by the faculty.

In the event that the student does not have the opportunity to perform a required procedure on an actual patient, program policy may permit the procedure to be performed as a *simulation*. This provision may be made for infrequent or limited volume procedures. In this situation, the student must accurately demonstrate all of the tasks included in the procedure just as was described previously for when performance occurs. The only difference is that the procedure is not performed on an actual patient. A phantom patient or a live substitute patient takes the place of the actual patient. When a live substitute patient is involved in the simulation, *no radiographic exposure is to be made under any circumstances*.

The standards of quality for educational programs for radiographers are provided in the "Standards for an Accredited Educational Program in Radiologic Sciences," often referred to as the "Standards," adopted in 1996 by the Joint Review Committee on Education in Radiologic Technology. The "Standards" document is used for program development and evaluation and includes criteria for program accountability.

The "Standards" document for radiography programs provides for the appropriate supervision of students. Until a student achieves and documents competency in any given procedure, all clinical assignments are carried out under the direct supervision of a qualified practitioner (radiographer). The parameters of *direct supervision* require that the qualified practitioner (1) review the request for examination in relation to the student's achievement, (2) evaluate the condition of the patient in relation to the student's knowledge, (3) be present during the examination, and (4) review and approve the radiographs.

Indirect supervision means that the qualified practitioner reviews, evaluates, and approves the procedure as for direct supervision and is immediately available to assist students regardless of the level of student achievement. "Immediately available" is interpreted as the presence of a qualified practitioner adjacent to the room or location where a radiographic procedure is being performed. This availability applies to all areas where ionizing radiation equipment is in use.

In support of professional responsibility for the provision of quality patient care and radiation protection, unsatisfactory radiographs are repeated only in the presence of a qualified practitioner, regardless of the student's level of competency.

RESOURCES

Physical Facilities

Imaging facilities must be of a sufficient number to accommodate the students enrolled in the radiography program and to provide a variety of procedures for each student's clinical performance continuum. A variety of equipment should be available to produce diagnostic images during trauma or emergency, bedside, surgical, abdominal, gastrointestinal, genitourinary, musculoskeletal, and head and neck procedures. Additionally, equipment used for computed tomographic, ultrasonographic, neuroradiologic, cardiovascular, and interventional procedures should also be available for the educational opportunities they present.

Program Officials

A number of individuals work together to assist the student in understanding and accomplishing the goals and objectives of the program. Included are the program director, clinical coordinator (in many programs), clinical instructor, medical director or advisor, didactic faculty, and the clinical staff. Figure 4–2 illustrates a sample organizational chart for a radiography program.

The *program director* works full-time in organizing and administering the radiography program. This individual is responsible for the didactic and clinical effectiveness of the program. Program directors must be credentialed by and in good standing with the American Registry of Radiologic Technologists, or they must possess equivalent qualifications, have a baccalaureate degree or higher, and be proficient in such areas as curriculum design, program administration, program evaluation, instruction, and counseling.

If a program uses four or more clinical education facilities or has more than 20 enrolled students, a *clinical coordinator* must be among the program's officials. This individual works closely with the program director in ensuring program effectiveness through a regular schedule of coordination, instruction, and evaluation. Like the program director, the clinical coordinator must also possess appropriate professional credentials.

The *clinical instructor* has the unique opportunity to directly influence the professional development of the radiography student. Of all of the program's officials, this individual works intimately with the student in one-on-one observation, instruction, and evaluation. The clinical instructor should also possess the appropriate professional credentials.

These program officials must possess current knowledge regarding medical imaging procedures as well as competence in instructional and evaluation techniques.

The *medical director* or *advisor* works in consultation with the director in establishing goals, objectives, and standards for program quality. The medical director or advisor must be a diplomate of the American Board of Radiology or must have suitable equivalent certification and possess a current license to practice medicine.

Additionally, many programs are supported by a number of individuals responsible for teaching general education, professional, and technical courses within the radiography curriculum. These *didactic faculty members* are individually qualified to teach the appropriate course work. They work closely with the program director in ensuring coordination and integration of course content with the program's goals and objectives.

Members of the *clinical staff* work in assisting the clinical instructor in one-on-one observation and instruction of radiography students. In addition to meeting patient needs, these dedicated professionals are committed to sharing their knowledge and expertise with student radiographers, their future colleagues.

Major Clinical Education Policies

All participants in clinical education—faculty, clinical staff, and students—need a complete and accurate understanding of the process by which students are instructed and evaluated in the clinical setting. A clinical education handbook, student handbook, or clinical education guide is vital in providing consistent written information for all parties. The resultant benefit is improved integration of the didactic and clinical aspects of the radiography curriculum. To

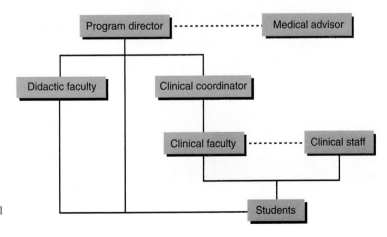

FIGURE 4–2. Sample organizational chart for a radiography program.

this end, program faculty members should develop timely policies, procedures, rules, regulations, and guidelines that are applicable to clinical education. It is appropriate to briefly discuss examples of these policies.

SUPERVISION

The activities of student radiographers must be monitored by an appropriately credentialed clinical staff member. Until a student demonstrates competence in a given diagnostic procedure, all of the student's clinical assignments must be directly supervised (Fig. 4–3). The parameters for direct and indirect supervision were described previously. These strict requirements serve to protect the student from being used inappropriately to replace paid staff. There should never be a time when a student radiographer is not supervised either directly or indirectly. Until the student completes all of the program's published academic and clinical requirements, supervision by a qualified practitioner must occur.

PERFORMANCE OF ACTUAL EXAMINATIONS

In a competency-based clinical education and evaluation system, the student proceeds at his or her own pace. The timing and length of

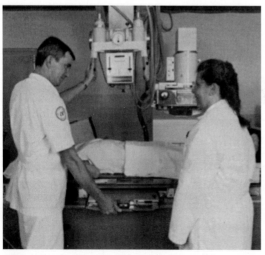

FIGURE 4–3. Students need direct supervision by a qualified radiographer prior to demonstrating competency for a procedure.

the observation and assistance phases of clinical education are variable. Because most radiography programs must work within the framework of an academic grading period (semester or quarter), policies may exist that specify a suggested pace for procedure performance and proficiency.

PERFORMANCE OF SIMULATIONS

A simulated clinical procedure is designed to re-create an actual, real-life diagnostic examination. Simulations may involve mannequins, artificial body parts, or dramatizations (using live simulated patients). Program policy may stipulate what specific procedures may be simulated and when. Only a minor portion of the total number of clinical evaluations should be completed as simulations.

AVOIDANCE OF USING STUDENTS TO REPLACE STAFF

Students in an accredited program for radiographers should *never* substitute for, or assume the responsibilities of, regular staff. After demonstrating competency, students may perform procedures under direct or indirect supervision as determined by a qualified practitioner.

COMPLETION OF EVALUATIONS

Written examinations (paper and pencil tests) are frequently used to evaluate cognitive skills. Practical examinations utilizing a checklist or rating scale are often used to evaluate psychomotor skills. Oral examinations or direct observations may be used to evaluate affective behaviors. A combination of these evaluations is commonly used to determine the student's overall level of clinical skill and performance. Program policy determines the timing and weight of all clinical evaluations as well as the specific method by which clinical grades are achieved and documented.

RADIATION PROTECTION PRACTICES

A radiation monitoring device is a part of the professional radiographer's uniform. Program policy may specify when and where this monitor is to be worn and the procedure to be followed if a monitor is lost or needs to be replaced. Program policy regarding the holding of patients during radiographic procedures should also be specifically documented.

PROFESSIONAL ETHICS

The Code of Ethics of the American Registry of Radiologic Technologists (Appendix E) reflects the rules and standards that govern the conduct of professional technologists. Student radiographers should strive to understand, appreciate, and value these standards. To this end, program faculty should outline the standards of ethics required for all radiography students. Violations of published standards may result in disciplinary action.

PROFESSIONAL APPEARANCE

The program's policy regarding professional appearance outlines the acceptable uniform for the student radiographer. Identifying name badges, patches, and radiation-monitoring devices are also a part of the professional uniform. Generally, extremes are to be avoided when it comes to jewelry, hair styles, and cosmetics. Specific guidelines and program requirements should be available in the published student handbook.

ATTENDANCE

The program provides clinical schedules that indicate the actual dates and times for all clinical experiences. Students should also be informed of schedule variations such as breaks, vacation periods, and holidays. In the event that a student is unable to participate in a scheduled clinical activity because of personal business or illness, it is important that program procedure be followed regarding notification of the designated program faculty or staff. Absenteeism and tardiness are ofen documented and may result in disciplinary or other actions.

PREGNANCY

Because of the potential radiation hazard to the fetus, particularly during the first trimester,

pregnancy should be reported to the program director or radiation safety officer in accordance with program policy or government recommendations. It is recommended that a pregnant student discuss her situation with her physician. The program's officials will review the program's policy with the student, describing possible options. The pregnancy may result in rescheduling of classes or clinical experiences, other temporary inconveniences, and a delay in the completion of the program. This topic is discussed in detail in Chapter 8.

DISCIPLINARY PROCEDURES

Students in radiography programs are required to abide by the policies and procedures of the sponsoring institution, the program, and the clinical education centers. Students are also expected to abide by the Code of Ethics of the American Registry of Radiologic Technologists. Failure to adhere to these may result in disciplinary action against the student. The specific steps in the disciplinary procedure, which are usually detailed in the student clinical education handbook, may include oral and written warnings. A repetition of infractions may result in suspension or dismissal from the program. Serious infractions, including, but not limited to, a threat to patient safety, gross insubordination, the disclosure of confidential information, falsification of records, cheating, theft, willful damage of property, and substance abuse, may result in immediate dismissal from the program. In all cases, students have the right of due process and the right to appeal all unfavorable evaluations, disciplinary actions, suspensions, and dismissals.

Progressive Clinical Development

Student clinical progress occurs when goals and objectives are clearly outlined, didactic information is integrated with the appropriate clinical experiences, and timely and objective evaluations occur.

THE PROCESS

The highlights of each clinical course are provided through a review of the course description. The description often includes the department code, course number, course title, number of credits, and the mandatory corequisite or prerequisite courses. In two or three sentences, a brief glimpse of the course is achieved. The clinical courses should be sequential, with each clinical course building on the previous ones.

The program faculty must determine what is to be learned in each clinical course. This information is then linked to the didactic material presented and to the clinical experiences available to the student during a given period. The course outline or syllabus usually includes such information as course title and instructor, time and location of the clinical education course, a brief overview of the course, clinical competencies, specific goals and objectives, the schedule of clinical rotations and activities, grading procedures, and references. This document should be distributed to all clinical instructors and students so that all parties are thoroughly familiar with the clinical course requirements and expectations.

Performance objectives are descriptions of observable student behaviors. These are required for all of the clinical courses in the radiography curriculum. Objectives are provided for (1) the student's scheduled orientation experiences (ie, darkroom and film file areas); (2) routine radiographic procedures; and (3) imaging specialties, such as pediatric, surgical, mobile, tomographic, and mammographic procedures. Objectives should also be provided for scheduled observations in specialty areas such as computed tomography, ultrasonography, radiation therapy, nuclear medicine, magnetic resonance imaging, and cardiovascular interventional imaging.

The first clinical education course may be structured to orient the new student to the radiology department. Students are often given assignments to observe, assist, and perform specific activities as indicated by the objectives for this course. Areas of assignment may include the darkroom or other film-processing area, the radiology office, patient transport areas, and the various fluoroscopic and radiographic rooms.

Subsequent clinical courses may emphasize the performance of specific radiographic procedures. Students will be required to evaluate the request for the given radiographic procedure, prepare the radiographic room before the patient's arrival, provide complete and accurate patient instructions, properly position and care for the patient, set the appropriate exposure factors, provide protection from unnecessary radiation, evaluate the processed radiographic image, and appropriately discharge the patient. The student's ability to completely handle the radiographic procedure should gradually improve as the weeks and months proceed. Eventually, the student should be able to pick up speed in doing procedures and should be able to organize the activities to be completed in an assigned radiographic area.

A number of instructional methods are effective in teaching clinical course content. First, the clinical instructor may use *demonstrations* to assist the students in seeing the proper way to perform the various aspects of the radiographic examination (Fig. 4–4). This may occur in a laboratory or practice setting as well as with actual patients. The student may be asked to perform a *return demonstration*, in imitation of the instructor's actions and manner. At a later time, a *discussion* of the performance events should occur. This provides the instructor and the student an opportunity to critique the performance and to make mental and written notes of its strengths and weaknesses. Instructors often use additional methods to enhance the learning process and to facilitate learning.

ASSESSMENT

The clinical instructor may determine that some aspects of the radiographic procedure in-

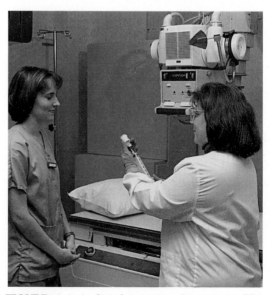

FIGURE 4–4. A clinical instructor demonstrates filling a syringe.

volve the assessment of the student's knowledge or comprehension, or perhaps the ability to apply, analyze, synthesize, or evaluate. These are the levels within the cognitive domain of learning. Measurement of the learning that has occurred within these categories usually involves an objective test of some kind: multiple choice, matching, or true or false.

A number of cognitive and psychomotor behaviors are involved in performing a radiographic procedure, including the following:

- Assessing the requisition
- Preparing the radiographic room for performance of the procedure
- Caring for the needs of the patient
- Performing the radiographic procedure
- Providing radiation protection for the patient
- Manipulating the exposure factors
- Evaluating the radiographic image
- Manipulating specialized equipment

These behaviors are assessed by the clinical instructor's use of direct, objective observation and are documented through the use of rating scales, checklists, critical incident forms, and anecdotal notes.

Behaviors involving attitudes and values are also among those considered by instructors in assessing the progress of the student's clinical development. Instructors may wish to assess the student's ability to (1) communicate effectively with staff and patients, (2) perceive patient needs, (3) display maturity and confidence, (4) follow through with clinical responsibilities in a reliable and conscientious manner, and (5) display an interest in professional literature and organizations.

As with the psychomotor area, these behaviors require the use of direct objective observations, documented through the use of rating scales, checklists, critical incident forms, and anecdotal notes.

Summary

Clinical education is a necessary component of the radiography curriculum. It provides a structured and ordered mechanism for the student to develop and refine important skills needed in a variety of one-on-one, direct interactions with the patient. A correlation between the didactic and clinical portions of the curriculum must occur for clinical education to be successful. This correlation includes a successful weaving and integration of cognitive, psychomotor, and affective behaviors during observation, assistance, and performance of actual radiographic procedures.

The standards of quality for the educational program are described in a document called the "Standards for an Accredited Educational Program in Radiologic Sciences."

Appropriate supervision for students in radiography programs is essential. Direct supervision is required until a student achieves and documents competency for a given procedure, and indirect supervision is necessary once competency has been achieved and documented. In either situation, unsatisfactory radiographs should be repeated only in the presence of a qualified practitioner.

In an effort to ensure a complete and accurate understanding of the clinical education process, a number of major clinical education policies and procedures are developed and implemented by the program officials. These usually include policies regarding appropriate supervision, procedure performance, evaluations, radiation protection practices, professional ethics, attendance, pregnancy, and disciplinary procedures.

Progressive clinical development occurs when valid and achievable goals and objectives are clearly outlined, correlated with corresponding cognitive information, integrated with the appropriate clinical experiences, and objectively and promptly assessed. This progressive development is achieved through the use of clinical course descriptions, outlines, performance objectives, and the appropriate content.

Important judgments are made after the assessment of a variety of cognitive, psychomotor, and affective behaviors. They are vital in assisting the student to ultimately assume the role of professional radiographer.

◀R REVIEW QUESTIONS

1 Clinical procedures and activities are performed in what setting?
   a) classroom
   b) hospital
   c) laboratory
   d) library

2 Cognitive learning includes:
   a) attitudes, values, and beliefs
   b) physical actions, neuromuscular manipulations, and coordination

c) assistance, observation, and performance
d) knowledge, reason, and judgment

3 How does a qualified practitioner directly supervise a student radiographer?
a) by reviewing the request in relation to the student's achievement
b) by evaluating the condition of the patient in relation to the student's knowledge
c) by being present while the student conducts the examination
d) by reviewing and approving the radiographs
e) all of the above

4 A student's unsatisfactory radiographs must be repeated in the presence of a qualified practitioner because:
a) students are not instructed in how to repeat films
b) quality patient care and radiation protection must be ensured and provided
c) the qualified practitioner is responsible for all unsatisfactory radiographs
d) patient preference mandates it

5 Which program official often provides one-on-one instruction and evaluation of students?
a) program director
b) clinical coordinator
c) clinical instructor
d) medical director/advisor

6 Which program official regularly schedules students to work in the clinical setting when department staff are unavailable?
a) program director
b) clinical coordinator
c) clinical instructor
d) medical director/advisor
e) none of the above

7 Disciplinary action may be initiated against a student if which serious infraction occurs?
a) disclosure of confidential information
b) falsification of records
c) cheating
d) intoxication
e) all of the above

8 An instructor may use which format to measure cognitive behaviors?
a) rating scale
b) critical incident form
c) anecdotal note
d) multiple-choice test
e) none of the above

9 Affective behaviors influence one's ability to:
a) comprehend
b) analyze
c) synthesize
d) evaluate
e) none of the above

10 If a radiography student is to competently perform radiologic procedures, that individual must:
a) observe a qualified radiographer
b) develop and refine the appropriate skills and behaviors
c) help and support a qualified radiographer as much as possible
d) simulate as many radiographic procedures as possible

BIBLIOGRAPHY

Ford CW: Clinical Education for the Allied Health Professions. St. Louis, CV Mosby, 1978.
Ford CW, Morgan MK: Teaching in the Health Professions. St. Louis, CV Mosby, 1976.
Roberts GH, Carson J: The roles instructors play in clinical education. Radiol Tech 63:28, 1991.
Standards for an Accredited Educational Program in Radiologic Sciences. Chicago, IL, The Joint Review Committee on Education in Radiologic Technology, 1996.
Student Handbook. Gary, IN, Indiana University Northwest, Radiologic Technology Program, 1997.

CHAPTER 5

RADIOLOGIC SERVICES ADMINISTRATION

Gail A. Nielsen, BSHCA, RT(R), FAHRA

We can show that the number of lives that have been saved by x-rays since their discovery by Roentgen is as great as the number of lives that have been taken in all of the wars that have been fought since that time.

A.H. COMPTON, NOBEL LAUREATE IN PHYSICS AND DISCOVERER OF THE COMPTON EFFECT, 1927

The Hospital Environment
Hospital Organization
Organizational Transition in the 1990s
Radiology Organization
Subdepartments of Radiology
Administrative Director of Radiology
Medical Director
Department Chair

Other Health Care Settings
Clinics
Physician Offices
Imaging Centers
Mobile Imaging
Emergency Care Centers
Outpatient Surgical Centers
Industry and Research

Management Functions
Planning
Organizing
Staffing
Directing
Controlling
Coordinating

Regulating Agencies and Committees
External
Joint Commission on Accreditation of
Healthcare Organizations
State Health Departments
Nuclear Regulatory Commission
Occupational Safety and Health
Administration
Mammography Accreditation
Internal
Safety Committee
Infection Control Committee
Radiation Safety Committee
Pharmacy and Therapeutics
Committee

Characteristics of Good Employees

Summary

OBJECTIVES

On completion of this chapter, the student will be able to:

1 Provide an overview of the administration of a hospital radiology department and the structure of hospital organization.
2 Describe how the radiology department fits into the hospital world.
3 Appreciate the role of the radiology administrator.

4 Define the organization of a hospital and a hospital department of radiology or medical imaging.
5 Explain the functions of management including planning, organizing, staffing, directing, controlling, and coordinating.
6 Discuss the transition from traditional functions of management to the requirements of managing radiology in the current health care environment.
7 Describe regulating agencies that affect radiology.
8 Discuss the characteristics of desirable applicants for employment in radiology imaging.

GLOSSARY

Board of Directors or Governing Board: group of people authorized by law to conduct, maintain, and operate a hospital for the benefit of the public and whose legal and moral responsibility for policies and operations of the hospital are not for personal benefit of the members

Certificate of Need (CON): certificate approved by a local (state) review board permitting hospitals to construct new or additional facilities, open new services, or make large purchases—a condition required for reimbursement by Medicare

Chief Executive Officer (CEO): person appointed by the board of directors who has full accountability for the entire hospital

Clinical Support Services: services to provide the components of patient care that collectively support the physician's plan for diagnoses and treatments

Continuous Quality Improvement (CQI): system of development in the workplace for daily improving performance at every level in every operational process by focusing on meeting or exceeding customer expectations

Department: unit of the hospital with specific functions or specialized skills such as housekeeping, surgery, radiology, or accounting

Department Chair: physician who represents a department or service to the formal organization of the medical staff and who has voting privileges on the executive committee of the medical staff

Human Resources Department (Formerly Personnel): department of the hospital responsible for recruiting, selecting, supporting, and compensating employees; maintaining skills, quality, and motivation; collective bargaining; and occupational health and safety

Joint Commission on Accreditation of Healthcare Organizations (JCAHO): national organization of hospitals and other health care providers; it offers its members inspection and accreditation of the quality of operations

Medical Director: physician who has responsibility for the operation and quality of a hospital department or service; he or she is responsible for policies and procedures and day-to-day operations of his or her department

Medical Staff: formal organization of physicians authorized to admit and attend to patients within a hospital; they have authorized privileges, bylaws, elected officers, and various committees and activities (*see medical director, department chair, and service chief*)

Mission Statement: statement of an organization that summarizes its intent to provide service in terms of the services it offers, the intended recipients of services, and a description of the level of cost

Occupational Safety and Health Administration (OSHA): federal agency that enforces standards for safety in the workplace; it conducts inspections and directs levy of fines for noncompliance with rules

Radiology Department: organization of a hospital or medical clinic that provides imaging through medical technologies such as x-ray, general diagnostics, nuclear medicine, and ultrasonography; sometimes known as medical imaging

Service Chief: physician head of a hospital service

Third-Party Payers: insurance companies, Medicare, Medicaid, and other commercial companies who are the payers of medical expenses for the patient

Total Quality Management (TQM): management of quality in the workplace from a perspective of total involvement of every employee

The Hospital Environment

HOSPITAL ORGANIZATION

Hospitals are a central part of one of the nation's largest industries, the health care industry, offering a broad range of services provided by increasingly expensive personnel, equipment, and technology. The complexity of a hospital can be compared to that of a town or city in which people work together in mutually supportive functions. For example, the building, or plan, of a hospital provides space, electricity, plumbing, and roadways that require upkeep and maintenance. A hospital employs persons in 20 or more different professions and an equal number of trades; these people require physical supports such as food service and payroll. Supplies are needed, which are purchased from outside the hospital or produced from within the organization. As a city does, a hospital requires policies, procedures, administrative staff, rules, regulations, traffic laws, and plans.

The hospital-city analogy can be carried further to compare the governance and organization of a hospital to that of a city. Citizens are central to a city and patients are central to a hospital. To ensure that its citizens are protected and to provide services necessary to living and conducting business, a city is organized through its governmental body. In a similar fashion, the hospital is organized through a board of directors and administrative staff to carry out the hospital's mission.

Hospitals have a direct relationship to the community in which they reside. This can be compared to the relationship a city has with the county or state within which it is located. This relationship should be mutually supportive and beneficial. Single hospitals have merged into multihospital groups, similar to the way nearby cities merge activities first and later combine governance.

The medical staff and employees of a hospital find a correlate with the city's skilled and trained persons who provide services to other citizens. Volunteers in both scenarios enable many tasks to be performed at reasonable cost to the central customers. In the hospital setting, volunteers and the auxiliary organizations provide many hours of service, compassion, and assistance, in an embodiment of the spirit of cooperation central to the best in human living.

The **mission statement,** or charter, is the driving and guiding force that outlines the organization's reason for existence and defines what should be done and how. But the comparison between a hospital and a city stops here. Not every citizen of a city is charged with carrying out the city's mission or charter or fully understands its meaning. But because every function of a hospital should be focused on its mission, all of its members should be familiar with the mission. The mission statement summarizes the hospital's intent to provide service in terms of the intended recipients of service, the type of care or services, and the level of quality and cost expected. If the citizens of a city can be compared to a hospital's patients, the city's elected officials, magistrates, and other civil servants might be compared to the variety of hospital employees who are organized to provide services.

The organizational chart of a hospital demonstrates how the functions within the institution are carried out by its employees in an organized and logical manner. Governance of a hospital begins with the **board of directors or governing board,** which is authorized by law to operate a hospital. The board employs a **chief executive officer (CEO)** or president and defines how the operation of the hospital is maintained and conducted. The primary restriction imposed on individual board members is that their governance may not afford them personal benefit. The CEO or president then sets in place a formal reporting structure for the organization and interacts with the medical staff to ensure coordination and quality of patient care and services.

In the organizational chart in Figure 5–1, the line of communication between the medical staff and CEO is a broken line, indicating communication but not control. The **medical staff** is the formal organization of physicians within a hospital with authorized privileges, bylaws, elected officers, committees, and organized activities. Radiologists fit into the formal organization of the medical staff; they either perform on a contractual basis to provide and supervise specific services or serve as paid employees of the institution.

A hospital is composed of many **departments** and services organized to provide care and **clinical support services** to its patients and clients.

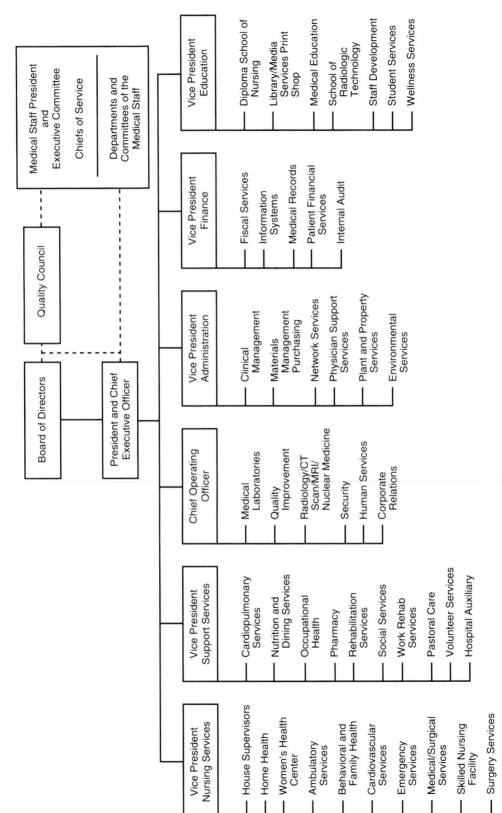

FIGURE 5-1. Organizational chart.

While most of a hospital's departments are interrelated, some of these departments and services are directly dependent on each other. For example, all patient care services depend on the admissions department for information regarding the patients being served. Nursing, the medical staff, billing offices, and other departments rely on the medical records department for retaining records of patients and maintaining the patients' histories in charts. The **human resources department** is responsible for the recruitment, retention, and compensation of all employees who work in the hospital. Business offices handle the financial functions of the hospital, including billing patients and insurance companies, paying for equipment and supplies, and maintaining strict accounting practices. Besides nursing, medical laboratories, and radiology, other departments that support patients include pastoral care, pharmacy, cardiopulmonary services, rehabilitation services (such as physical therapy), nutritional services, social services, and medical clinics.

The radiology or medical imaging department plays an important role in the care of the patient. The quality of care provided to the patient by radiology (or any department) is directly related to the quality of the coordination and cooperation that exists between the department and all of the other departments and services that make up the organization.

ORGANIZATIONAL TRANSITION IN THE 1990s

Social and economic conditions of the late 1980s and early 1990s have caused vast changes in health care organizations, forcing them to alter their organizational structures. Economic hardships and total quality management both have been influential in eliminating middle-management positions in many hospitals and radiology departments. These changes have continued throughout the 1990s as changes in reimbursement escalated cost reductions and downsizing. Figures 5–2 and 5–3 demonstrate the vertical and horizontal organizational structures that represent changes occurring in health care, as well as other industries, in the 1990s. The vertical structure depicted in Figure 5–2 demonstrates a more top-heavy organization, with more layers of senior administration staff. Following reorganization, many hospital organizations resemble the flatter horizontal structure in the example in Figure 5–3. An example of continued downsizing can be seen if the positions in Figure 5–1 are altered to eliminate the chief operating officer and vice president of administration.

The matrix structure pictured in Figure 5–4 has been useful in some hospitals as well as other industries attempting to strategically manage products and services that cross departmental boundaries. An example of matrix management structure that could affect radiology departments is when a manager of outpatient services or women's services interacts with many department managers in the hospital to be certain that maximum quality of care and efficiency is maintained for all patients who enter the hospital for that service.

The women's services manager would likely consult with the radiology manager about gyne-

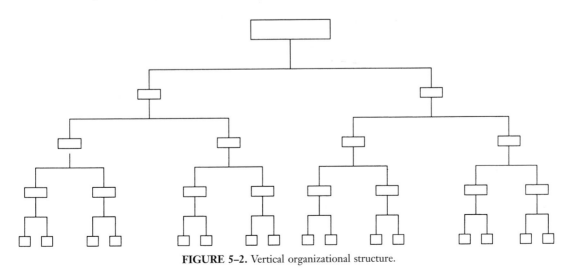

FIGURE 5–2. Vertical organizational structure.

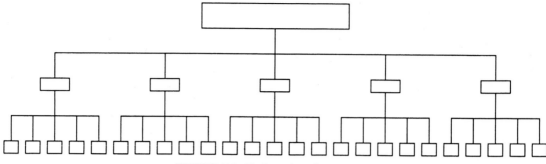

FIGURE 5–3. Horizontal, or flat, structure.

cologic and obstetric ultrasonography and mammography. The outpatient services manager would consult with the radiology manager on patient waiting time and the flow of patients from one department to the next (eg, emergency department, electrocardiography, laboratory, radiology); other managers would consult in a like manner.

RADIOLOGY ORGANIZATION

Similar to the organization of a hospital, the formal structure of a **radiology department** is a subset of the larger organization. The radiology department has the same focus on the hospital mission to serve patients and has needs similar to those of the larger organization—personnel, information, supplies, equipment, space, electricity, plumbing, upkeep, and maintenance.

Subdepartments of Radiology

Larger radiology departments are often divided into subdepartments or sections such as radiography, diagnostic medical sonography, nuclear medicine, and radiation therapy/oncol-

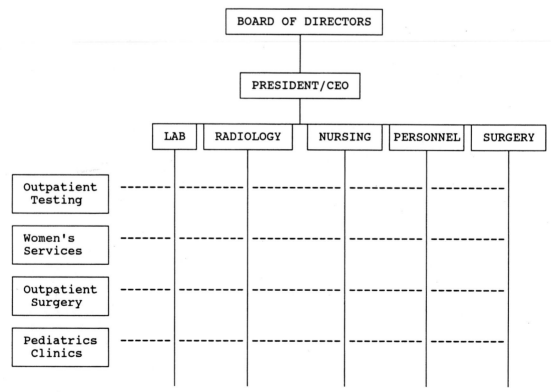

FIGURE 5–4. Matrix structure.

ogy (Fig. 5–5). Depending on the size of the facility, each of the subdepartments may be organized as a department within itself with separate budgeting, reporting structure, and staffing. Examples of this include nuclear medicine and ultrasonography departments or emergency radiologic services that may be independent of the main radiology department. Both centralized and decentralized radiology services have advantages and disadvantages. Each facility develops its reporting structure to best meet the apparent needs of the patients and physicians while attempting to maximize the potential of its managers and technical staff.

Administrative Director of Radiology

Organization of the radiology department begins with an administrative director who reports to senior hospital administration and who has direct responsibility and authority for operation and organization of the department. Key traditional responsibilities of the administrative director of radiology include staffing, planning, educating, supervising, organizing, coordinating, communicating, maintaining safety, and minimizing hazards in the workplace.

The many changes facing the health care industry of the 1990s have brought to all adminis-

trators and specifically those in radiology new challenges that require new skills and responsibilities, including

- managing limited resources
- leading
- coaching
- managing and directing change
- analyzing opportunities
- developing market plans
- analyzing administrative data
- negotiating and managing contracts for purchase of equipment and supplies and for maintaining equipment
- justifying budgets
- managing capital assets and contracts
- planning facilities to maximize use of space and efficiency
- recognizing and managing legal risks
- conducting customer relations
- specifying and managing information systems
- understanding organizational politics
- recruiting, retaining, and developing qualified employees in the face of shortages of radiology professionals
- delegating responsibilities effectively
- networking other departments and professional organizations

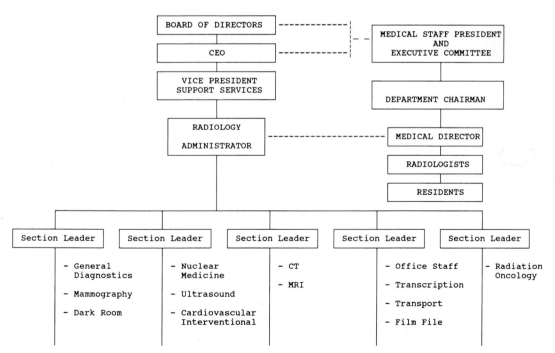

FIGURE 5–5. Example of radiology department structure.

- maintaining technical proficiency
- strategic planning

Medical Director

The radiology administrator has a responsibility to communicate with the medical director, department chairman, and service chief to ensure coordination of medical staff activities with the activities and policies and procedures of the department. Considerable variation occurs from one hospital to another in the relationship between the administrative director and the medical director of radiology. In some institutions, the administrator reports directly to the medical director; in others, the medical director has little responsibility for day-to-day operations, staffing, and organization. In most cases, the **medical director** has responsibility for overseeing the quality of patient care, approving policies and procedures, and recommending improvements to quality of care, equipment purchases, and technology acquisition. According to the **Joint Commission on Accreditation of Healthcare Organizations (JCAHO),** the medical director is responsible for all quality-improvement activities, although he or she may delegate responsibilities to the administrative director.

Department Chair

The medical director of radiology may also serve as department chair. The **department chair** of radiology is the department's link to the formal organization of the medical staff. He or she serves on the executive committee and other standing and ad hoc committees. Whereas a medical director has responsibility for a department or subdepartment, in some facilities the chair has responsibility for the full range of services and is directly responsible to participate in the medical staff organization. Considerable variation occurs from institution to institution in the title and responsibilities of the radiologist head of Radiology Services and its subdepartments. Whether the title is medical director, chair, or **service chief,** the primary responsibility is quality patient care.

Radiologists may practice alone or in groups. Within groups, the larger the number of radiologists, the more formal the group's own organizational structure. Partnerships may be established that may or may not include all of the radiologists working together by agreement.

When radiologists first become part of a practicing group of radiologists, they may work as employees or junior partners before becoming full partners. The function of the group's organization is to run the business of the group, which includes billing patients for services, managing and paying employees, managing group investments and benefits plans, and serving as a mechanism for decision making.

Other Health Care Settings

In recent decades, the provision of radiology services has changed from primarily hospital based to include many other settings. Among the newer settings are physicians' offices, clinics, free-standing imaging centers, manufacturing plants, research centers, outpatient surgical centers, mobile imaging centers, and veterinary medicine.

CLINICS

Imaging in clinics includes a range of modalities from radiography for orthopedic services to all modalities for major outpatient health care settings. Technologists may perform a variety of procedures and other functions or, in larger clinics, may specialize in specific procedures. Clinics may be owned or operated by physicians or by university medical centers, hospitals, or for-profit organizations.

PHYSICIAN OFFICES

Often, physicians' offices may be similar to clinics, but they are organized as the homebase of a single physician or a group of physicians. The radiologic services offered vary from basic x-ray procedures to a full range of services including ultrasonography, computed tomography, nuclear medicine, magnetic resonance imaging, and vascular or interventional procedures.

IMAGING CENTERS

Imaging centers may be owned by hospitals, medical centers, radiologists, other physicians, or nonmedical investors or corporations. They may be free-standing or associated with a clinic, physicians' office, or other medical center. The difference between a clinic and an imaging center is primarily that a clinic provides patient care by nonradiologist physicians as its primary function. The imaging center's primary function is diagnostic imaging; however, some imaging centers provide basic laboratory tests, electrocardiograms, and other diagnostic testing in addition to imaging procedures.

MOBILE IMAGING

The 1980s saw the development of a large array of imaging modalities on wheels. Mobile services provide better access to care in remote areas and, in the case of high-priced technologies such as magnetic resonance imaging and lithotripsy, allow facilities to share the expense of providing access. Although the same basic skills are required of technologists and sonographers in these settings, new challenges are presented in the constant travel and interaction with medical facilities with diverse expectations and personalities.

EMERGENCY CARE CENTERS

In the 1980s, a variety of free-standing emergency or urgent care centers sprang up in America to provide quick access in emergency situations. Shopping centers were among the many locations in which these centers were developed. Although many did not survive, some centers remain and meet important needs in their locations. Most of these centers provide primary general diagnostic radiographic procedures.

OUTPATIENT SURGICAL CENTERS

During the 1990s, managed care and other forces influencing reduced costs in health care stimulated movement toward less inpatient hospital care and more outpatient services. Surgical procedures are increasingly performed outside the traditional hospital setting. Radiology services in surgery centers represent yet another opportunity for technologists who are willing and ready to change.

INDUSTRY AND RESEARCH

Less well-known settings in health care for radiology services, primarily x-ray, are those in industry and research. In recent years, health care entered industry to protect the health of workers and lower the cost of health care. Some workplaces have their own clinics to monitor and safeguard the health of the workers. Employers are also seeking to reduce the cost of their employees' health care by negotiating lower costs with preferred hospitals, clinics, and physicians.

Management Functions

The primary functions of management include *planning, organizing, staffing, directing, controlling, and coordinating.* In the course of performing these functions, the radiology administrator communicates with a wide range of clients, customers, employees, service providers, manufacturers, other departments, senior administration, and medical staff, as well as the community at large. As organizational transitions occur, the skills of communication take on a far greater significance. In the past, an administrator of any department or service could operate independently while focusing primarily on his or her own department. In the 1990s, new skills of communication are required to improve quality, enhance coordination, and lower the costs of doing business.

Similarly, the functions of management are evolving from the traditional roles of directing and controlling employees to leading, coaching, and supporting employees. The influence for this change comes from the movement toward **Continuous Quality Improvement (CQI), Total Quality Management (TQM),** or process improvement.

The concept of quality improvement moved from industry to health care in the 1980s. The impetus was derived from both the need to reduce the costs of providing health care and the rising expectations of patients, physicians, and third-party payers of Medicare bills. When an institution focuses on quality or process improvement, it undergoes a cultural revolution, evolving over a number of years into a customer-focused organization. Employees are organized into work teams and trained to evaluate their work processes to reduce errors and simplify work. "Doing the right things right the first time" and "meeting and exceeding the customer's expectations" become facility-wide objectives under the quality mission. The cost savings resulting from CQI are discovered through in-depth analysis of work processes and elimination of redundant, unnecessary, and outdated work details. Improvements in productivity and efficiency may reduce the costs of doing business and may encourage employee ownership in the workplace.

Radiology departments involved in CQI or process improvement study work functions within the department such as patient waiting time and report turn-around time. Perhaps even more significant to the overall success of the hospital are the CQI or process improvement activities conducted between multiple departments. An example of this would be the review of emergency services to reduce length of stay in the emergency department. Laboratory, radiology, admissions, and nursing services all have an impact on the time required to diagnose and treat a patient in the emergency department. As these departments begin to look at each other as internal customers, they begin the cultural change of a quality focus.

PLANNING

A primary management function is the process of deciding in advance what is to be accomplished. *Planning* charts a course of action for the future that enables coordinated and consistent fulfillment of goals and objectives. Without planning, activities occur at random. With planning, activities are assigned to specific employees with the skills and knowledge to achieve results.

Planning focuses attention on objectives and emphasizes efficiency and consistency. It also offsets uncertainty and change through thinking about the future and creating contingencies for what can be imagined or foreseen as well as promoting economical operation and minimizing costs.

An example of planning in a radiology facility is the activities and forethought required to maintain sufficient supplies to accomplish the volume of radiologic procedures without expending unnecessary dollars to support a large inventory of x-ray film. Planning is also critical to maintaining a sufficient number of properly qualified technologists to accomplish a variety of procedures in many different subspecialties.

Starting new services, efficiently performing growing or changing procedure volumes, and managing work during leaves of absence (eg, maternity leaves or vacations) involve considerable planning skills, which vary directly with the size of the facility.

Other examples of areas in which planning is critical include developing and educating radiology employees, orientating new employees, replacing expensive radiology equipment, interpreting the hospital's goals and objectives for the accomplishment of work in the radiology department, and developing policies, procedures, guidelines, and methods for carrying out goals and objectives of the hospital and department.

ORGANIZING

Once objectives, policies, procedures, and methods are defined through planning, administrators must define ways of carrying out those objectives. *Organizing* is the development of a structure or framework that identifies how people do their work. The division of work is essential to efficiency because it defines responsibility and authority.

Through the organizing function, the administrator defines what activities are to be performed, how they are grouped together, who has the responsibility, and who has the authority for carrying out the work. The framework created by the organizing function can be demonstrated through organizational charts like those in Figures 5–2 through 5–5 for a hospital and a radiology department.

STAFFING

Staffing involves getting the right people to do the work and developing their abilities so they can do the work better. Because work cannot be accomplished without people, and the quality of work is directly related to the quality of skills of the people involved, staffing is often viewed as critical.

The tools used by administrators to carry out their staffing functions are job descriptions and specifications, structural interviews, performance appraisals, the budget, wage or salary scales, orientation programs, and, most significant, the human resources department. Staffing functions include recruiting qualified employees, retaining quality employees, orientating and developing competent employees, identifying short- and long-term labor needs, and developing specifications for job qualifications.

DIRECTING

Directing involves the stimulation of effort needed to perform the required work. Activities of directing include giving orders and promoting an understanding of what is to be done. Supervising activities relate to training, developing, and guiding employees. Through the function of leading, an administrator or supervisor inspires or influences employees to contribute toward the accomplishment of goals and objectives. Motivating works to encourage independent participation.

Within the function of directing, an administrator or supervisor uses communication skills to clarify and ensure understanding not only of the work to be accomplished but also of the rationale of why and how it should be accomplished. An example of how supervisors direct through good communication is the discussion of policies and procedures. When employees understand the rationale for policies, they are more likely to enforce and support them.

While directing, an administrator or supervisor often finds it necessary to delegate work to others. The ability to delegate well is a learnable skill that includes informing, guiding, educating, reviewing, evaluating, and giving feedback. Student radiologic technologists learn their clinical skills through a form of delegation. Work performed by others is assigned to them, and they are entrusted with the technical accuracy, patient safety, and a measure of efficiency necessary to complete radiologic procedures. It is important that the clinical instructor or registered technologist in charge of the student understand the educational development and proficiency of the student being assigned to complete a procedure. The supervisor of a delegated task must achieve a balance that permits independence of student action to maximize the learning experience while maintaining the quality of the procedure for the patient.

For students being delegated work in patient care, the issue of responsibility versus authority is often perplexing. Unless it is well defined for students in the clinical setting, it may not be clear that a certain measure of authority is also

delegated with the responsibility of caring for patients. Examples of situations in which this is important include the student's authority to direct patients to follow instructions for activities such as procedure preparation, movement through the facility, and radiation safety. Students should also be instructed in their authority to report and solve problems, and to adhere to ethical standards.

The transition in management previously described also affects the function of directing. Under the old concept of directing, some administrators or supervisors barked orders or issued directives. Under the new concepts of management, administrators and supervisors employ the tactics of guiding, persuading, and coaching employees.

CONTROLLING

Just as students need instructors to observe, test, measure, and guide their educational progress, the hospital needs administrators to review daily, weekly, monthly, or annually the activities and resources it uses to provide care to patients. *Controlling* defines performance standards or guidelines used to measure progress toward the goals of the organization. Once the plans and goals of the hospital are formed, measures must be developed to determine whether each department or section is achieving success toward those goals. The mechanism used for reporting the defined measures creates a formal process of feedback and flow of information. The feedback can then be used to make adjustments if needed to keep operations or expenses moving in the right direction.

The controlling process can be described in four steps: (1) establishing methods of achieving planned goals and objectives, (2) defining standards and measures to give feedback on progress, (3) measuring and reporting progress, and (4) taking action to correct variations from the expected standards. An example of controlling for radiologic technology students is the use of testing in the educational program:

1 One of the goals is the successful completion of the registry examination.
2 Defining standards is the development of curriculum, and measures are the tests used to check student progress in learning.
3 Test taking and reporting define student progress.

4 Taking action to correct deficiencies in learning helps the student to move toward the successful registry examination.

In the typical radiology department, control measures may include monitors such as monthly expense and revenue reports, weekly reports of employee performance, inventory of supplies, radiation safety, and quality of equipment operation.

Standards of controlling are often discussed as either managerial or technical. The standards used to control managerial functions include policies and procedures, rules, and other reports of operations or "people functions." Standards for hiring personnel with specific job skills and credentials fall into this category. Technical standards refer more to safety and equipment operation such as processor sensitometry, radiation protection reports, and other measures of equipment quality control. Technical standards would then include those that govern the more technical functions such as equipment operation (quality control), and the specific routines for radiographic positioning and exposure.

COORDINATING

While performing each of the other functions of management, synchronization of efforts must occur. *Coordinating* is a process by which the manager achieves orderly group activities and unity of effort by workers who are fully aware of a common purpose. In carrying out coordinating activities, an administrator communicates with other areas to facilitate work information and flow. Representing the department and being a spokesman for the department to the organization or outside the organization are critical administrative functions requiring political sensitivity to the needs of both the department and the hospital.

Optimal coordination requires superior skills in the critical areas of presentation, debate, analysis, and articulation. For example, the coordination required to bring a new service such as mobile lithotripsy to a community hospital includes at least the following departments or individuals:

- Financial management department for assistance or approval of the proposed financial plan for the project
- Hospital administration for project approval
- Board of directors for project approval

- Physicians for arranging case scheduling
- Medical staff to keep them informed of the arrival of the new service
- Human resources department if new employees are needed or changes in job descriptions or salaries are involved
- Supervisors to inform and train employees for the new service requirements
- Plant services to plan for the location and docking of the lithotripsy truck on the hospital campus and provision of electrical, water, and phone connections
- Service providers to coordinate the schedules of arrival and departure for the purpose of scheduling patients
- Surgery services for provision of anesthesia and monitoring equipment and nurses
- Nursing services for required assistance with patient care
- Postanesthesia recovery services to care for patients after treatment
- Purchasing services to ensure availability of new supplies

The success and speed with which a new service (such as the example used here) is developed are directly related to the skills of the administrator coordinating the project and to the cooperative spirit of the interacting departments.

Regulating Agencies and Committees

The operation of a radiology department is regulated by external agencies as well as by the governing body of the hospital. External regulating agencies include both voluntary and required regulation. Whereas government agencies usually impose required regulations on health care institutions, other regulating groups such as the JCAHO are voluntary, paid membership regulators that apply guidelines to measure quality or safety. An example of an involuntary regulating activity that is becoming tied to reimbursement is accreditation of mammography services for reimbursement by Medicare. Although participation in some external regulating agencies is voluntary, reimbursement is becoming more dependent on satisfactory compliance with their guidelines.

EXTERNAL

External regulators and agencies that affect radiology operations today include the following:

Joint Commission on Accreditation of Healthcare Organizations

The JCAHO regulates the quality of care provided to patients and the way the organization is supervised and operated. JCAHO guidelines include the assignment of responsibilities within the hospital, the development of policies and procedures for safety, and the management of continuously improving quality. Hospitals voluntarily subscribe to membership in the JCAHO, which conducts on-site visits to check hospital compliance with established guidelines.

State Health Departments

State regulatory agencies such as the state boards of health define rules to protect the health and safety of the patients or clients served by health care facilities.

The **Certificate of Need (CON)** is a certificate of authority or permission granted by a state review board allowing a hospital or other health care entity to construct new facilities, develop new services, or purchase expensive equipment or technologies. The rules for cash expenditures, which vary from state to state, were developed in an attempt to control the rising costs of health care through control of duplication of services.

Nuclear Regulatory Commission

Radiation regulating agencies include the Nuclear Regulatory Commission (NRC) and state licensing agencies for control of equipment and technologists. A state board of health may require licensure of radiologic technologists or may leave the regulation of users of ionizing radiation to the voluntary jurisdiction of the individual health care facility. These regulating groups conduct inspections and levy fines for noncompliance with regulations, which vary from state to state. In most states, the NRC duties have been phased into state agencies such as the department of health or department of radiation safety.

Occupational Safety and Health Administration

The Occupational Safety and Health Administration (OSHA) is the federal agency that establishes standards for safety in the workplace. Some of the critical concerns of OSHA in radi-ology include handling and disposal of hazardous materials, universal precautions for protection of employees from infectious diseases, and eye protection from processing chemicals.

Mammography Accreditation

The certification of administrative, professional, and technical aspects of mammography services is provided by the American College of Radiology (ACR), the Food and Drug Administration (FDA), and various state health departments. The ACR provides voluntary accreditation while the FDA certification is required for reimbursement by Medicare. Many states now also certify mammography equipment and services and in some cases have authority to inspect on behalf of the FDA.

INTERNAL

In addition to external agencies, there are also internal committees that regulate operations in a radiology department.

Safety Committee

Hospitals are required by the JCAHO to have a Safety Committee that directs education of employees on safety policies and procedures and ensures safe operations of the facility for patients and employees. Safety committees regulate such things as storage and removal of hazardous or contaminated materials; physical control of chemical, radiation, and biologic hazards; special cleaning and emergency procedures; inspection of facilities to identify hazards; and correction of hazardous conditions.

Infection Control Committee

The Infection Control Committee regulates infection control policies and procedures and conducts epidemiologic studies for patient and employee protection.

Radiation Safety Committee

The Radiation Safety Committee, required by the NRC or state radiation governing body and the JCAHO, regulates hospital activities for radiation safety and nuclear medicine activities. Radiation safety committees define safe handling of radioactive materials and policies for care of patients exposed to radiation. Policies and procedures used in the case of radiation accidents are also within the responsibilities of radiation safety committees.

Pharmacy and Therapeutics Committee

The Pharmacy and Therapeutics (P&T) Committee is a required committee of the hospital medical staff that reviews drugs and their use in the hospital. In most hospitals, the P&T Committee reviews drugs used in radiology and their protocols for use, such as ionic or non-ionic contrast media. The direct control of hazards and safety in a radiology department is the responsibility of the radiology administrator, who writes policies and procedures, keeps records, and arranges for training in safety for all employees in the department.

Characteristics of Good Employees

When radiology administrators and supervisors set out to hire new employees, they would like to find many characteristics in the new hiree, but two specific criteria stand out in the minds of most administrators. The prospective radiology employee should have a good knowledge of the required technical skills and superior skills in interactive relationships.

Many administrators believe they can assist the new employee who has a solid technical knowledge base to grow and acquire a broader range of technical skills, but people skills depend more on long-term training, instincts, and personality development. The employee with strong interpersonal skills cooperatively enhances patient care and work flow, thereby increasing his or her value to the workplace.

One of the most important concepts that employees in any organization or business should understand is that the customer writes the paychecks. Even in health care organizations, the hospital, clinic, or office cannot survive or succeed without a steady supply of customers who use the services provided and pay for those services. In past decades, health care facilities depended on physicians to refer patients to them. In recent years, however, patients have begun to exert influence about where they will obtain service, even to the point of changing physicians when they are dissatisfied. It there-

fore becomes crucial for every employee to consider that both physicians and patients indirectly write their paychecks. If clients are dissatisfied, they can easily carry their money down the street to a facility that provides better service. Payers are also scrutinizing satisfaction of their health plan members and hold the facility accountable through contractual arrangements. In the 1990s, health care providers are beginning to recognize new customers in the insurance companies and other **third-party payers** that now contract with health care providers for the best quality, lowest cost service.

In 1991, the Association of Educators in Radiological Sciences (AERS), in conjuction with the American Healthcare Radiology Administrators (AHRA), conducted a survey of radiology administrators that revealed that when hiring a recently graduated technologist, the most important skills desired were knowledge of the technical aspects of the job, customer service skills for dealing with patients, and interpersonal communication skills for dealing with coworkers, physicians, and other departments.

The same survey revealed that the most common reasons for a technologist to be disciplined, reprimanded, or terminated were poor interpersonal skills, lack of technical knowledge, and poor customer service skills. The AERS survey recommended that educators in radiologic technology programs heed the advice of radiology administrators in developing customer service–oriented technologists with interpersonal communication skills. The message for students of radiologic technology is to seek direction and personal development in sensitivities to patients and coworkers. In 1996, Akroyd and Wold surveyed AHRA members' perceptions of needed workplace skills and the ability of radiography graduates to perform them. Results indicated that the skills of students may need development. Problem-solving and critical thinking, patient care skills, and customer satisfaction skills were among the top eight areas in need of development.

Quality service and communication skills are as important as technical skills in the preparation of students for future employment. Quality service can be defined as doing the right things right the first time and meeting or exceeding the customer's expectations.

Radiology administrators expect employees (including students as prospective employees) to take personal responsibility for their own motivation to seek out personal development in basic communication skills. Radiologic technologists and students should seek to

- develop an ability to see their work from the patient's or physician's point of view
- develop their skills in handling customer complaints
- practice service with a smile
- react as if the customer were always right
- remember that the patients and physicians write the paychecks
- strive to meet or exceed the expectations of all patients and physicians

An opportunity in which the student radiologic technologist can work on developing desirable people skills is through routine clinical practice. Although technical skills can be readily learned and proficiency can be proved, the interaction with each and every patient offers a new opportunity for problem solving. Each difficult patient improves the student's ability to meet or exceed the next patient's expectations. When student technologists become discouraged performing another routine chest radiograph, they should consider that the skills in interpersonal relationships are built patient by patient and that each offers an opportunity to do it better than before.

Yet another area of opportunity for developing people skills is through interaction with employees in departments outside radiology. With each interaction, the student technologist is an ambassador of the department of radiology, an emissary of the department administrator and even the hospital president. Future cooperation and efficiency are built step by step through brief encounters in the workplace. When an investment is made in cooperation and mutual support, the dividends are paid back in many forms. When patients observe cooperative interactions between employees, it enhances their perception of the quality of the facility and the value they receive in the service provided. Perhaps the most obvious payback to the technologist is in the satisfaction realized in working in a supportive and cooperative environment. Every encounter or interaction between two employees makes an investment—either enhancing or destroying the satisfactory environment.

Within the radiology department, students should be offered additional opportunities to learn the details of operations through involvement in all departmental functions. Transporting patients, filing films, processing requisi-

tions, assisting radiologists, and assisting technologists are all important activities that develop well-rounded perspectives of the importance of all radiology employees. Students are well advised to take advantage of every opportunity to become knowledgeable, empowered employees serving and solving problems for every customer, because this will be the hallmark of both successful institutions and the sought-after employees of the future.

Summary

With an understanding of how a radiology department functions within the framework of a hospital organization, the student radiologic technologist can better relate to the cooperation and interaction required to deliver quality care to patients.

The field of radiology has broadened in recent decades to include other health care settings such as clinics, imaging centers, and mobile imaging. With the new radiologic settings, the knowledge requirements for technologists continue to include solid technical skills; a higher demand, however, is placed on superior interpersonal skills.

The basic functions of management apply to all hospitals, departments, subdepartments, and work units. Each is required to plan and organize work, staff with workers, direct the work to be done, control the quality and outcome, and coordinate activities of workers within the unit as well as with workers and others outside the work unit. The organization of workers within a health care facility, such as a hospital, is developed to provide service to its primary customers: the physicians and their patients.

Health care facilities, providers of diagnostic services, and users of ionizing radiation and other medical devices are regulated by mandatory and state agencies, plus voluntary agencies to ensure the safety of patients, workers, and others in the workplace. In addition to external agencies, radiology departments must comply with internal safety committees and maintain policies and procedures for patient and employee safety.

Because radiology services provide a unique service in diagnosis and treatment, those services are usually organized within the facility under a departmental structure within which the student radiologic technologist is expected to learn and become proficient. Each activity of the student in radiology, whether directly related to developing technical skills or indirectly related to developing interpersonal skills, is an important activity that will prepare the student for future success in his or her chosen profession.

◀R REVIEW QUESTIONS

1 The driving and guiding force that outlines the reason for the existence of a hospital is its:
a) CEO
b) medical director
c) mission statement
d) JCAHO

2 The board of directors employs (_____) who interacts with the medical staff to ensure coordination and quality of patient care and services:
a) an insurance agent
b) a radiology chairman
c) a vice president of nursing
d) a president or CEO

3 Forces causing hospitals to reorganize include:
a) state regulators
b) economic hardships
c) Total Quality Management
d) JCAHO

4 When an organization focuses on quality, it:
a) undergoes a cultural revolution
b) prohibits employees from participating in groups
c) encourages employees to focus on one department to the exclusion of others
d) lowers workers' perceptions of patient or physician expectations

5 The management function that charts a course of action for the future to enable coordinated and consistent fulfillment of goals and objectives is:
a) coordinating
b) planning
c) communicating
d) setting goals

6 The management function that involves the development of a structure or framework that identifies how people do their work is:
a) staffing
b) planning
c) organizing
d) coordinating

7 The management function that involves getting the right people to do the work and developing their abilities is:
a) staffing
b) organizing
c) directing
d) describing

8 Performance standards or guidelines used to measure progress toward the goals of the organizations are defined as:
a) employee evaluations
b) feedback
c) controlling
d) JCAHO guidelines

9 The internal hospital committee that ensures safe operations for the facility for both patients and employers is the:
a) Safety Committee
b) Certificate of Need
c) Hazardous Chemicals Group
d) Radiation Safety Committee

10 Besides acquiring a strong knowledge of technical skills, a radiologic technology student should develop:
a) a broader range of procedural abilities
b) referrals of patients from physicians
c) skills in magnetic resonance imaging, computed tomography, ultrasonography, and nuclear medicine
d) superior skills in interactive relationships

BIBLIOGRAPHY

Akroyd D, Wold B: Managers' perceptions of radiographer skills: Current and future needs. Radiol Manage 18(3): May/June, 1996.

Bouchard E: Radiology Management: An Introduction. Denver, Multi-Media Publications, 1983.

Callaway WJ: Graduate technologists and customer service: A 1991 survey. Radiol Manage 14(2):50, 1992.

Deming WE: Out of Crisis. Boston, Massachusetts Institute of Technology, Center for Advanced Engineering Study, 1986.

Donabedian A: The quality of care: How can it be addressed? JAMA 260:1743, 1988.

Gillem TR: Deming's 14 points and hospital quality: Responding to the customer's demand for the best value health care. J Nurs Qual Assur 3:70, 1988.

Griffith JR: The Well-Managed Community Hospital. Ann Arbor, Health Administration Press, 1987.

Joint Commission on Accreditation of Healthcare Organization: Transitions: From QA to CQI: Using CQI Approaches to Monitor, Evaluate, and Improve Quality. Joint Commission on Accreditation of Healthcare Organization, Oak Brook Terrace, IL, 1991.

Juran JM: Juran on Planning for Quality, New York, Free Press, 1988.

King B: Better designs in half the time. Methuen, MA, GOAL/QPC, 1989.

Leebov W: The Quality Quest: A Briefing for Health Care Professionals. Chicago, American Hospital Publishing, 1991.

Leebov W: Patient Satisfaction: A Guide to Practice Enhancement. Medical Economics Books, 1990.

Leebov W: Health Care Managers in Transition: Shifting Roles and Changing Organizations. San Francisco, Jossey-Bass Publishers, 1990.

Leebov W: Effective Complaint Handling in Health Care. Chicago, American Hospital Publishing, 1990.

Peters TJ, Waterman RH Jr: In Search of Excellence. New York, Warner Books, 1984.

Peters T, Austin N: A Passion for Excellence. New York, Warner Books, 1986.

Pichert JW, Miller CS, Hollo AH, et al: What health professionals can do to identify and resolve patient dissatisfaction. J Qual Improve 24(6): June, 1998.

Rakich JS, Longest BB, O'Donovan TR: Managing Health Care Organizations. Philadelphia, WB Saunders, 1977.

Rosenthal JS: Customer focus: The competitive edge. Administr Radiol 8(6):34, 1989.

Schwartz H: Managing radiology in the 1990s: Part 2. Appl Radiol 19:20, 1990.

Stockburger W: Radiology Administration: A Business Guide. Philadelphia, JB Lippincott, 1989.

Tobin E: Patient feedback. Administr Radiol 10(7):51, 1991.

Wesolowski CE: Let's put "care" back into health care. Radiol Manage 12(3):49, 1990.

CHAPTER 6

RADIOGRAPHIC IMAGING

Jane A. Auger, MD

Four factors . . . contribute to the quality of the . . . radiograph: First, distortion; second, detail; third, contrast; fourth, radiographic density. . . .

PROFESSOR ED. C. JERMAN, THE FATHER OF RADIOLOGIC TECHNOLOGY
AN ANALYSIS OF THE END-RESULT: THE RADIOGRAPH. RADIOLOGY 6:59-62, 1926.

OBJECTIVES

On completion of this chapter, the student should be able to:

1 Discuss primary, secondary scatter, and remnant radiation.
2 Describe the fundamentals of image production.
3 Discuss radiographic quality in terms of density, contrast, recorded detail, and distortion.
4 List the major factors that influence radiographic quality.
5 Differentiate sharpness of detail from visibility of detail.
6 Perform basic calculations using milliampere seconds, inverse square law, density maintenance, and 15% rule formulas.
7 Compare film/screen imaging, fluoroscopic imaging, and digital imaging.

GLOSSARY

Attenuation: process by which a beam of radiation is reduced in energy when passing through tissue or other materials

Central Ray: theoretical center of a beam of radiation

Contrast: difference between adjacent densities in a radiograph

Density: degree of darkening of exposed and processed photographic or radiographic film

Distortion: misrepresentation of the true size or shape of an object

Dynamic: with motion

Grid: device consisting of thin lead strips designed to permit primary radiation to pass while reducing scatter radiation

Half-Value Layer: amount of filtration necessary to reduce the intensity of the radiation beam to half its original value

Intensifying Screen: layer of luminescent crystals placed inside a cassette to more efficiently expose x-ray film

Inverse Square Law: mathematical law that describes the relationship between radiation intensity and distance from the source of the radiation

Kilovoltage Peak (kVp): measure of the potential difference, which controls the quality of x-ray photons produced in the x-ray tube

Latent Image: invisible image that is stored in photographic film after exposure but before processing

Milliampere Seconds (mAs): measurement of milliamperage times seconds, which controls the quantity of x-ray photons produced in the x-ray tube

Penetrating Ability: ability of an x-ray beam to pass through an object, controlled by the kilovoltage peak of the beam

Penumbra: fuzzy border of an object as imaged radiographically

Photon: particle, or packet, of radiant energy

Positive Beam Limitation (PBL): automatic collimation system used on diagnostic x-ray units

Primary Radiation: x-ray beam after it leaves the x-ray tube and before it reaches the object

Radiolucent: permitting the passage of x-rays or other forms of energy with little attenuation

Radiopaque: not easily penetrable by x-rays or other forms of radiant energy

Recorded Detail: representation of an object's true borders

Relative Speed: relative measurements of the speed of a radiographic film and intensifying screen system

Remnant Radiation: radiation resulting after the x-ray beam exits the object

Resolution: a measurement of the recorded detail on a radiograph

Secondary Scatter Radiation: radiation produced from x-ray photon interactions with matter in such a way that the resulting photons have continued in a different direction

Source-to-Image Distance (SID): the distance between the source of the x-rays (usually the focal spot of the x-ray tube) and the image receptor (usually a film cassette)

Static: unmoving

Umbra: true border of an object as imaged radiographically

Image Production

When x-rays were discovered in 1895, the medical community almost immediately realized the value of this discovery. It was now possible to see within the human body. In the intervening years, it has become the task of the radiologic technologist to capture the image produced by x-rays in a format allowing for storage and repeated viewing. Despite the almost daily advances within the field of radiology, the basic mechanism of image production has not changed a great deal. A beam of x-rays, mechanically produced by passing high voltage through a cathode ray tube, traverses a patient and is partially absorbed in the process. The x-ray photons that are able to exit the patient are intercepted by an interpretation device, called an *image receptor*. There are three major classifications of diagnostic radiographic imaging based on the type of image receptor used: film/screen radiography, fluoroscopic imaging, and digital or computerized imaging.

A beam of x-ray photons is generated by the careful selection of technical exposure factors by the radiographer and exits the x-ray tube during an exposure. This beam of photons, before it interacts with the patient's body, is called **primary radiation**. When the primary beam passes through a patient, the individual packets of energy, or **photons**, interact with the various materials that make up the human body.

Depending on the characteristics of these materials, the energies of the photons are lessened by differing degrees as they pass through matter. The resulting beam that is able to exit from the patient is called exit or **remnant radiation**. It is this remnant radiation that produces a photographic image on radiographic film or other recording medium.

Along the way, an x-ray photon may interact with the body's matter in such a way that the resulting photon continues its travel in a different direction. This type of radiation may or may not be able to reach the film, but it does not carry any useful information. **Secondary scatter radiation** is the term generally used to describe this type of nondiagnostic radiation. **Attenuation** is the process by which the nature of the primary radiation is changed (partially absorbed) as it travels through the patient. The x-ray beam is attenuated differently depending on the type of body tissue irradiated. For example, bone tissue, being more densely packed and made of harder material, attenuates the beam to a greater degree than does soft tissue of the same thickness. It is this difference in attenuation that allows for the formation of radiographic images.

In describing the relative ease with which x-ray photons may pass through matter of different types, two terms are commonly used. **Radiolucent** materials allow x-ray photons to pass through comparatively easily, as translucent panes of glass allow the passage of light. **Radiopaque** materials are not easily traversed by x-ray photons, just as panes of frosted glass do not allow the full amount of light to pass through. Thus, bone is described as a relatively radiopaque tissue, whereas air is described as relatively radiolucent.

Film/Screen Radiography

THE IMAGING CHAIN

Once the attenuated beam has exited the patient as the remnant radiation, the information it carries about the types of tissue it has traversed must be translated from an energy message to a visual image that can be viewed and stored. X-ray photons have the ability to produce changes in photographic film. For this reason, some people do not like to put a loaded camera through the x-ray baggage check machine at the airport. Special film, manufactured to be particularly sensitive to x-radiation and certain colors of light radiation, is used to capture the energy message carried by the remnant

beam and to convert it into an image. After the energy strikes it, the film must be processed before an image can be seen. A useful analogy is that of regular photographic film, in which the camera is loaded with the film, which then receives the light reflecting off the subject. When the roll of film is finished, it is rewound into a light-tight canister, developed, and printed. The printed image can then be viewed and stored. The image is not visible before processing because it is stored in a form that is not visible.

Radiographic film is similar. The remnant x-ray photons carry an energy representation of the object of interest that strikes the film emulsion, causing a transfer of energy. This image is stored in the emulsion until it is processed. This invisible image is called the **latent image**. Once the film has been processed, a visual image appears. The correct term to describe an image produced by x-ray photons on a piece of film is *radiograph*.

Historically, the film emulsion was exposed directly by x-ray photons. Each piece of information on the radiograph was put there by an x-ray photon. This required a great deal of radiation, particularly for large, dense body parts. It was discovered that certain crystals *luminesce*, or emit light, when struck by x-ray photons. In addition, this luminescence was at a greater than one-to-one correspondence, meaning that for every x-ray photon that hit a crystal, hundreds of light photons might be produced. By adjusting the emulsion of the radiographic film to be sensitive to the color of light emitted by a particular crystal, the photographic effect of the x-ray beam can be multiplied or intensified, resulting in the use of lower amounts of x-radiation to produce an image. **Intensifying screens** are thin layers of cardboard or polyester coated with layers of luminescent phosphor crystals. The screens are mounted in a cassette, and the film is placed inside. Typically, modern radiographic film has an emulsion coating on both sides and is known as *duplitized* or double-emulsion film. Duplitized film is meant to be used with two intensifying screens for the most efficient performance. It is estimated that over 99% of the photographic effect on a film/screen radiograph is due to screen light, with the remaining effect due to the direct action of x-ray photons. Most general-purpose radiography is performed using this kind of film/screen system. Film/screen combinations may be manipulated to provide differing radiographic quality criteria where necessary. The entire path of a beam of x-radiation is shown in Figure 6–1.

PROCESSING

Radiographic film is similar to photographic film in that it has a silver-based emulsion. Incoming photons of light or x-ray energy are able to excite the crystals holding the silver in place, causing a rearrangement of electrons. This excited arrangement produces the latent image. To produce a manifest image from the latent image, the excited state of the emulsion components must be relaxed. This is accomplished through a sequence of chemical reactions known collectively as *processing*. As in photographic film processing, the film must be developed, fixed, washed, and dried. Originally, each step was performed manually, which was

time-consuming and messy. Moreover, if not done properly, it could produce variable results. *Automatic processing* has allowed these steps to be compressed into about 90 seconds, with more uniform radiographs resulting. In an automatic processor, the film is carried through the chemical solutions by a series of rollers. It passes through the developer, fixer, and wash tanks, and then through the dryer compartment. The film that exits the dryer is ready to be viewed, interpreted, and then stored (archived) for later use.

TECHNICAL EXPOSURE FACTORS

Radiographic quality is directly controlled by the radiographer. Selection of the proper exposure factors for each individual examination is necessary to produce a high-quality diagnostic

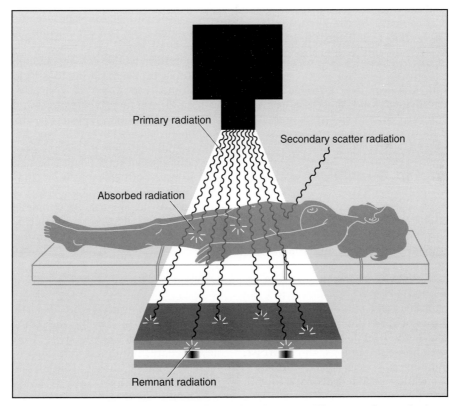

FIGURE 6–1. The path and attenuation of a beam of x-radiation. (1) The primary beam exits the x-ray tube. (2) The beam enters the patient, where the individual x-ray photons' energies are altered (attenuated) by their passage through body tissues of varying characteristics. (3) The attenuated, or remnant, beam exits the patient, carrying with it an energy representation of the body tissues traversed. (4) The x-ray photons in the remnant beam strike the phosphor crystals of the intensifying screens, causing them to emit many light photons for each incident x-ray photon. (5) The light photons photographically expose the film emulsion, resulting in an invisible latent image.

radiograph. The exposure factors under the control of the radiographer, often referred to as "technique," include the following, which are often called the *prime factors*:

1 *Milliamperage (mA)* is a measure of the electrical current passing through the x-ray tube. **Milliampere seconds (mAs)** is the parameter that controls the amount of radiation produced by the x-ray tube; it is the product of milliamperage times seconds. It directly controls the *quantity* of x-ray photons produced. Time (in seconds) is a measure of the duration of the exposure.

2 **Kilovoltage peak (kVp)** is a measure of the electrical pressure (potential difference) forcing the current through the tube. It affects the energy *quality* of the x-ray photons produced.

3 **Source-to-image distance (SID)** is the standardized distance between the point of x-ray emission in the x-ray tube (the focal spot) and the image receptor. It affects the relative intensity of the radiation as it reaches the film and affects the geometric properties of the image. It is also known as *focal-film distance* or *target-to-film distance*.

Other factors that can be controlled by the radiographer include focal spot size, primary beam configuration, quantity and quality of scatter, and the speed of the image receptor.

Radiographic Quality

Once processed, the finished radiograph must be evaluated for technical quality. A radiograph must exhibit proper quality to be deemed diagnostic and should demonstrate all of the desired information within the range of acceptance. Overall, the acceptance characteristics of a radiograph, termed *radiographic quality factors*, fall into two main divisions: photographic qualities and geometric qualities. Photographic qualities include **density**, the overall blackening of film emulsion in response to photons, and **contrast**, the visible difference between adjacent densities. Geometric qualities include **recorded detail**, the distinct representation of an object's true borders, or edges, and **distortion**, the misrepresentation of the true size or shape of an object. Each of these factors contributes to the overall radiographic quality.

Good radiographic quality is achieved by a proper balance between the photographic and geometric properties of an image. The geometric properties allow the size, shape, and edges of the object of interest to be accurately represented, whereas the photographic properties allow these carefully reproduced characteristics to be seen.

By way of illustration, imagine that you are trying to take a snapshot of an ornately carved stone. You want every detail to be captured on film, so you take extra trouble to focus carefully. To make certain of success, you make three exposures, each at a different setting. When the film has been processed and printed, you examine your three photos. One photo is perfectly exposed, and you are able to see every important detail in the carving. The second is too dark, and it is hard to make out any detail. The third is too light, again making it impossible to see the details of the carving. Consider the two poorly exposed photos. Just because a photograph is too dark or too light, does that mean that good detail sharpness is not present? These problems of overexposure and underexposure affect the *visibility* but not the *sharpness* of the detail.

You return to the carving, intending to use the proper exposure setting to get more photos. This time, you forget to properly focus the camera, or you move while pressing the shutter. The resultant photograph has beautiful photographic properties but is fuzzy and blurred. This photo could be said to possess good visibility but poor sharpness of detail. The desired image should have both characteristics (Fig. 6–2).

When evaluating radiographs, sharpness and visibility of detail must be examined to assess overall quality. The photographic factors that control visibility of detail are considered first.

DENSITY

While commonly being described as the overall darkening of a film in response to light or x-ray photons, radiographic density can be described technically as a comparison of the light transmitted through the film to the light incident on the film.

When a radiograph is viewed on a viewbox, it is obvious that the incident light is transmitted more easily through the light gray areas than through the darker areas. Those darker areas that block the transmission of light are said to have greater radiographic density. Although it can be easily measured scientifically,

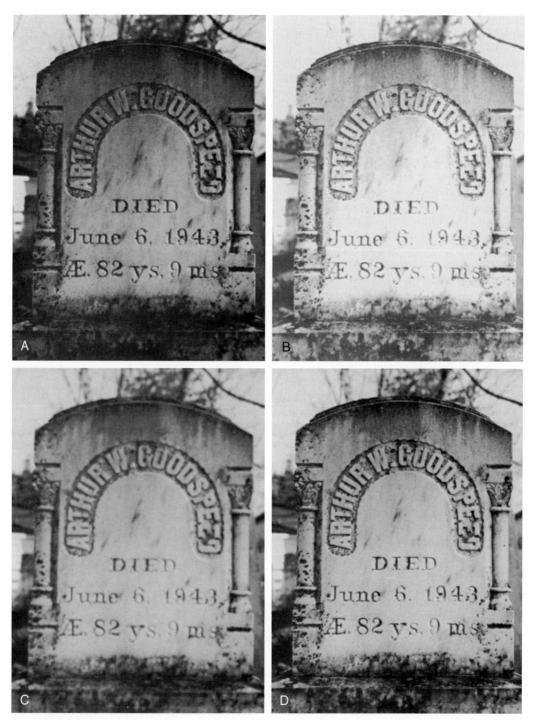

FIGURE 6–2. Different-quality photographs of a gravestone: too dark *(A)*, too light *(B)*, out of focus *(C)*, perfect *(D)*.

density is a more often a subjective measurement, judged by the human eye. A radiograph must possess the proper density to present adequate visibility of detail to the viewer, in the same way that a photograph should not be overexposed or underexposed to do justice to its subject.

In many instances a radiologist's use of the term *density* refers to anatomic density and not to radiographic density. A report noting "an increased density in the right lung field" should be interpreted to mean that the lung tissue is denser. The radiographic density in such an area would therefore be decreased because the denser tissue would absorb more of the x-ray beam.

Density is affected by many variables, including patient size and tissue composition, milliampere seconds, kilovoltage peak, distance, beam modification (collimation, filtration, grids), film/screen combinations, and processing.

Patient Factors

Diagnostic radiography makes use of the differential attenuation of a beam of radiation by various types of body tissue. In this way, information may be gained about the anatomy, physiology, and pathology of many of the body's organ systems. The degree to which the radiation is attenuated depends on tissue characteristics such as cell composition, relative atomic number, thickness, and cell density. Additionally, pathologic conditions can change the way in which the radiation is attenuated. A thick, dense tissue with a relatively high atomic number, such as bone, attenuates the beam to a greater degree than does a thin, less dense tissue with a low atomic number, such as fat. Bone prevents the easy passage of the x-ray photons; therefore, bone is represented as a light color, or an area of decreased radiographic density, on the radiograph.

Because radiography is actually the investigation of tissue characteristics, it makes sense to attempt to standardize all other factors affecting radiographic quality so that the subject is the only variable. Technique charts, automatic exposure control, accurate positioning, and standard imaging protocols are useful in this regard.

Milliampere Seconds

The greater the quantity of x-ray photons generated, the greater the resultant density on the radiograph. This is a direct relation. Increasing the number of x-ray photons produced increases radiographic density. *Milliampere seconds is the chief controlling factor of exposure and density.* Milliampere seconds controls the number of electrons that flow from cathode to anode in the x-ray tube. This in turn controls the number of x-ray photons produced. Milliampere seconds is the product of milliamperage and time. Any combination of milliamperage and time producing equivalent milliampere seconds values should produce equivalent exposures and therefore densities. This is known as milliampere seconds reciprocity.

$$mA \times time = mAs$$

Example

---

100 mA $\times$ 1/10 second = 10 mAs
200 mA $\times$ 1/20 second = 10 mAs
300 mA $\times$ 1/30 second = 10 mAs

The milliampere seconds, milliamperage, and time factors are all directly related to density. These effects can also be stated as follows:

Increasing milliampere seconds increases density.

Decreasing milliampere seconds decreases density.

The radiographs in Figure 6–3 illustrate these effects.

Example

---

100 mA $\times$ 1/10 second = 10 mAs = density A
200 mA $\times$ 1/10 second = 20 mAs = increases density A
100 mA $\times$ 1/5 second = 20 mAs = increases density A

Kilovoltage Peak

In addition to the number of x-ray photons produced and how many seconds the exposure lasts, the relative strength of the photons must be considered. An x-ray photon of very low energy would have difficulty passing through dense body tissue. Conversely, this same low-energy photon would pass easily through less

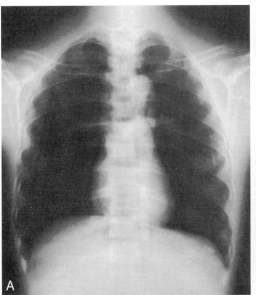

120 kVp at 2.5 mAs (100 mA and 0.025 second)

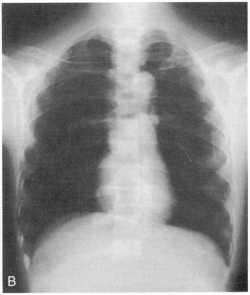

120 kVp at 2.5 mAs (160 mA and 0.016 second)

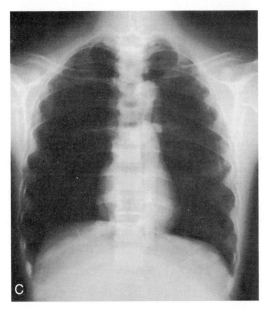

120 kVp at 5.0 mAs (160 mA and 0.032 second)

FIGURE 6–3. Radiographs showing the influence of milliamperage and time on density: *A* and *B*, same milliampere seconds with different milliamperage and time settings; *C*, double the milliampere seconds.

dense tissue. This is referred to as the **penetrating ability** of an x-ray beam. Each average body part can be shown at best advantage by using an optimal kilovoltage peak setting as a guideline.

The kilovoltage peak setting predicts the highest energy level, or the *peak*, possible for the photons within that beam. Most of the photons are in fact below the peak kilovoltage, covering a range from zero to peak value, depending on the electrical supply. The x-ray beam is described as polyenergetic or heterogeneous for this reason.

The relation between kilovoltage peak and exposure is not as that simple as of milliampere seconds. As kilovoltage peak increases, exposure increases but not in a direct proportion. The rule of thumb to account for the change in exposure relative to change in kilovoltage peak is called the 15% rule:

Increasing kilovoltage peak 15% will double exposure.

Decreasing kilovoltage peak 15% will halve exposure.

Example

---

60 kVp at 50 mAs produces an image with a given exposure. What effect would a change to 69 kVp have on the exposure?

$$15\% = 0.15 \text{ and } 9/60 = 0.15$$

Changing from 60 to 69 kVp represents a 15% increase.

$$69 - 60 = 9 \text{ and } 9/60 = 0.15 \text{ or } 15\%$$

Therefore, the exposure is doubled.

It is also possible to use this rule to change kilovoltage peak while maintaining the same exposure. This is done by changing the milliampere seconds to compensate for the exposure change caused by the change in kilovoltage peak. To change kilovoltage peak while maintaining the same exposure:

Increase kilovoltage peak 15% and halve milliampere seconds.

Decrease kilovoltage peak 15% and double milliampere seconds.

Example

To maintain the original exposure, what new milliampere seconds is necessary when changing from 60 kVp and 50 mAs to 69 kVp?

$$69 - 60 = 9 \text{ and } 9/60 = 0.15 \text{ or } 15\%$$

Because the kilovoltage peak increased 15%, the milliampere seconds must be halved to maintain the original exposure:

Original milliampere seconds = $50/2 = 25$ mAs

The radiographs in Figure 6–4 illustrate these effects.

Distance

A beam of radiation obeys many of the same laws that light does. If a flashlight is projected onto a wall, the relative intensity of the light increases as it is moved closer to the wall. *The intensity increases as the distance decreases.* As the flashlight is moved farther away from the wall, *the intensity decreases as the distance increases.* This is described as an *inverse relation*.

The same relation holds true for an x-ray beam. If all other factors are equal, the farther the photons have to travel, the less chance they have of reaching the film because of the divergence of the beam (Fig. 6–5). This means that the same exposure factors used at a greater distance would result in a radiograph of decreased density. When the effect of distance on beam intensity is measured, it is found to be related to the distance squared, rather than having a one-to-one correspondence. In other words, if the distance is doubled, the intensity decreases to one fourth of the original. This relation is described by the **inverse square law**: The intensity of a beam of radiation is inversely proportional to the square of the distance from the source. The mathematical expression of the inverse square law is:

$$\frac{I_1}{I_2} = \frac{D_2{}^2}{D_1{}^2}$$

where: I_1 = original intensity
I_2 = new intensity
D_1 = original distance
D_2 = new distance

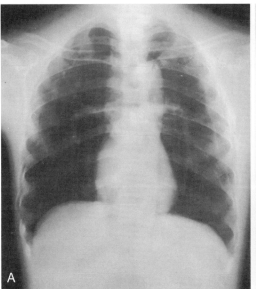

120 kVp at 1.2 mAs

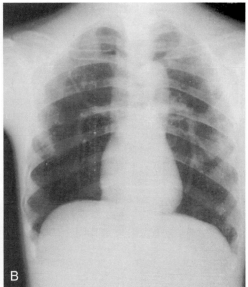

103 kVp at 1.2 mAs

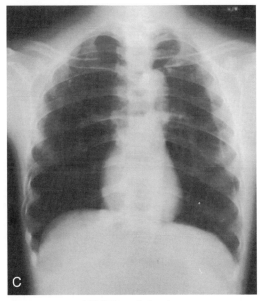

103 kVp at 2.4 mAs

FIGURE 6–4. Radiographs showing the influence of kilovoltage peak on density. *A,* Acceptable radiograph; *B,* 15% decrease in kilovoltage peak with no change in milliampere seconds; *C,* 15% decrease in kilovoltage peak with double the milliampere seconds to maintain the same density as in film *A.*

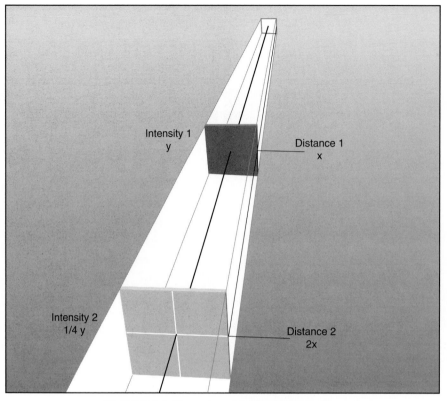

FIGURE 6–5. Illustration of the inverse square law.

Example

If the intensity of the beam is 40 R/min (R = roentgen, a unit of radiation exposure) at the original distance of 40 cm, what will the intensity be if the new distance is 20 cm?

$$\frac{I_1}{I_2} = \frac{D_2{}^2}{D_1{}^2}$$

$$\frac{40}{x} = \frac{20^2}{40^2}$$

$$\frac{40}{x} = \frac{1^2}{2^2}$$

$$\frac{40}{x} = \frac{1}{4}$$

$$x = 160 \text{ R/min}$$

Notice that decreasing the distance by half causes the intensity to increase by a factor of 4.

The inverse square law describes the effect of a change in distance on beam intensity, but frequently the radiographer would like to be able to compensate for a necessary change in distance. This may be accomplished by using a conversion of the inverse square law known as the *density maintenance formula*. This formula is actually a direct square law. The mathematical expression of the density maintenance formula is:

$$\frac{mAs_1}{mAs_2} = \frac{D_1{}^2}{D_2{}^2}$$

where: mAs_1 = original milliampere seconds value
mAs_2 = new milliampere seconds value
D_1 = original distance
D_2 = new distance

Because milliampere seconds, milliamperage, and time are all directly proportional to beam intensity, this formula may be used to derive any of these three factors.

Example

If a radiograph produced at 72 inches SID using 20 mAs must be repeated at 36 inches

SID, what new milliampere seconds setting is necessary to maintain the same radiographic density?

$$\frac{mAs_1}{mAs_2} = \frac{D_1{}^2}{D_2{}^2}$$

$$\frac{20}{x} = \frac{72^2}{36^2}$$

$$\frac{20}{x} = \frac{2^2}{1^2}$$

$$\frac{20}{x} = \frac{4}{1}$$

$$4x = 20$$

$$x = 5 \text{ mAs}$$

Beam Modification

Anything that changes the nature of the radiation beam, apart from the factors already discussed, is referred to as *beam modification*. The beam may be modified before it enters the patient, in which case it is called *primary beam modification*, or after it exits the patient, in which case it is generally known as *scatter control*.

The primary beam may be adjusted by changing filtration and beam limitation. *Filtration* is the use of attenuating material, usually aluminum, between the x-ray tube and the patient. This serves mainly to prevent the inclusion of very-low-energy nondiagnostic x-ray photons in the primary beam in order to decrease patient exposure. As more material is placed in the path of the beam, the resultant intensity decreases. For example, a bare lightbulb glows with a certain intensity. Placing a paper shade over the bulb filters out some of the light, thereby reducing its intensity. With all other factors equal, the same exposure factors used with 4 mm of filtration would produce a radiograph with less density than if used with only 2 mm of filtration.

The amount of attenuating material required to reduce the intensity of a beam to half the original value is referred to as the **half-value layer**. Because aluminum is the most common material used for filtration in diagnostic radiography, half-value layer is usually expressed in terms of millimeters of aluminum equivalency (mm Al/Eq).

Beam limitation is the use of devices to confine the x-ray beam to the area of interest, thereby reducing exposure to body parts other than those under examination. In addition to patient protection, beam limitation dramatically affects radiographic quality. During the transit of an x-ray photon through matter, there is a high probability that the photon will collide with an atom. This collision may result in a change in direction as well as a decrease in the energy of the photon. This scattered photon is virtually useless from a diagnostic standpoint and contributes only to patient dose. This type of photon is usually described as *secondary scatter radiation*. If secondary scatter radiation reaches the film, it is not carrying information. Scattered photons that strike the film emulsion degrade the quality of the image by contributing radiographic densities known as *fog*.

By limiting the size and shape of the primary beam to the area of interest, we are decreasing the probability of the production of secondary scatter radiation. Scatter can never be eliminated, but its effect can be lessened. In fact, scatter accounts for a large percentage of the density of any radiograph. By restricting the primary beam and decreasing scatter, we are in effect subtracting photons from the remnant beam. Therefore, a decrease in scatter causes a decrease in density.

Devices used to limit the size and shape of the primary beam include aperture diaphragms, cones and cylinders, and variable aperture collimators. The collimator is the device most familiar to radiographers. It consists of adjustable pairs of lead shutter leaves that allow for the use of various size rectangular fields. **Positive beam limitation (PBL)**, often referred to as *automatic collimation*, is an electronic interlock system that is required in the United States. It automatically collimates the beam to the size of the film placed in the Bucky tray, the cassette holder tray within the x-ray table.

Grids

Despite the careful use of primary beam modification, once the beam enters the patient, secondary scatter radiation is produced. As stated previously, the more scatter allowed to reach the film as fog density, the poorer the appreciation of the details. A **grid** is a device that is designed to remove as many scattered photons exiting the patient as possible before they reach the film. A grid consists of thin lead strips interspersed with spacing material. The grid is placed between the patient and the film to intercept scattered photons, which by definition have been diverted from their original paths. The more lead contained in a grid, the better its ability to remove scatter from the remnant beam. Decreasing the amount of scatter enhances the radiographic contrast. However, the additional lead in the grid also requires higher exposure factor settings, which increases the radiation dose to the patient.

Grids are described according to *grid ratio*, the ratio of the height of the lead strips to the distance between them. Grid ratios commonly range from 5:1 to 16:1, with the higher ratio grid able to remove more photons from the beam. Because the grid reduces the number of photons reaching the film, it also causes a decrease in density. All other factors being equal, if the same exposure factors are used with a 5:1 grid and a 10:1 grid, the 10:1 grid produces an image with less density.

Film/Screen Combinations

The most common image receptor is a combination of intensifying screens that emit a specific color light and radiographic film that is sensitive to the same color. This matching of colors is called *spectral matching*, and it controls the efficiency of the image receptor. Using a mismatched combination results in an image receptor that does not make the greatest use of the incident x-ray photons. The careful selection of the correct film/screen combination is essential to good radiographic quality.

Image receptor efficiency is often described in terms of speed. A fast system requires less radiation to produce a certain radiographic density than does a slow system, but slower systems generally produce crisper details. System speed ratings are based on an arbitrary average **relative speed** of 100, and commonly range from 50 to 1200. The higher the relative speed number, the less radiation required to produce a given density. However, the higher-speed film/screen combinations also produce an image with less recorded detail.

Processing

Inaccurate processing is responsible for destroying many carefully exposed radiographs. Processing errors that affect density generally fall into two major categories: underdevelopment and overdevelopment. Chemical changes in the film emulsion are responsible for changing the latent image into the manifest image. If the temperature of the chemical solutions is too hot, there is an increase in density, known as *chemical fog*, on the radiograph. If the temperature is too cool, there is a decrease in density as a result of insufficient chemical activity.

Automatic processing appears to be easy but in fact requires rigorous quality control to ensure consistent results. A difference of only 0.5 degrees can produce a visible change in density.

CONTRAST

The second photographic property to be considered is *contrast*. Contrast is the visible difference between adjacent radiographic densities. An object may be accurately represented on a radiograph, but if it cannot be distinguished from the objects surrounding it, it will not be adequately appreciated by the eye. The visibility of detail is enhanced by the use of proper contrast. Contrast can be understood by recalling the story of the little boy who was asked to draw a picture in art class. After laboring for some time, he presented the teacher with a sheet of completely white paper. The puzzled teacher asked what the picture was supposed to represent, to which the little boy replied, "It's a white horse eating marshmallows in a snowstorm." Of course, because there was no contrast between the different densities, the teacher failed to see the same image as the child.

Contrast is affected by many factors, including patient factors, kilovoltage peak, milliampere seconds, beam modification, film/screen combinations, contrast media, and processing.

Patient Factors

As described in the section on density, the tissues that make up the human body attenuate the beam of radiation to differing degrees. This differential attenuation is the basis for radiographic contrast. If two objects represented on a radiograph have similar tissue densities, they produce similar radiographic densities. This is often the case in radiography of the abdominal organs. It would be difficult to distinguish details within these similar densities. This is an example of a body part with low subject contrast. Other body parts possess high subject contrast. In radiography of the chest, the bony tissue of the ribs has much greater tissue density than does the surrounding air-filled lung tissue.

The resulting radiographic densities likewise are different and easily distinguishable.

Kilovoltage Peak

Control of the penetrating ability of the radiographic beam allows the radiographer to manipulate radiographic contrast. More energy is required to penetrate bony tissue than soft tissue. For this reason, some technique charts are based on an optimal kilovoltage peak level for a particular body part. *Kilovoltage peak is the chief controlling factor of contrast.*

The terminology used to describe radiographic contrast can be confusing. Contrast is a comparison of all the various densities represented on a radiograph. These densities fall into a range from darkest to lightest gray. This range of gray tones is known as the *scale of contrast.* The fewer gray tones, the greater the difference between individual densities. Consider the difference between maximum and minimum densities (D_{max} and D_{min}). In Figure 6–6, if the 60

kVp strip goes from D_{max} to D_{min} in five steps, whereas the 120 kVp strip goes from D_{max} to D_{min} in more steps, there will be less difference between the individual density steps in the 120 kVp strip than in the 60 kVp strip.

Radiographs with relatively few gray tones between minimum and maximum densities are said to possess *high contrast, short scale contrast,* and *narrow latitude.* Radiographs with greater numbers of gray tones between minimum and maximum densities are said to possess *low contrast, long scale contrast,* and *wide latitude.* Remember that contrast is a relative measure. There are no absolute standards of high or low contrast, only comparisons between radiographs.

The effect of kilovoltage peak on scale of contrast is that increasing kilovoltage peak (the penetrating ability of the beam) lowers contrast. A higher energy beam tends to penetrate everything in its path more easily and thus produces a wider range of gray tones. Table 6–1 outlines these relations.

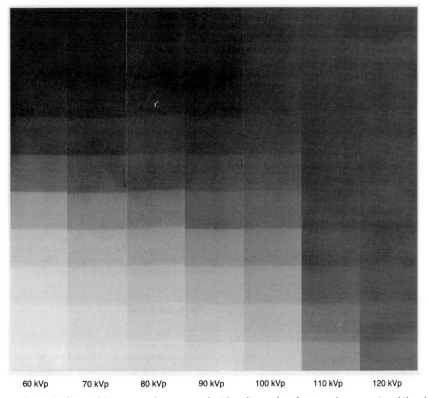

| 60 kVp | 70 kVp | 80 kVp | 90 kVp | 100 kVp | 110 kVp | 120 kVp |

FIGURE 6–6. Radiographic contrast demonstrated with radiographs of step wedges at various kilovoltage peak settings to show variations in the number of shades of gray, also known as the scale of contrast.

TABLE 6–1. Terms Used to Describe Contrast Relationships

Few Gray Tones	Many Gray Tones
Minimum to maximum relatively quickly	Minimum to maximum slowly
High contrast	Low contrast
Short scale contrast	Long scale contrast
Narrow latitude	Wide latitude
Lower kilovoltage peak value	Higher kilovoltage peak value

Milliampere Seconds

Because milliampere seconds is responsible for the production of densities on the radiograph, it is considered to be a secondary influence on contrast. Changing milliampere seconds affects contrast by changing the relative density readings of minimum and maximum. However, changing milliampere seconds has no effect on the penetrating ability of the beam. *No increase in milliampere seconds or density can compensate for inadequate penetration.*

Beam Modification

Whether through filtration, collimation, or the use of grids, the purpose of beam modification is scatter control. Scattered radiation allowed to reach the film produces nondiagnostic densities referred to as *fog*. Removal of these fog densities results in the loss of some specific gray tones. Decreasing the number of gray tones by definition causes a move toward higher contrast. *Anything that decreases scatter increases contrast.*

Film/Screen Combinations

Screens and film are manufactured to produce a particular scale of contrast. Systems may be purchased to complement the inherent subject contrast of a particular area. Some common specialty systems include mammographic, chest, and extremity film/screen systems. In theory, the faster the system, the higher the contrast. Film/screen system choices are made by department managers and radiologists, and are often standard within a department.

Contrast Media

In areas of low subject contrast, it is sometimes possible to enhance the inherent contrast through the use of contrast media. A contrast medium is a substance that attenuates the beam to a different degree than the surrounding tissue. Examples of contrast media used in radiography include barium and iodine compounds and air. Filling the stomach and intestine with barium compound allows these structures to be visualized and examined radiographically. An intravenous injection of iodine compound is filtered by the kidneys, allowing the examination of the urinary tract as it is excreted. Because the contrast medium introduces an additional subject density to the body, technical factors, particularly kilovoltage peak, must be adjusted for adequate penetration.

Processing

As previously discussed, inappropriate processing can necessitate that a carefully performed radiographic examination be repeated. Underdevelopment and overdevelopment change the range of visible densities on the finished radiograph. This in turn degrades the radiographic contrast.

RECORDED DETAIL

The sharpness with which an object's borders and structural details are represented on a radiograph is referred to as *recorded detail*. It is also described as *sharpness of detail, definition,* and **resolution**. Sharpness of detail is complemented by visibility of detail. Good radiographic quality requires a proper balance of the two.

The chief factors affecting recorded detail include motion, object unsharpness, focal spot size, source-to-image distance, object-to-image distance, and material unsharpness.

Motion

The most common cause of radiographic unsharpness is motion. Patient motion may be voluntary or involuntary, and is best controlled by short exposure times. Voluntary motion may be controlled by the use of careful instructions to the patient, suspension of patient respiration during exposure, short exposure times, and judicious use of appropriate immobilization devices. Involuntary motion, such as that caused by the heartbeat and the peristaltic movements of the intestines, is best controlled by the shortest exposure time possible. Equipment motion, such as the vibration of the tabletop during a table grid exposure, may also be decreased by the use of short exposure times.

Object Unsharpness

The fundamental problem in radiography, as in photography, is that of attempting to represent a three-dimensional object on a two-dimensional film. Objects that undergo radiography do not consist of straight edges and sharp angles. There is a basic unsharpness to the image of a three-dimensional object that cannot be eliminated. It is possible to lessen the effect of this inherent loss of detail by adjusting those factors over which we have control: focal spot size, source-to-image distance, and object-to-image distance.

Focal Spot Size

Imagine the beam from a penlight-size flashlight. The light beam is relatively narrow and causes a sharp, well-defined shadow of an object placed in its path. Compare this with the shadow of the same object produced by a floodlight. If all the distances are the same, the image produced by the narrower beam will be sharper than that produced by the wider beam. In the x-ray tube, the width of the beam is controlled by the selection of the small or large focal spot. In general, the small focal spot is used when fine detail is required, as in radiography of small bones. The large focal spot is used for most general radiographic examinations. Figure 6–7 illustrates how the focal spot size is controlled by the configuration of the x-ray tube target.

Source-to-Image Distance

In addition to its effect on the intensity of a beam of radiation, the distance from the focal spot to the image receptor is also a major influence on the size and sharpness of the image. Because a beam of radiation diverges from the source in the same fashion as light, the flashlight may again be used to illustrate the point. If an object is positioned close to a blank wall (the image receptor) and the flashlight is held at a distance from the object so that a shadow is visible, a fuzzy border around the true shadow becomes obvious. The fuzzy border is called **penumbra**, and it obscures the true border, or **umbra**. If the flashlight is positioned closer to the object, as distance decreases, the penumbra around the true shadow increases. If the flashlight is positioned farther from the object, the penumbra decreases, causing the image to appear sharper (Fig. 6–8).

In radiography, the greater the SID, the better the recorded detail. Because radiographic rooms and equipment are not currently built to accommodate extremely long focal film distances, SIDs are standardized so that the degree of penumbra is at least a known factor. The most common SID is 40 inches, but some procedures such as chest radiography use a 72-inch SID. There are exceptions to these standards, but the focal film distance of an examination should always be indicated to allow for calculation of image unsharpness.

Object-to-Image Distance

The flashlight experiment is used to observe what happens to penumbra when the OID, also known as the object-film distance, is varied. When the object is moved closer to the image receptor, penumbra decreases and image sharpness increases (Fig. 6–9). As the object is moved farther from the receptor, penumbra increases and sharpness decreases. Thus, it can be said that the smaller the OID, the better the recorded detail. Many of the objects that must be radiographed are structures located deep within the body. It is often impossible to get them close to the film. Therefore, control over OID often depends on the radiographer's knowledge of anatomy and positioning.

Material Unsharpness

In addition to the inherent unsharpness of the objects that undergo radiography, the equipment that is used also contributes to the unsharpness of the image. Films and screens both have characteristics that affect their abilities to accurately represent an image. Film/screen combinations must be carefully chosen to provide adequate recorded detail. In general, faster systems produce greater unsharpness of detail.

DISTORTION

Distortion is the misrepresentation of the true size or shape of an object. Size distortion is more commonly known as *magnification*, and

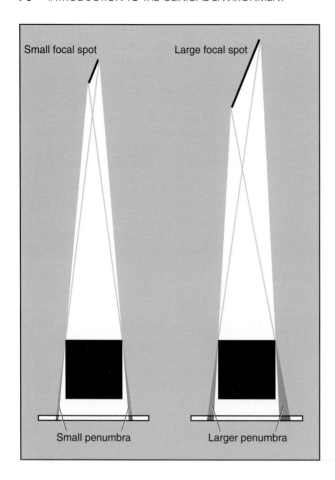

FIGURE 6–7. Effective focal spot size.

shape distortion is sometimes referred to as *true distortion*.

Size Distortion

Magnification of the radiographic image is unavoidable but may be controlled to a certain extent by the use of proper exposure factors. The major influences on magnification are SID and OID.

The size of the image and the size of the light field covered by the flashlight vary with the distance from the source. If the distance decreases, magnification increases. Magnification decreases as SID increases (see Fig. 6–8). The use of standardized SIDs allows the radiologist to assume that a specific magnification factor is present on all films. For this reason, it is extremely important to note any deviation from the standard SID.

Varying the OID also influences the magnification of the resultant image. If a flashlight is kept at a standard distance and the object is moved closer to the receptor, the magnification of the image decreases. If the object is then moved farther from the receptor, magnification increases. Magnification decreases as OID decreases. In terms of recorded detail and magnification, the best image is produced with a small OID and a large SID (see Fig. 6–9).

Shape Distortion

The misrepresentation of the shape of radiographic image is called shape distortion or true distortion. It is controlled by the alignment of the beam, part, and image receptor. Influencing factors include *central ray angulation* and *body part rotation*.

The beam of radiation diverges from the source in an approximate pyramid shape (see Fig. 6–5). This means that the photons in the center of the beam are traveling along the straightest pathway, and those at the beam's periphery are traveling at an angle. The straight, central portion of the beam is referred to as the

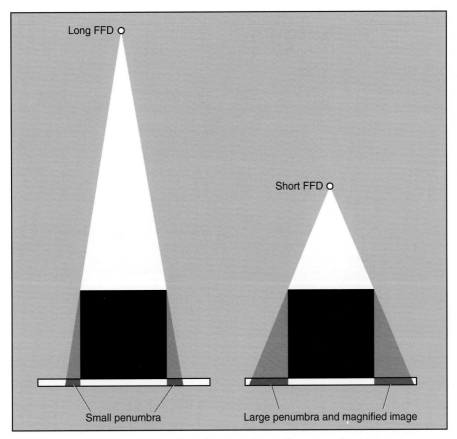

FIGURE 6–8. The effect of source-to-image distance on sharpness.

central ray. The most accurate representation of an object results from the passage of photons in a straight line through the area of interest. This is the reason for the emphasis on central ray entrance and exit points in positioning instructions.

When the central ray is angled, the relationship between the beam, part, and image receptor is altered. A sphere that is imaged by a straight perpendicular beam is represented as a circular image. An image of the same sphere, when imaged by an angled beam, appears as an oval. Objects may appear to be elongated or foreshortened (Fig. 6–10).

Because the structures of the body do not lie in exact 90-degree perpendicular relationships to one another, central ray angulation is used in many radiographic examinations to help demonstrate specific anatomic details.

Changing the orientation of the body part undergoing radiography also affects the relation of the beam, object, and image receptor. If the object of interest is superimposed on another object, the resulting image is difficult to evaluate. By rotating or obliquing the body, the object of interest can be projected free from the interference of the overlying object. Frequently, a combination of part rotation and central ray angulation is used to best demonstrate anatomic details free from superimposition by overlying structures (Fig. 6–11).

Fluoroscopic Imaging

Fluoroscopic examinations often involve a combination of imaging processes. The fluoroscopic image itself is a **dynamic**, or moving, image as opposed to a **static** radiographic image. An analogy is that of a movie compared with a snapshot.

The fluoroscopic examination is usually divided into two portions: viewing a physiologic event in real time (as it occurs) and archiving images for later review. Modern fluoroscopic units are constructed so that the x-ray tube may

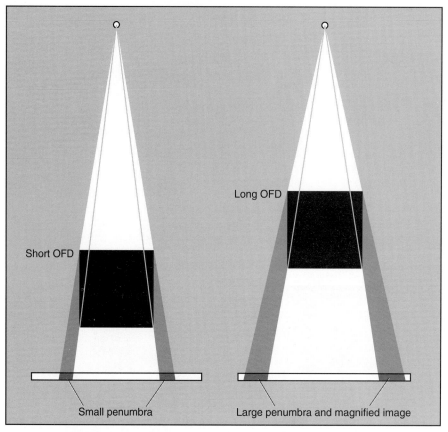

FIGURE 6–9. The effect of object-to-image distance on sharpness.

be located either over or under the x-ray table. Opposite the tube is the image intensifier unit, a device that intercepts the attenuated beam as it exits the patient. The image intensifier is the actual image receptor in this case, as opposed to the film image receptor previously described. When the x-ray photons reach the image intensifier, they are transformed into an electronic image. This image is then displayed on a television monitor for viewing. The radiologist is able to view a physiologic event (eg, the passage of barium compound through the stomach) and observe abnormalities in function.

While observing the dynamic image, the radiologist frequently wishes to preserve an image as a record of the dynamic examination. There are a variety of image-archiving methods available. Spot filming is still the most common method of achieving this end. For spot films, the fluoroscopic unit changes instantaneously to radiographic mode for the duration of the exposure. A regular film/screen cassette is placed in the image intensification device and is

exposed to the remnant beam at the desired time. These spot film radiographs are then processed, viewed, and stored as any other radiograph. Roll or cut filming uses rolled or cut radiographic film of 70, 90, or 105 mm widths to record one image at a time in much the same fashion as with cassette spot filming. The difference is that the roll or cut film is exposed by the light from the image intensifier tube image instead of from the fluoroscopic x-ray tube. This permits less total radiation dose to the patient. The film is then developed and mounted for viewing and storage. Cinefluororadiography uses movie film to record dynamic images for later viewing with a projector, and videotaping allows the dynamic television image to be recorded.

Digital Imaging

With the advent of computerized medical technology, diagnostic imaging is advancing to-

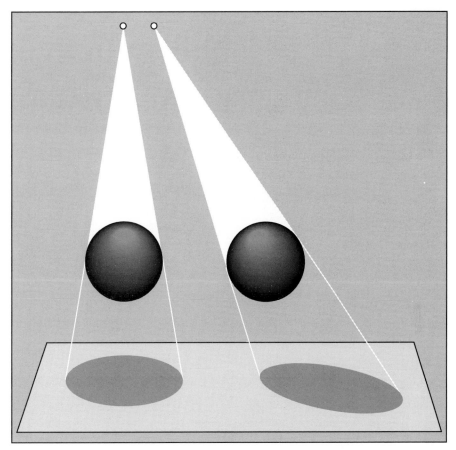

FIGURE 6–10. The effect of central ray angulation.

ward a filmless system. In the current image chain, a wide range of problems may occur at any point between the patient exposure and the finished radiograph. As previously indicated, mistakes in processing have ruined many radiographic examinations. In digital imaging, film is replaced by computerized sensing and storage devices as the image receptor. Thus, processing errors do not affect the diagnostic properties of the image. The image receptors in digital modalities operate in a similar fashion to that described for fluoroscopy. The attenuated beam of x-ray photons exits the patient and is intercepted by the image receptor device. These devices vary according to the specific imaging modality, but all cause the x-ray photon energy to be transformed into a digital electronic signal. This signal carries the diagnostic information and must be displayed for viewing and interpretation on cathode ray tube monitors. During viewing, the operator may change the appearance of the displayed image by simply

instructing the computer as to how many shades of gray to include in the picture matrix. Images can be made darker or lighter with no further exposure to the patient. If the operator wishes, an image from the cathode ray tube can be recorded on radiographic film to be stored as a hard copy record. Most examinations are simply stored in digital form, on magnetic or optical disk or on tape. Storing the raw data allows the operator to recall the original information at a later date for further manipulation.

Digital radiographic imaging is currently used in computed tomography, as well as in imaging modalities that do not use x-radiation, such as ultrasonography, nuclear medicine, and magnetic resonance imaging. Digital subtraction angiography is one application of digital x-ray technology. It uses digital computer imaging to record and manipulate radiographic images produced by a fluoroscopic unit, usually as part of an angiographic procedure. Digital radiography systems are being developed that will allow

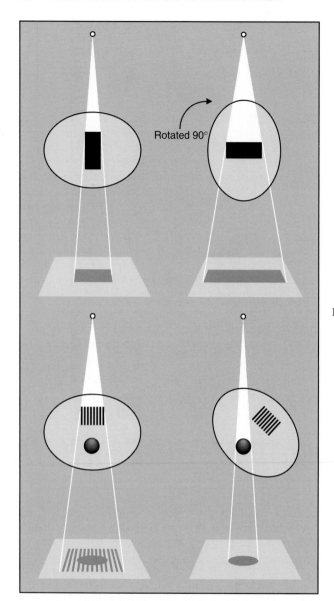

Rotated 90°

FIGURE 6–11. The effect of body part rotation.

filmless imaging in all aspects of diagnostic radiography. These systems use halide crystal screens that, when struck by an incident beam of x-radiation, store a latent image. Following stimulation by laser, the screens emit light that is then detected by photomultiplier tubes. The photomultipliers change the light into an electronic signal, which is the digital image. Within the next decade, digital imaging will become more common and affordable for all aspects of radiography. The replacement of film as the primary recording medium will revolutionize the field of radiography and will serve to de-

crease radiation exposure to both patient and radiographer.

Summary

A radiograph of good quality must possess a proper balance of photographic properties (density and contrast) and geometric properties (recorded detail and distortion). Of the many factors contributing to radiographic quality, the radiographer must be able to manipulate technical factors such as milliampere seconds, kilovoltage peak, and focal film distance; choose and operate appropriate imaging equipment and accessories; and use proper positioning and patient care skills to obtain a high-quality diagnostic radiograph. Most diagnostic radiographic examinations use some combination of film/screen imaging, fluoroscopic imaging, and digital imaging. Advances in digital imaging technology have allowed a slow move away from film as the exclusive recording medium.

◀R REVIEW QUESTIONS

1 The process by which a beam of x-ray photons is altered as it passes through matter is known as:
   a. density
   b. attenuation
   c. fog
   d. processing

2 The beam of radiation as it exits the x-ray tube and before it reaches the patient is:
   a. primary radiation
   b. secondary scatter
   c. remnant radiation
   d. potential difference

3 The chief controlling factor of radiographic contrast is:
   a. milliampere seconds
   b. source-to-image distance
   c. object-to-image distance
   d. kilovoltage peak

4 What milliampere seconds value would result using the 500 mA setting at 0.25 seconds?
   a. 12.5 mAs
   b. 20 mAs
   c. 125 mAs
   d. 2000 mAs

5 Which of the following sets of technical factors would produce the *greatest* radiographic density?
   a. 300 mA, 1/10 second, 36 SID/inches
   b. 200 mA, 1/10 second, 40 SID/inches
   c. 100 mA, 1/10 second, 40 SID/inches
   d. 200 mA, 1/10 second, 72 SID/inches

6 A radiograph is made using 40 mAs at 40 inches SID. If the film must be repeated at 72 inches SID, what milliampere seconds value is necessary to maintain the same density?
   a. 12 mAs
   b. 13 mAs
   c. 120 mAs
   d. 130 mAs

7 The 15% rule helps explain the effect of _____ on exposure.
   a. grids
   b. milliampere seconds
   c. source-to-image distance
   d. kilovoltage peak

8 Which of the following is *not* a radiographic contrast medium?
   a. barium compounds
   b. air
   c. iodine compounds
   d. water

9 The most common cause of radiographic unsharpness is:
   a. motion
   b. material unsharpness
   c. increased object-to-image distance
   d. decreased source-to-image distance

10 Which of the following uses *x-radiation* to produce a digital computer image?
   a. ultrasonography
   b. nuclear medicine
   c. computed tomography
   d. magnetic resonance imaging

BIBLIOGRAPHY

Burns EF: Radiographic Imaging: A Guide for Producing Quality Radiographs. Philadelphia, WB Saunders, 1992.
Bushong S: Radiologic Science for Technologists. 6th ed. St. Louis, CV Mosby, 1997.
Carlton R, Adler A: Principles of Radiographic Imaging: An Art and a Science. 2nd ed. Albany, NY, Delmar Publishers, 1996.
Carroll Q: Fuchs' Principles of Radiographic Exposure, Processing and Quality Control. 5th ed. Springfield, IL, Charles C Thomas, 1993.
Cullinan AM: Producing Quality Radiographs. Philadelphia, JB Lippincott, 1987.
DeVos DC: Basic Principles of Radiographic Exposure. 2nd ed. Philadelphia, Lea & Febiger, 1995.
Lauer OG, Mayes JB, Thurston RP: Evaluating Radiographic Quality: The Variables and Their Effects. Mankato, MN, Burnell Company Publishers, 1990.

CHAPTER 7

RADIOGRAPHIC AND FLUOROSCOPIC EQUIPMENT

Scott T. Gregory, MS, RT(R)

Radiographic equipment is only a link in a system of which the end purpose is to make available a record . . . for interpretation by the physician. . . . A system is only as strong as its weakest link, . . . the radiographer must understand the x-ray equipment to operate it properly.

THOMAS THOMPSON
A PRACTICAL APPROACH TO MODERN IMAGING EQUIPMENT, 1985

Manipulation of Radiographic Equipment
Generic Components
X-ray Tube
Collimator
X-ray Table
Control Console
  Power
  Kilovoltage Peak
  Milliamperage
  Time
  Milliamperage Seconds
  Exposure

Tube Stands
Controls for Tube Movement
Wall-Mounted Bucky System and
  Cassette Holders
Alignment Concepts

Manipulation of Fluoroscopic Equipment

Manipulation of Mobile Equipment

Summary

OBJECTIVES

On completion of this chapter, the student will be able to:

1 Explain radiographic equipment manipulation.
2 List the generic components of a radiographic system.
3 Locate the x-ray tube in a radiographic room.
4 Describe the purpose of the collimator and its controls.
5 Describe various types of radiographic tables and how they are operated.
6 Identify the major controls on the radiographic system control console.
7 Describe various types of radiographic tube stands and how they are manipulated.
8 Describe the various planes of x-ray tube movement and how they are controlled.
9 Explain the purpose of the upright wall Bucky system and cassette holder.
10 Discuss the concept of alignment of the various radiographic system components.

11 Describe the movement of the fluoroscopic tower.
12 Describe the types of mobile x-ray systems.

GLOSSARY

Anode: positive electrode of the x-ray tube

Bucky Mechanism: grid that is an integral part of the x-ray table, located below the tabletop and above a cassette tray; it decreases the amount of scatter radiation reaching the film, which increases contrast, and it moves during exposure so that no grid lines appear on the radiograph

Cassette: lightproof holder for x-ray film, containing front and back intensifying screens between which the film is placed; it is usually backed with lead to prevent back scatter

Cathode: negative electrode of the x-ray tube

Collimator: diaphragm or system of diaphragms made of an absorbing material; it is designed to define the dimensions and direction of a beam of radiation

Fluoroscope: device used for examining deep structures by means of x-rays; it consists of a screen covered with crystals on which are projected the shadows of x-rays passing through the body situated between the screen and the source of irradiation

Fluoroscopy: examination by means of the fluoroscope

Longitudinal: lengthwise; along the long axis

Spot Film Device: equipment that permits the radiologist to obtain static radiographs during a dynamic fluoroscopic examination

Transverse: placed crosswise; situated at right angles to the long axis of a part

Tube Angulation: pivoting the tube at the point where it is attached to its support

Vertical: perpendicular to the plane of the horizon

X-ray Tube: device that produces x-rays

Manipulation of Radiographic Equipment

A primary role of a radiographer is the manipulation of expensive, high-technology x-ray equipment. The mechanical aspects of a radiographic examination must be mastered early by the new student. It is important to become as comfortable as possible with the physical manipulation of the x-ray equipment. Once this is accomplished, the beginning radiographer can concentrate on the other important skills that must be learned, such as patient care, requisition information, positioning, technique, and film quality. Generally speaking, a student who masters the essential skills of equipment manipulation early does well in the more professional aspects of radiography. On the other hand, a student who struggles and fails to quickly learn to handle the x-ray equipment often has trouble moving to more advanced skills.

GENERIC COMPONENTS

A first step in mastering equipment manipulation is being able to identify the generic components of a radiographic system. A beginning radiographer who has visited a radiology department can be overwhelmed by how different each radiography room looks. The differences are similar to those found in automobiles, which are manufactured with seemingly endless variations in outward appearance. There are different models, sizes, body styles, dashboard layouts, and instruments. However, each one has a motor, steering column, brake pedal, speedometer, fuel gauge, and so forth. The same is true of different types of radiographic equipment. They appear different in shape, size, and layout, but they all have common components. The new student should be able to visit different x-ray rooms at their clinical sites and identify these generic (common) components: x-ray tube, collimator, x-ray table, control console, and tube stand (Fig. 7–1).

X-RAY TUBE

The **x-ray tube** is the part of the radiographic system that produces the x-rays. It is made of glass similar to that used in old television and radio tubes and is encased in a sturdy metal housing, which is usually a cylinder with a large electrical cable attached at each end. The x-ray tube's primary components are the **anode** and the **cathode** (see Fig. 8–1). A tube

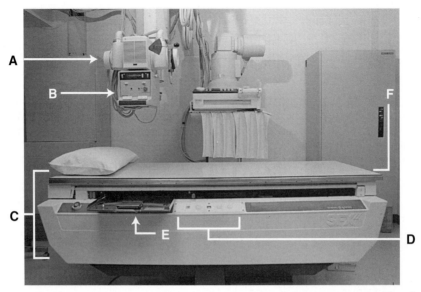

FIGURE 7–1. The generic components of diagnostic radiographic equipment: x-ray tube *(A)*, collimator *(B)*, radiographic table *(C)*, top and tilt controls *(D)*, Bucky tray for cassette and film *(E)*, moving table top *(F)*. The tube is suspended from an overhead tube stand and the control console is behind a leaded wall.

stand supports the x-ray tube and allows the radiographer to position it as needed over and around the patient.

The radiographer controls the electrical energy that is supplied to the x-ray tube through the two large electrical cables. The tube converts this electrical energy into x-rays and heat in a manner similar to energy conversion in a light bulb. Electrical energy that is supplied to a light bulb is converted into light and heat. With an x-ray tube, the radiographer controls the number and energy of the x-rays produced by adjusting the amount of electrical energy going into the tube. This is done at the radiographic system's control console.

These controls move lead shutters or plates that block a portion of the x-ray beam. As an aid to adjusting the size of the x-ray beam, the operator uses a light source to project a representation of the x-ray field onto the patient. This collimator light is turned on by the radiographer so that the size of the x-ray field corresponds to the anatomic part to be radiographed. The collimator light automatically shuts itself off after a short time. Many radiographers refer to collimators as *shutters* and the act of adjusting the collimator as *coning* or *collimating*. The use of these words as verbs—for example, "I'm going to collimate [or cone] on the lateral position"—always indicates decreasing the size of the x-ray field.

Most x-ray machines are equipped with an automatic collimation system known as *positive beam limitation*. This feature allows the x-ray unit to detect the size of the film the radiographer is using and to automatically limit the x-ray field size to that film size. The positive beam limitation system is required by federal law to operate within set accuracy limits. It is a violation of federal standards to permit the x-ray beam to expose patient tissue without creating an image. For example, collimating to a 12×12 inch area when using x-ray film that is only 10×12 inches is against the federal standards. Most collimators are also equipped with a tape to measure the distance from the tube to the x-ray film.

COLLIMATOR

Attached directly below the x-ray tube is an x-ray beam–limiting device called a **collimator** (Fig. 7–2). The collimator controls the size and shape of the x-ray field coming out of the x-ray tube. The radiographer determines the size of the x-ray field by adjusting two controls on the front or sides of the collimator, one for the length and one for the width of the rectangular x-ray field.

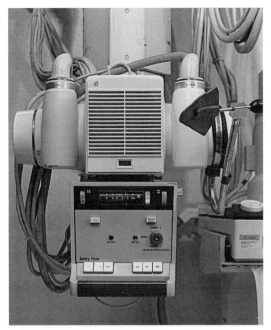

FIGURE 7–2. X-ray tube collimator with control switches for various tube movements.

X-RAY TABLE

The x-ray table is the most obvious and recognizable component of the radiographic system. The size, shape, and location of the controls for the tables vary from manufacturer to manufacturer. X-ray tables are classified as tilting or nontilting, free-floating or stationary top, and adjustable or nonadjustable height.

A tilting table can be angled as shown in Figure 7–3. There are basically two types of tilting tables. A 90–90 table can tilt from the horizontal position to a complete vertical position in either direction. A 90–30 table can tilt to a complete vertical position in one direction and to a 30-degree tilt in the other direction. Table tilt is controlled by a switch located at table or floor level on the long side of the table. The switch is usually depressed in the direction of the desired tilt. Keeping the switch depressed tilts the table to its maximal permitted degree of tilt. Releasing the switch stops the tilting action, allowing the radiographer to set the table to any desired angle. Both tilting and nontilting tables may have additional features, including a moving tabletop, a cassette tray (often called a Bucky tray), and a group of buttons or switches for tabletop movement and tilt control (see Fig. 7–1).

Most x-ray tables have movable tabletops that may be motorized or free-floating. Most can be moved in two directions so the radiographer can move the tabletop rather than the patient. Floating tabletops have a switch that controls a locking mechanism. If it is turned off, the radiographer can move the top manually. Motorized tops have switches that drive the tabletop in the direction desired. The controls for the tabletop or table tilt are usually located at the end or center of the working side of the x-ray table. The **Bucky mechanism** is located directly beneath the tabletop. It is designed to hold the x-ray **cassette** (film holder) stationary and to keep it centered to the x-ray tube. It also serves as the holder for the radiographic grid, which is positioned underneath the tabletop so that it forms a top to the Bucky tray when it is pushed completely into the table (Fig. 7–4). The tray is pulled out from the table, and the cassette is placed in the tray and locked into place. The Bucky mechanism can be manually moved the entire length of the table and then locked into place. A beginning radiographer should take time to practice operating the various x-ray tables and Bucky trays before attempting to position any patients.

CONTROL CONSOLE

The control console of a radiographic system is like the cockpit of an airplane. It is the device

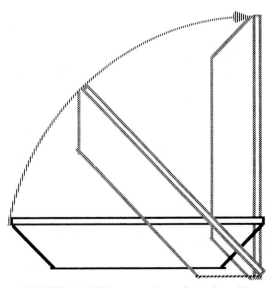

FIGURE 7–3. Tilting or angling radiographic table.

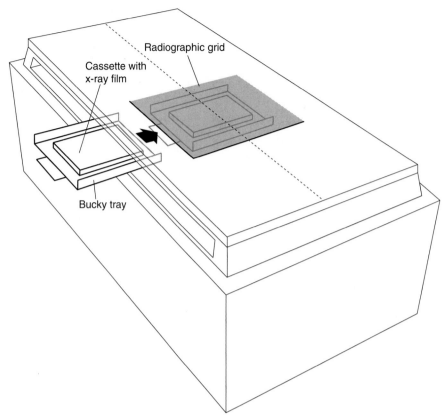

FIGURE 7–4. Bucky tray holding a cassette containing x-ray film. The Bucky tray is centered to the x-ray tube underneath a radiographic grid.

that gives the operator command of the x-ray machine. Accordingly, it is one of the most complicated components of the radiographic imaging system. The first encounter with an unfamiliar control console can be intimidating even for an experienced technologist. There is tremendous variation in how control consoles look between manufacturers and even between different models from the same manufacturer. Control consoles have evolved from basic knobs, push buttons, switches, and meters to sophisticated computer screens with digital readouts. Most radiology departments have a variety of control consoles from different manufacturers (Fig. 7–5).

One of the first hands-on skills that a beginning radiographer may be asked to perform is setting the proper exposure factors on the control console. The console has five generic controls that the new student must learn. These are the main power, kilovoltage peak (kVp), milliamperage (mA), timer, and rotor-exposure switch. The selection of kilovoltage peak, milli-

amperage, and time is collectively referred to as *technique selection*. On many units, milliamperage and time are combined into a factor known as milliampere seconds (mAs), which is simply milliamperage × time in seconds.

Power

The first challenge when encountering an unfamiliar control console is how to turn on the x-ray machine. The main power switch supplies power to the radiographic system. Turning the power on does not activate x-ray production. The power device is usually clearly marked on the control console and is usually either a switch or a push-button device.

Some x-ray units require power to be activated both at the control console and at a main power box equipped with a high-voltage circuit breaker.

Kilovoltage Peak

Kilovoltage peak is indicated as kVp. One kilovolt is equal to 1000 volts. The kilovoltage

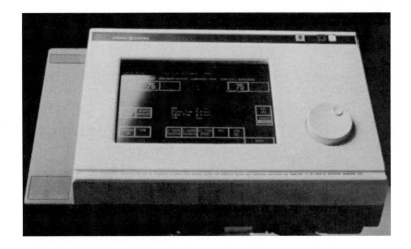

FIGURE 7–5. Example of a radiographic control console. (Courtesy of General Electric Medical Systems.)

peak indicates the amount of voltage selected for supply to the x-ray tube. Control consoles may range from 30 to 150 kVp. Some control consoles have major and minor kilovoltage peak controls. The major kilovoltage peak control allows the radiographer to change kilovoltage peak settings in increments of 10 (ie, 50, 60, 70, 80 kVp). The minor kilovoltage peak control allows the radiographer to select between two major settings in increments of 1 or 2 kVp. For example, if 85 kVp is selected, the major kilovoltage peak knob is set to 80 kVp, the minor kilovoltage peak knob is set at 5 kVp, the total is then 85 kVp. The newer control consoles have digital readouts in which major and minor kilovoltage peak settings are obtained with one selector, similar to changing channels on a television set with a digital remote control. The actual selection control may be a touch button or panel, touch-screen on a computer, or a dial (Fig. 7–6). On digital readout units, these controls may simply be arrows going up and down or left and right. The exposure factor is decreased by a down or left arrow and increased by an up or right arrow (Fig. 7–7).

Milliamperage

Milliamperage is often displayed as mA. One milliampere is equal to one thousandth of an ampere. It indicates the amount of current supplied to the x-ray tube. Control consoles may range from 10 to 1200 mA. Milliamperage is usually selectable in increments of 100 (ie, 200, 300, 400 mA) up to the maximum value. Most routine diagnostic radiography is done between 100 and 400 mA.

kVp

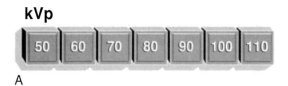

A

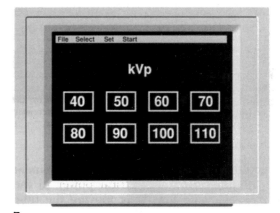

B

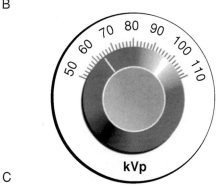

C

FIGURE 7–6. Radiographic console selection controls may be touch buttons or panels *(A)*, computer touch-screen *(B)*, or dials *(C)*.

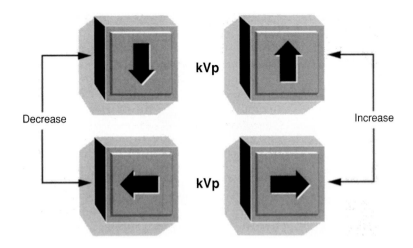

Decrease

Increase

FIGURE 7–7. Selection controls may be up and down arrows or left and right arrows. The factor is decreased with a down or left arrow. The factor is increased with an up or right arrow.

Time

By selecting a time setting in seconds, the radiographer determines how long x-rays will be produced. Depending on the type of equipment, time settings can range from 0.001 to 6 seconds, often in increments of at least 25% (ie, 0.1, 0.13, 0.16, 0.2, 0.25, 0.5). For example, increasing the time setting from 0.2 second to the next highest setting of 0.25 second is a 25% increase in time.

Milliampere Seconds

Some radiographic imaging systems do not permit independent selection of milliamperage and time. These units use a control that combines these two factors. Milliampere seconds (mAs) are calculated by multiplying the milliamperage chosen by the time selected. This represents how many x-rays will be produced for how long. For example, 100 mA × 0.2 second is 20 mAs.

Exposure

After the x-ray exposure factors are selected and the patient, x-ray tube, and other equipment for the examination are all properly prepared, an exposure must be made. The device that begins the exposure is called the *rotor-exposure switch*. It is usually a hand-held push button or trigger-type switch connected to the control console by a telephone-type extension cord. The rotor-exposure switch actually contains two different switches that are mechanically interlocked so that one must be activated before the other. The first switch that is activated is the rotor, or prep, switch. The rotor switch causes the anode to rotate and prepares the x-ray tube for the exposure factors that have been selected. The preparation process usually takes 1 to 2 seconds; when the x-ray tube is ready, the equipment gives the radiographer an audible or visual indication, or both. After the tube is properly prepared, the second switch is activated to begin the exposure. A timer automatically ends the exposure. According to federal regulations, the termination of the exposure must be indicated both audibly and visually.

Activating the rotor-exposure switch is a skill that the beginning radiographer must master early. One common mistake that beginning students make is to start the exposure too soon before the rotor switch has done its job. The x-ray machine will not allow the exposure until the x-ray tube is ready. The beginner must get the feel for the rotor switch and try not to initiate the exposure switch until this tube preparation process is complete. Many manufacturers recommend complete depression of both switches simultaneously. This allows the exposure to occur as soon as the tube is ready. All units include electronic interlocking circuits that prevent an exposure from occurring until the rotor has reached full speed. The rotor speed can be heard immediately before the "ready" light comes on on most units.

Another common error for the new student is releasing the exposure switch too quickly. This ends the exposure too soon. This is especially a problem with longer exposure times. To avoid ending the exposure too soon, the student must get into the habit of not releasing the exposure switch until the audible tone or light message indicates that the timer has terminated the exposure.

TUBE STANDS

The tube stand is the device that supports and permits the x-ray tube to be moved in different directions. There are many types of tube stands. The floor-mounted tube stand has a steel column that runs along a track on the floor. A floor-to-ceiling or floor-to-wall system has a second track that runs along the wall or ceiling. An overhead suspension system has the x-ray tube attached to an overhead track that runs between rails on the ceiling. A third type has the tube attached and integrated with the table (Fig. 7–8).

The basic tube movements that the beginning radiographer must master are longitudinal, transverse, vertical, and tube angulation (Fig. 7–9). These basic movements can usually be accomplished with most tube stands, but they differ significantly in the degree of movement permitted. The directions of tube travel are given from the position of the technologist at the side of the x-ray table. **Longitudinal** travel is moving the x-ray tube lengthwise to the technologist's left or right, or toward the patient's head or feet. **Transverse** travel is moving the tube at right angles across the table. In other words, moving the tube toward or away from the technologist, or from right to left over the patient. **Vertical** travel is moving the tube up toward the ceiling or down toward the floor. **Tube angulation** is pivoting the tube at the point where it is attached to its support. For example, angulating the tube that is facing the tabletop to a position in which it is facing a wall is a 90-degree tube angulation.

CONTROLS FOR TUBE MOVEMENT

Most x-ray tube housings have a set of handlebars that are located between the x-ray tube and the collimator. The radiographer grips the handlebars and releases the appropriate locks to move the x-ray tube in the direction desired. For the longitudinal, transverse, vertical, and tube angulation movements, a corresponding switch is located between or on the handlebars; each switch locks or unlocks the corresponding movement. For example, if the radiographic system is energized and all the tube movement switches are in the locked position, the tube cannot be moved. If the vertical switch is moved to the unlocked position, the tube can be moved toward the ceiling or the floor. Locks for each of the tube movements are controlled independently, allowing the operator to make adjustments in one plane at a time. Some units also have a single switch that takes all the locks off. Shutting off the electrical power to the entire radiographic unit disengages all locks and permits free travel of the tube in any direction. It is extremely important not to force the movement of the tube with the locks on. If the tube does not move easily, the proper lock must be released. A beginning radiographer should get a feel for x-ray tube movement by shutting off the electrical power to the entire unit and practicing moving the tube with all electromagnetic locks turned off. Patients may quickly lose confidence in a student's abilities if they observe difficulty in handling a simple task like moving the x-ray tube.

In addition to the electrical locks, x-ray tubes can have manual locks. The tube stand that is attached to an overhead track allows rotation of the tube around the vertical tube column (Fig. 7–10). These movements are often controlled by a manual lock that is released by hand.

WALL-MOUNTED BUCKY SYSTEM AND CASSETTE HOLDERS

Many radiographic rooms have a special unit that allows the technologist to obtain radiographs of standing patients. The two primary devices are a simple wall-mounted film cassette holder and a wall-mounted Bucky system.

A simple wall-mounted cassette holder is a mechanical device that allows the radiographer to place a cassette in an adjustable holder. The cassette holder mechanism is attached to a two-rail system that permits the cassette to move up and down. A locking mechanism controlled by a knob secures the cassette at the appropriate height (Fig. 7–11).

A wall-mounted Bucky unit is similar to a miniature table that is attached to the wall. It has a surface similar to a tabletop. Beneath this surface is a Bucky mechanism. The tray is manually pulled out, and the cassette is placed in the tray and locked into place. The entire Bucky mechanism can be manually moved after releasing a locking mechanism that permits the radiographer to move it along a vertical plane. A

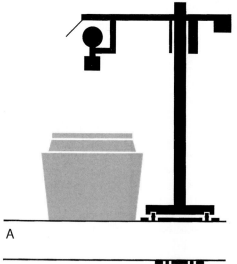

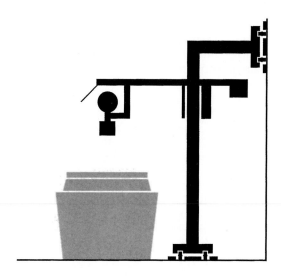

FIGURE 7–8. Tube stands. *A*, Floor mounted; *B*, floor to wall or ceiling; *C*, overhead suspension; *D*, table supported.

A

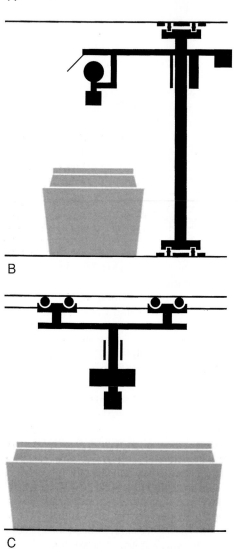

B

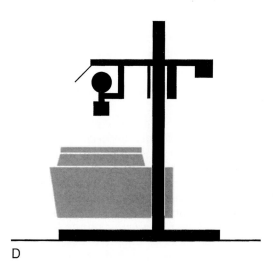

C

D

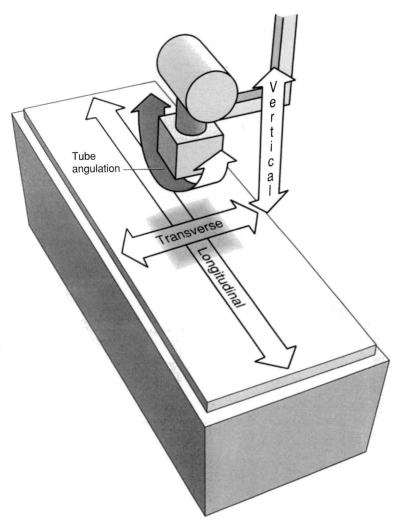

FIGURE 7–9. The basic movements of a typical diagnostic radiographic tube stand: longitudinal, transverse, vertical, tube angulation.

control knob or lever operates a manual locking mechanism that permits vertical movement. Wall-mounted Bucky units typically permit only vertical movement, although some can be tilted into a horizontal position for radiography of the head and extremities.

ALIGNMENT CONCEPTS

The major responsibility of the radiographer is proper manipulation of the various components of the radiographic system to provide a quality image or radiograph of the anatomic area of interest. This is accomplished by proper alignment of the various components of the

radiographic system to that anatomic area of interest. The concept of proper alignment is important to the student radiographer. The x-ray tube, tabletop, and Bucky mechanism all move separately. The student must quickly learn to align the x-ray tube with the center of the cassette within the center of the Bucky tray or a quality radiograph will not be produced. Students often center the x-ray tube and then, while trying to perfect the alignment during the examination, move the tube transversely. To avoid this error, the new student should approach the x-ray table and center the tabletop. The x-ray tube should then be centered over the table, locked transversely, and kept locked. After centering the tabletop, the student radiographer the image intensifier as part of a device called the *fluoroscopy carriage*. As the radiologist moves the entire unit and activates the x-ray tube, a dynamic image is displayed on a television monitor.

When the image-intensification unit is not in use it may be parked out of the way to allow the radiographer to perform routine radiography with the overhead x-ray tube. The beginning radiographer should learn how to move the image intensifier to a safe position to perform fluoroscopic procedures and to move it out of the way to perform radiographic procedures us-

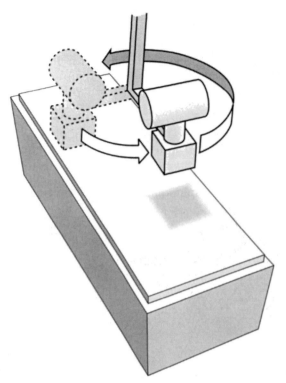

FIGURE 7–10. Tube rotation around the vertical tube column.

should leave it locked on center and manually move the patient. Moving tabletops are advantageous to experienced radiographers and patients in pain, but they can lead to errors for beginning radiographers.

Manipulation of Fluoroscopic Equipment

The equipment discussed so far produces static images. Radiographs provide an image of anatomic structures at a given time. They are not designed for the study of structures that are in motion. The presentation of a continuous or dynamic radiographic image is referred to as **fluoroscopy**.

A **fluoroscope** appears similar to a radiographic system but with some additional equipment components (Fig. 7–12). Added to the table is an image-intensification unit and another x-ray tube located under the table. During fluoroscopy, the radiologist moves the image intensifier over the patient. The x-ray tube is usually located under the table and moves with

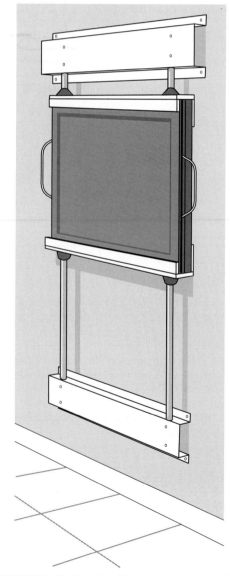

FIGURE 7–11. Simple wall-mounted cassette holder.

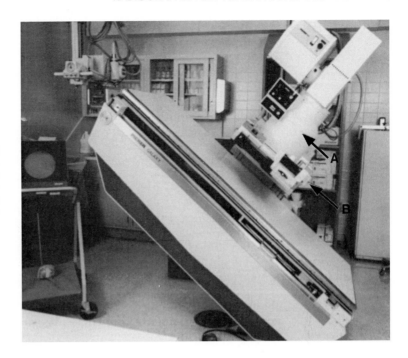

FIGURE 7–12. Radiographic and fluoroscopic unit set up for fluoroscopy: image intensifier *(A)*, fluoroscopy carriage unit *(B)*. The x-ray tube is underneath the table in alignment with the image intensifier.

ing the overhead x-ray tube. There is usually an interlock switch that allows the radiographer to move the image intensifier transversely from a parked position. The units are extremely fragile and expensive and must be handled carefully. Some image intensifiers are designed to shift back enough to clear the area directly over the patient for the overhead x-ray tube. These units do not have to be removed from the fluoroscopic carriage for storage.

Once put into position over the table, the image intensifier can be moved in all planes with a handlebar type of switch that works similar to a joystick on a computer. Moving the handlebar switch in one direction causes the entire carriage (both image intensifier and x-ray tube) to move as one.

A major component of the fluoroscopy tower is the spot film device (Fig. 7–13). The **spot film device** permits the radiologist to obtain static radiographs during a dynamic fluoroscopic examination. The spot film device contains a mechanical conveyor that accepts a variety of cassette sizes. The cassette is placed in a conveyor and automatically transfers to its parked position behind a lead shield outside the radiation field. When the radiologist makes a radiographic exposure, the conveyor moves the cassette from its protected position into the exposure field. The x-ray tube under the table

exposes the cassette and film. The cassette is then removed for processing or returned by the conveyor to its parked position for additional exposures. Depending on the equipment, exposure formats vary. The formats range from a single exposure on the entire film to a series of exposures (as many as 12) on different parts of the film. Most spot films are one on one (the entire film as one image), two on one (the film divided horizontally or vertically to form two images), or four on one (the film divided into quarters to form four images).

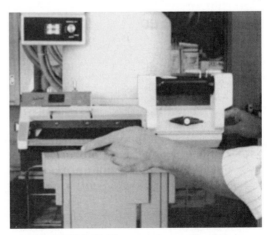

FIGURE 7–13. Fluoroscopic spot film device.

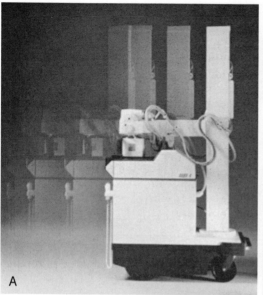
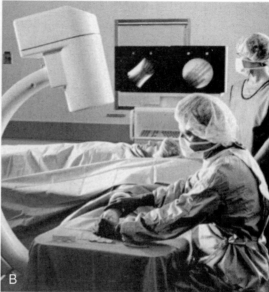

FIGURE 7–14. Mobile units: radiographic *(A)*, fluoroscopic C-arm *(B)*. (Courtesy of General Electric Medical Systems.)

Manipulation of Mobile Equipment

It is often necessary to take radiographic equipment to the patient. This may be at the patient's bedside, in the surgical suite, or in the emergency department. There are numerous types of mobile radiographic and mobile fluoroscopic x-ray systems (Fig. 7–14).

These systems are similar in components and manipulation principles to the equipment that is located in the radiology department. Although many units are motor driven, many must be physically pushed. A beginning radiographer should practice moving the mobile radiographic and fluoroscopic equipment until a measure of ability has been achieved. As with stationary units, it is important to practice the various tube movements and their mechanical or electric interlocks.

Summary

A beginning radiographer can be overwhelmed by the initial complexity of radiographic and fluoroscopic equipment. New students need to master the components of the radiographic system and how they operate. Familiarity with the x-ray tube, collimator, x-ray table, control console, and tube stand is important. The mechanical aspects of collimation, control console operation, and the manipulation of the Bucky mechanism, tube stand, table, and image intensifier are essential skills that must be mastered early by a beginning radiographer. The student must become as comfortable as possible with the mechanical aspects of the x-ray examination process. Students who do well in the clinical aspects of radiography are those who early on master the mechanics of equipment manipulation.

◀R REVIEW QUESTIONS

1 The device that produces radiation is the:
   a. collimator
   b. Bucky tray
   c. x-ray tube
   d. cassette

2 The component that gives the operator control of the exposure factors (technique) is the:
   a. control console
   b. fluoroscope
   c. spot film device
   d. x-ray tube

3 Milliamperage is usually selectable in increments of:
a. 10
b. 100
c. 250
d. 500

4 The primary components of the x-ray tube are:
a. kilovoltage peak and milliamperage
b. milliamperage and time
c. diode and triode
d. anode and cathode

5 The component that controls the size and shape of the x-ray field is the:
a. x-ray tube
b. collimator
c. anode
d. spot film device

6 The device that holds the x-ray cassette in place under the x-ray table is the:
a. Bucky tray
b. foot switch
c. wall-mounted Bucky unit
d. grid

7 The control that permits x-rays to be produced is:
a. kilovoltage peak
b. milliamperage
c. rotor-exposure
d. timer

8 The component that supports and permits the x-ray tube to be moved in different directions is the:
a. tube stand
b. Bucky mechanism

c. spot film device
d. collimator

9 Pivoting the x-ray tube at the point at which it is attached to its support is:
a. collimation
b. vertical travel
c. coning
d. tube angulation

10. The component that allows the radiologist to take radiographs during a fluoroscopic procedure is the:
a. spot film device
b. collimator
c. cassette
d. control console

BIBLIOGRAPHY

Bushong SC: Radiologic Science for Technologists. 6th ed. St. Louis, CV Mosby, 1997.

Carlton R, Adler AM: Principles of Radiographic Imaging: An Art and a Science. 2nd ed. Albany, NY, Delmar Publishers, 1996.

Chesney D, Chesney M: X-ray Equipment for Student Radiographers. 4th ed. Boston, Blackwell Scientific Publications, 1994.

Curry TS, Dowdey JF, Murray RC: Christensen's Introduction to the Physics of Diagnostic Radiology. 4th ed. Philadelphia, Lea & Febiger, 1990.

Forester E: Equipment for Diagnostic Radiography. Boston, MTP Press, 1985.

Hendee WR, Chaney EL, Rossi RP: Radiologic Physics, Equipment and Quality Control. Chicago, Year Book, 1977.

Seeram E: X-ray Imaging Equipment. Springfield, IL, Charles C Thomas, 1985.

Sprawls P: Principles of Radiography for Technologists. Rockville, MD, Aspen Publications, 1990.

Stockley SM: A Manual of Radiographic Equipment. New York, Churchill Livingstone, 1986.

CHAPTER 8

BASIC RADIATION PROTECTION AND RADIOBIOLOGY

Karen Jefferies, BS, RT(R)

Today I was reading about Marie Curie: she must have known she suffered from radiation sickness

> She died a famous woman   denying
> her wounds
> denying
> her wounds came from the same source as her power

ADRIENNE RICH
"POWER," THE DREAM OF A COMMON LANGUAGE: POEMS 1974–1977

OBJECTIVES

On completion of this chapter, the student will be able to:

1 Identify the sources of ionizing radiation.
2 Describe the units used to measure radiation exposure.

3 Describe the nature of ionizing radiation.
4 Explain the ways in which ionizing radiation interacts with matter.
5 List the permissible limits of exposure for occupational and nonoccupational workers.
6 Explain the reason for the varying sensitivity of body cells to ionizing radiation.
7 Describe the ways in which the entire body responds to varying amounts of radiation.
8 Discuss the various methods used to protect the patient from excessive radiation.
9 Discuss the various methods used to protect an occupational worker from excessive radiation.
10 Describe several devices used to detect and measure exposure to ionizing radiation.

GLOSSARY

ALARA: Mnemonic: to keep all radiation exposure as low as reasonably achievable

Becquerel (Bq): unit of radioactivity in the SI system, equal to one disintegration per second

Classic Coherent Scattering: interaction with matter in which a low-energy photon (below 10 keV) is absorbed and released with its same energy, frequency, and wavelength but with a change of direction

Compton Effect (scattering): interaction with matter in which a higher-energy photon strikes a loosely bound outer electron, removing it from its shell, and the remaining energy is released as a scattered photon

Curle (Ci): unit of radioactivity, defined as the quantity of any radioactive nuclide in which the number of disintegrations per second is 3.7×10^{10}

Germ Cell: cell of an organism whose function it is to reproduce its kind (ie, ovum or spermatozoon)

Gray (Gy): unit in the SI system used to measure the amount of energy absorbed in any medium; 1 Gy equals 100 rads.

Kiloelectron Volt (keV): unit of energy equal to 1000 electron volts

Pair Production: interaction between matter and a photon possessing a minimum of 1.02 MeV of energy, producing two oppositely charged particles

Photoelectric Effect: interaction with matter in which a photon strikes an inner shell electron, causing its ejection from orbit with the complete absorption of the photon's energy

Rad (Radiation Absorbed Dose): unit used to measure the amount of energy absorbed in any medium; equal to 100 ergs of energy absorbed in 1 gram of material

Radiation: term applied to forms of energy emitted and transferred through matter

Rem (Radiation Equivalent Man): unit of dose equivalence; equal to the product of absorbed dose in rads and a quality factor

Roentgen (R): a unit of exposure in air; that quantity of x-radiation or gamma radiation that produces the quantity 2.08×10^9 ion pairs per cubic centimeter of air

SI Units: system of units based on metric measurement developed in 1948, used to measure radiation

Sievert (Sv): unit in the SI system used to measure the dose equivalence, or biologic effectiveness, of differing radiations; 1 Sv is equal to 100 rems

Somatic Cell: undifferentiated body cell

X-ray: a form of electromagnetic radiation traveling at the speed of light, with the ability to penetrate matter

Ionizing Radiation

Whenever a radiographer is applying ionizing radiation to produce a diagnostic film for the radiologist, it is important that he or she remember the great responsibility this carries. Exposure to radiation always involves a risk of biologic changes that cannot be ignored. The benefits of better diagnosis of disease outweigh the risk, however, as long as the radiographer is using sound judgment and always works to minimize the quantity of radiation the patient receives. The radiographer must also act to protect all individuals who come in contact with radiation from any unnecessary exposure. This includes himself or herself, the patient, and anyone else.

SOURCES OF IONIZING RADIATION

Although humans are exposed to radiation in everyday living, it is rarely given much thought. There are two basic sources of ionizing **radiation:** natural or background radiation, and man-made radiation. Background sources are those that occur spontaneously in nature and can be affected by human activity. These include cosmic radiation from the sun and other planetary bodies, and naturally occurring radioactive substances present on earth (such as uranium and radium), which can be inhaled or ingested through food, water, or air (radon or radiophosphorus). Sources of man-made radiation include the nuclear industry, radionuclides, and medical and dental exposures. The nuclear industry has contributed fallout from above-ground weapons testing, from accidents in nuclear power stations, and from disposal of byproducts from these plants. Exposure to radionuclides results from products containing radioactive elements, such as smoke detectors, exit signs, watch dials, and radiopharmaceuticals used in the diagnosis and treatment of disease. Finally, medical and dental exposure constitute the greatest source of man-made radiation. Because the radiographer is primarily responsible for the application of medical ionizing radiation to patients, it is important to understand the process by which x-rays interact with matter.

MAN-MADE RADIATION

Man-made ionizing radiation, or **x-rays** as they are more commonly called, is a form of electromagnetic radiation that travels at the speed of light. Unlike particulate radiation, which is a liberated portion of the atom capable of traveling for short distances and reacting with matter, x-rays are bundles of energy moving like waves in space, depositing their energy randomly. For x-rays to be produced, three things must be present: (1) a source of electrons, (2) a force to move them rapidly, and (3) something to rapidly stop that movement. These conditions are all met by the x-ray tube and its electrical supply (Fig. 8–1). The tube itself is composed of a cathode, or negative terminal, and an anode, or positive terminal, enclosed in a special glass envelope to maintain the vacuum necessary for optimal x-ray production. The filament in the cathode assembly is composed of thoriated tungsten, which provides the source of electrons. When kilovoltage (thousands of volts) is applied to the filament, it instantaneously accelerates the available stream of electrons toward the anode end of the tube. X-rays are produced when the electrons strike the anode, undergoing an energy conversion that produces both x-rays and heat. The resultant x-ray beam is heterogeneous; that is, it has many energies, measured in **kiloelectron volts (keV).** These x-rays, also known as the primary beam, are directed toward the patient through a win-

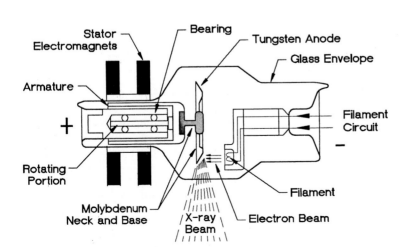

FIGURE 8–1. Rotating anode tube. (Reprinted with permission from Carlton R, Adler A: Principles of Radiographic Imaging: An Art and a Science. Albany, NY, Delmar Publishers, 1992.)

dow in the tube. Once the x-rays strike matter, three possibilities exist: (1) they can be absorbed; (2) they can transfer some energy and then scatter; or (3) they can pass through undisturbed.

INTERACTIONS OF X-RAYS WITH MATTER

There are five ways in which x-rays interact with matter: classic coherent scattering, photoelectric interactions, Compton scattering, pair production, and photodisintegration. Classic coherent scattering, photoelectric interactions, and Compton scattering occur within the diagnostic range of x-ray energies. Both Compton and photoelectric interactions directly influence the patient's and occupational worker's exposure. They are the way in which x-rays transfer their energy to living tissue. They constitute the basis for all patient exposure and the reason behind the need for protective measures.

Classic Coherent Scattering

X-rays that possess energy levels below 10 keV may interact with matter through **classic coherent scattering** (Fig. 8–2). Also known as coherent or Thomson scattering, classic coherent scattering occurs when an incoming x-ray photon strikes an atom and is absorbed, causing the atom to become excited. The atom then releases the excess energy in the form of another x-ray photon, possessing the same energy as the original photon, but proceeding in a different direction. This change in direction is known as scattering. Most of these scattered photons travel in a forward direction, stopping when they strike anything in their path. More importantly, classic coherent scattering results in no energy transfer to the patient.

Photoelectric Interactions

The second common interaction of x-rays with matter in the diagnostic range is the **photoelectric effect** (Fig. 8–3). Photoelectric effect occurs when an incoming x-ray photon strikes an inner shell electron and ejects it from its orbit around the atom, creating an ion pair. The atom, having lost an electron, is positively charged, and the released electron, referred to as the photoelectron, continues to travel until it combines with other matter. All the energy

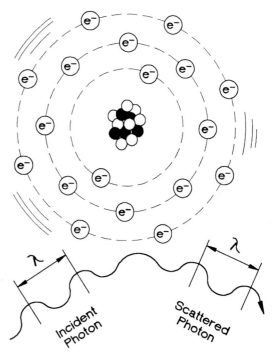

FIGURE 8–2. Classic coherent scatter interaction. (Adapted with permission from Carlton R, Adler A: Principles of Radiographic Imaging: An Art and a Science. Albany, NY, Delmar Publishers, 1992.)

from the photon is completely used up in this action; it is said that the energy is absorbed by the atom. Because complete energy absorption takes place in photoelectric interactions, this constitutes the greatest hazard to patients in diagnostic radiography.

Compton Scattering

The last interaction common to the diagnostic x-ray range is the Compton effect (Fig. 8–4). **Compton effect,** or Compton scattering, occurs when an incoming x-ray photon strikes a target atom and uses a portion of its energy to eject an outer shell electron. The remainder of the photon's energy proceeds in a direction different from the incoming photon. This results in a Compton or recoil electron, which travels until it combines with matter, and a photon of less energy that can react with the patient through further Compton interactions or photoelectric effects or that can exit the patient and reach imaging equipment or the occupational worker. This interaction is extremely important because most of the occupational worker's exposure to radiation comes from Compton scatter.

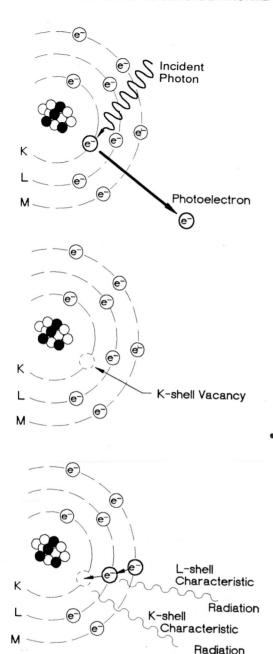

FIGURE 8–3. Photoelectric absorption interaction. (Adapted with permission from Carlton R, Adler A: Principles of Radiographic Imaging: An Art and a Science. Albany, NY, Delmar Publishers, 1992.)

Pair Production

The last two interactions that occur between ionizing radiation and matter require high-energy photons above 1 million electron volts (1 MeV). They are less relevant to diagnostic radi-

ography because the equipment used in the production of x-rays cannot produce photons that possess this energy.

For **pair production** to occur, an incoming x-ray photon must possess a minimum of 1.02 MeV of energy (Fig. 8–5). This photon does not interact with the surrounding electron orbits; instead, it approaches the nucleus of the atom and interacts with its force field. The photon disappears, and two particles—one negatively charged and termed a negatron and one positively charged and called a positron—replace it.

Each particle possesses half the energy (minimum, 0.51 MeV) of the original x-ray photon. The particles continue to travel, causing ionization, until the positron interacts with another electron, annihilates it, and produces two photons moving in opposite directions. Because the energy level necessary for pair production is at least 1.02 MeV, it does not normally occur in the diagnostic x-ray range.

Photodisintegration

X-ray photons possessing a minimum of 10 MeV of energy can interact directly with the nucleus of the atom, causing a state of excitement within the nucleus, followed by the emission of a nuclear fragment (Fig. 8–6). This process is referred to as *photodisintegration*, and does not occur in diagnostic radiography; it occurs in the nuclear industry.

UNITS OF MEASUREMENT

To quantify the amount of radiation a patient or occupational worker receives, a system of units has been developed. The units most commonly used since the 1920s are listed in Table 8–1. In 1948, a system of units based on metric measurement was developed by the International Committee for Weights and Measures. The SI units (Systeme International d'Unites) were officially adopted in 1985.

Roentgen (Coulombs per Kilogram)

The **roentgen (R)** is the measure of ionization in air as a result of exposure to x-rays or gamma rays. It is defined as the quantity of x-radiation or gamma radiation that produces the quantity 2.08×10^9 ion pairs per cubic centimeter (cc) of air, for a total charge of 2.58×10^{-4} coulombs per kilogram (C/kg) (coulomb is a quan-

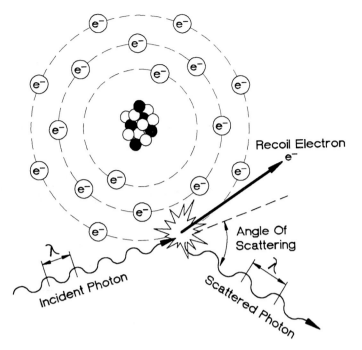

FIGURE 8–4. Compton scatter interaction. (Reprinted with permission from Carlton R, Adler A: Principles of Radiographic Imaging: An Art and a Science. Albany, NY, Delmar Publishers, 1992.)

tity of electric charge). The roentgen is restricted to measuring photons with energy below 3 MeV, and only exposure in air. It does not indicate actual exposure to individuals when absorbed. The roentgen has no equivalent in the SI units, since exposure may be directly expressed as coulombs per kilogram, and it is being phased out as a unit of measurement.

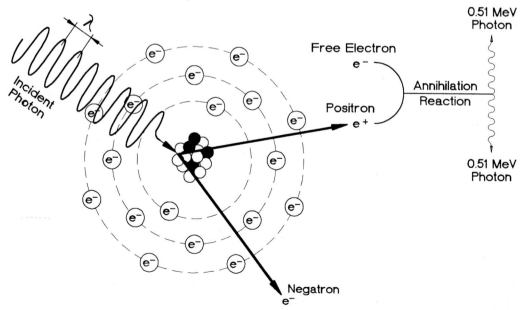

FIGURE 8–5. Pair production interaction. (Reprinted with permission from Carlton R, Adler A: Principles of Radiographic Imaging: An Art and a Science. Albany, NY, Delmar Publishers, 1992.)

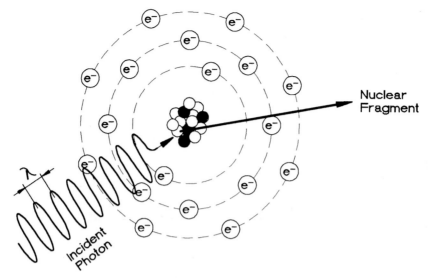

FIGURE 8–6. Photodisintegration interaction. (Reprinted with permission from Carlton R, Adler A: Principles of Radiographic Imaging: An Art and a Science. Albany, NY, Delmar Publishers, 1992.)

Rad (Gray)

The need for discussing absorbed dose resulted in the development of the rad. **The rad (radiation absorbed dose)** measures the amount of energy absorbed in any medium, defined as 100 ergs of energy absorbed in 1 g of absorbing material. The rad has been replaced by the **gray (Gy)** in the SI system, which is defined as 1 joule (J) of energy absorbed in 1 kg of material. The gray is 100 times larger than the rad; 1 Gy is equal to 100 rads.

Rem (Sievert)

Not all types of radiation produce the same response in living tissue. Alpha particles, neutrons, and beta particles may produce a different degree of biologic damage as compared to x-rays and gamma rays. To accurately express the biologic response of exposed individuals to the same quantity of differing radiations, the rem was developed. The **rem (radiation equivalent man)** is the unit of dose equivalence, expressed as the product of the absorbed dose in rad and a quality factor.

The quality factor varies, depending on the type of radiation being used. For example, the quality factor for x-rays is 1, so 1 rad of x-ray exposure equals 1 rem of dose equivalence (1 rad × 1 = 1 rem). However, the quality factor for fast neutrons is 10, so 1 rad of fast neutron exposure equals 10 rem of dose equivalence (1 rad × 10 = 10 rem). This means that neutrons are 10 times as biologically damaging as x-rays when their dose equivalents are compared. The rem has been replaced by the **sievert (Sv)** in SI units, which is defined as the product of the gray and the quality factor. The sievert is 100 times larger than the rad; 1 Sv is equal to 100 rem.

Curie (Becquerel)

Finally, the measure of the rate at which a radionuclide decays is referred to as *activity*.

TABLE 8–1. **Radiation Quantities and Units of Measurement**				
Quantity	**Traditional Unit**	**Definition**	**SI Unit**	**Definition**
Exposure in air	roentgen	2.08×10^9 ion pairs/cc	coulomb/kilogram	
Absorbed dose	rad	100 ergs/g	gray	1 J/kg
Dose equivalent	rem	rad × quality factor	sievert	1 J/kg
Activity	curie	3.7×10^{10} dps	becquerel	1 dps

The **curie (Ci)** is the unit of activity, equal to 3.7×10^{10} disintegrations per second (dps). The SI unit of activity is the **becquerel (Bq)**, defined as 1 dps. Therefore, 1 Ci equals 3.7×10^{10} Bq. These units are commonly employed in nuclear medicine and radiotherapy.

The traditional and SI units are compared in Table 8–1.

STANDARDS FOR REGULATION OF EXPOSURE

Because patients and workers exposed to radiation are at risk for biologic effects, it is important that limits are set to ensure safe practice for both the patient and the radiation worker. Guidelines and standards set by regulatory agencies must be followed. The Center for Devices and Radiological Health (DRH), under the direction of the Food and Drug Administration, sets and regulates the standards for radiation-producing equipment. It also continues to research possible ways of minimizing exposure to ionizing radiation. The National Council on Radiation Protection (NCRP) is a not-for-profit organization enacted by Congress in 1964 to collect and distribute information regarding radiation awareness and safe practice to the public. It cooperates with other organizations to constantly review the latest data on radiation units, measurements, and protection. The following information reflects the recommendations made by the NCRP, in cooperation with other organizations.

Effective dose limit recommendations have been set to minimize the biologic risk to individuals exposed. The concept of maximum permissible dose had been traditionally used to describe the maximum dose of ionizing radiation that, if received by an individual, carried a negligible risk of significant bodily or genetic damage. Maximum permissible doses were established for the occupational worker and the general population. These recommendations followed two theories; no-threshold and risk versus benefit (Fig. 8–7).

No-threshold indicates that no dose exists below which the risk of damage does not exist. Risk versus benefit governed the exposure to individuals when physicians ordered radiographic procedures. The benefit to the patient from performing those procedures far outweighed the risk of possible biologic damage. However, because current studies indicate that

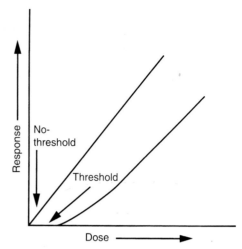

FIGURE 8–7. Graph indicating no-threshold versus threshold response to radiation.

an individual's dose should be kept *as low as reasonably achievable* **(ALARA),** and that no dose is considered permissible, the term *maximum permissible dose* is no longer acceptable. Instead, the NCRP has recommended certain *effective dose* limits, as summarized in Table 8–2.

The annual whole-body effective dose limit for the occupational worker is 50 mSv (5 rem). Before the NCRP issued their dose-equivalent limitations in 1987 and revised them in 1993 as effective dose limits, the lifetime accumulated whole-body dose equivalent was determined by the formula $5(N - 18)$ rem, where N equals the age of the worker in years. According to this formula, a 40-year-old occupational worker could have received $5(40 - 18)$, or 110 rem. Now, the recommended maximum accumulated whole-body effective dose limit is 10 mSv times age in years (or 1 rem $\times$ age in years). This same occupational worker may now accumulate only 1 rem $\times$ 40, or 40 rem (400 mSv), in his or her lifetime.

Anyone exposed to ionizing radiation not as a radiation worker is a member of the general population. The whole-body dose-equivalent limit for the general population is one tenth the occupational worker's annual limit, or 5 mSv (0.5 rem).

Biologic Response to Ionizing Radiation

Ionizing radiation, absorbed by matter, undergoes energy conversions that result in

TABLE 8–2. **Effective Dose Limit Recommendations**

Population and Area of Body Irradiated	Dose Limits	
	SI Unit	Traditional Unit
Occupational Exposures		
Effective dose limits		
Annual	50 mSv	5 rem
Cumulative	10 mSv × age	1 rem × age
Dose equivalent annual limits for tissues and organs		
Lens of eye	150 mSv	15 rem
Skin, hands, and feet	500 mSv	50 rem
Public Exposures (Annual)		
Effective dose limit		
Continuous or frequent exposure	1 mSv	0.1 rem
Infrequent exposure	5 mSv	0.5 rem
Equivalent dose limits for tissues and organs		
Lens of eye	15 mSv	1.5 rem
Skin, hands, and feet	50 mSv	5 rem
Embryo-Fetus Exposures (Monthly)		
Equivalent dose limit	0.5 mSv	0.05 rem
Education and Training Exposures (Annual)		
Effective dose limit	1 mSv	0.1 rem
Dose equivalent limit for tissues and organs		
Lens of eye	15 mSv	1.5 rem
Skin, hands, and feet	50 mSv	5 rem

Adapted from NCRP Report No. 116: Limitation of Exposure to Ionizing Radiation. Bethesda, MD, National Council on Radiation Protection and Measurements, 1993.

changes in atomic structure. These changes, when considered in light of living tissue, can have major consequences on the life of any organism. To understand the necessity of protecting oneself and the patient from exposure to radiation, a basic review of cellular biology and how radiation interacts with cells is important.

BASIC CELL STRUCTURE

The cell is the simplest unit of organic protoplasm capable of independent existence. Simple organisms are composed of one or two cells; complex organisms are multicellular, made of many cells. Although cells may differ from each other, depending on their primary function, their structures are similar. Most cells are divided into two parts: the nucleus and the cytoplasm (Fig. 8–8). The nucleus is separated from the rest of the cell by a double-walled membrane called the *nuclear envelope*. This membrane has openings, or pores, that permit other molecules to pass back and forth between the nucleus and the cytoplasm. Most importantly,

the nucleus contains the chromosomes, which are made up of genes. Genes are the units of hereditary information, composed of deoxyribonucleic acid (DNA). DNA, a double-stranded structure coiled around itself like a spiral staircase, is one of the molecules at risk when a cell is exposed to ionizing radiation.

The cytoplasm of the cell is separated from its environment by the cell membrane. It contains several organelles responsible for the metabolic function of the cell. The cytoplasm itself is primarily water, which can undergo changes when struck by ionizing radiation.

CELL TYPES

There are two types of cells: somatic cells and germ cells. **Somatic cells** perform all the body's functions. They possess two of every gene on two different chromosomes. Their chromosomes are paired, but each pair is different. Somatic cells possess a total of 46 chromosomes, or 23 pairs. They divide through the process of mitosis. **Germ cells** are the reproductive cells of an organism; they possess half the

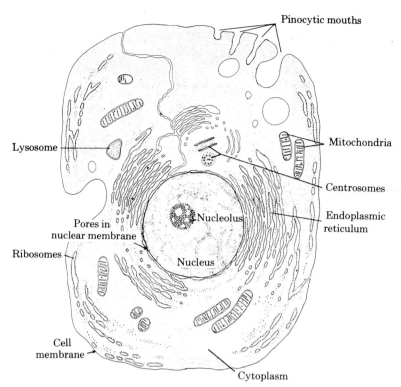

FIGURE 8–8. Diagram of a typical animal cell. (Reprinted with permission from Dorland's Illustrated Medical Dictionary. 27th ed. Philadelphia, WB Saunders, 1988, p 290.)

number of chromosomes as the somatic cells, for a total of 23. Germ cells reproduce through the process of meiosis.

THEORIES FOR CELLULAR ABSORPTION OF IONIZING RADIATION

When ionizing radiation is absorbed by a cell, there are two basic theories to explain this interaction. The first, known as the *direct hit theory*, occurs whenever any type of radiation transfers its energy directly to the key molecule it has struck, resulting in the formation of ion pairs or elevation to a higher, excited energy state. Although any important structure can be hit by radiation, serious consequences arise when radiation interacts with DNA. Breaks in the bases or phosphate bonds can result in rearrangement or loss of genetic information, which can injure or kill the cell as it continues through its life cycle.

The other interaction with ionizing radiation is by indirect hit: key molecules are affected by radiation depositing its energy elsewhere in the cell. Because cells are approximately 80% water,

indirect action occurs when water molecules are ionized. This action produces chemical changes within the cell that alter the internal environment, injuring the cell. This can result in eventual cell death.

TARGET THEORY OF ABSORPTION OF IONIZING RADIATION

Both direct and indirect interactions with ionizing radiation apply to the target theory of absorption of ionizing radiation. Simply stated, there exist certain molecules within a cell that are key to the continued viability or life of that cell. Some of these molecules exist in great number, others in limited supply. If damage occurs to a molecule in abundant supply, the effect to the cell may not be as detrimental since there are others to maintain the function of the cell. Injury to a molecule in limited supply, however, could be life threatening, since there is no immediate replacement. The term *target* is used to describe any critical molecule that has undergone some interaction with ionizing radiation, either directly or indirectly. The target whose damage has serious consequences to the life of the cell is DNA.

RADIOSENSITIVITY OF CELLS

To study the cell's response to radiation, a method of classification according to sensitivity was developed by Bergonie and Tribondeau in 1906. They determined that mitotic activity and specific characteristics of each cell affected how the cell manifested radiation damage. Cells are most sensitive to radiation during active division, when they are primitive in structure and function. Examples of radiosensitive cells include the basal cells of the skin, crypt cells of the small intestine, and germ cells. Cells resistant to radiation, being more specialized in structure and function, do not undergo repeated mitosis. These include nerve, muscle, and brain cells.

This theory was modified by Ancel and Vitemberger, who stated that all cells possess the same sensitivity to radiation; the time of expression of injury is what differs. This depends on mitosis and the external conditions in which the cell is placed. Therefore, rapidly dividing cells demonstrate the injury sooner and just look like they are more sensitive to radiation than those whose mitotic rate is slower. Organs composed of parenchymal cells that rapidly divide, such as skin or the small intestine, exhibit injury sooner than the esophagus or spinal cord, whose cells divide more slowly.

RESPONSE OF CELLS TO RADIATION

Cells respond to radiation in a number of ways: they die before beginning mitosis, delay entering mitosis, or fail to divide at their normal rate. Fortunately, cells also try to repair the damage sustained through absorption of ionizing radiation. This possibility depends on how sensitive the cell is to radiation, the type of damage sustained, the kind of radiation (particulate or electromagnetic), the exposure rate, and the total dose given. Incomplete repair can result in adverse biologic effects occurring after time has elapsed.

TOTAL BODY RESPONSE TO RADIATION

The total body response of any organism to radiation depends on the effect to all the systems of the body. Because every system is different in its sensitivity or resistance, the total body response at a particular dose is defined by the system most affected. This response, known as *acute radiation syndrome*, occurs only when the organism is exposed fully (total body) to an external source of radiation given in a few minutes. Only then does the organism develop the full set of signs and symptoms that define each syndrome.

There are three general stages of response for each acute radiation syndrome. The first is the prodromal stage, commonly referred to as the NVD (nausea, vomiting, and diarrhea) stage. The second stage is the latent period, in which the organism feels well. However, during this time, the body is undergoing biologic changes that will lead to the final period, the manifest stage. Now the full effects of the exposure are felt by the organism, leading to either recovery or death.

There are three radiation syndromes: bone marrow syndrome, gastrointestinal syndrome, and central nervous system syndrome. Bone marrow syndrome occurs between doses of 1 and 10 Gy (100 and 1000 rad). Total body exposure results in infection, hemorrhage, and anemia. Gastrointestinal syndrome results from doses between 10 and 100 Gy (1000 and 10,000 rad). Individuals experience massive diarrhea, nausea and vomiting, and fever when subjected to these doses. Central nervous system syndrome occurs at doses above 100 Gy (10,000 rad), with the individual experiencing convulsions, coma, and eventual death from increased intracranial pressure. Although these syndromes indicate serious, even lethal, consequences from exposure to radiation, it must be remembered that these doses are far greater than those received by the occupational worker or patient.

LATE EFFECTS OF RADIATION EXPOSURE

Other effects of radiation exposure are equally important. These are the late effects, which can develop over a long period after exposure. These effects result not only from high doses of radiation but from low doses administered over a longer time. Late effects are divided into two groups: somatic effects, which develop in the individual exposed, and genetic effects, which occur in future generations as a result of damage to the germ cells.

The two most frequently induced somatic effects are cataract formation and carcinogenesis. The lens of the eye is extremely sensitive to radiation, and studies have demonstrated the high incidence of cataract formation in laboratory animals exposed to radiation. Also, survivors of the explosion of the atom bomb developed cataracts.

The most important late somatic effect is cancer development. The first documented case was the hand of a radiographer in 1902. Early radiologists, technologists, and researchers developed skin cancer and leukemia from prolonged exposure to ionizing radiation. Watch dial painters developed osteosarcoma from ingesting radium when they put their paint brushes in their mouths to draw the tip to a point. Miners who inhaled radioactive dust while digging for uranium developed lung cancer. All these cases led to today's strict limitations on radiation exposure.

Long-term genetic effects result from germ cells whose DNA has been altered by radiation exposure. This means the effects are not seen in the individual exposed; instead, if an affected cell is fertilized and develops, they show up in future generations. These mutations—alterations in the DNA coding of the chromosome—are recessive. They appear only if the mutated cell is fertilized by another reproductive cell carrying the same mutation. This fact of genetics acts to minimize the appearance of possible radiation-induced changes.

Protecting the Patient

Although the patient must be exposed to ionizing radiation for a diagnostic image to be produced, care must be exercised to minimize the quantity of radiation exposure. The radiographer has the responsibility of maximizing the quality of the radiograph while minimizing the risk to the patient. Consequently, the concept of ALARA—as low as reasonably achievable—is used to guide technical factor selection when performing examinations on the patient. In particular, the cardinal principles of protection—time, distance, and shielding—can be used to minimize patient exposure.

TIME

When the radiographer minimizes the length of time a patient is placed in the path of the x-ray beam, he or she is applying one of the primary rules of protection. This is accomplished when the radiographer accurately applies the rules of radiographic technique to produce diagnostic images and uses technique charts to help determine the correct amount of radiation to direct toward the patient. The chances of repeated exposures are minimized, reducing the patient's time in the path of the x-ray beam.

DISTANCE

Another way to lessen patient dose is to maximize the distance between the radiation source and the patient. This serves to lessen the entrance or skin dose to the patient. This is not the most reasonable method to minimize patient dose, since the patient must be in the path of the ionizing beam for an image to be created. Also, increasing distance requires an increase in technical factors to create an acceptable image.

SHIELDING

The last rule of protection is to shield by placing some material over the reproductive organs (gonads) of the patient, whenever they are within 4 to 5 cm of the primary beam. This is particularly important when performing radiography on children and adults of reproductive age. Shields are made of lead, which has an atomic number of 82. Lead absorbs x-rays through the process of photoelectric effect, thereby minimizing patient exposure. The three basic types of shields are flat contact shields, shaped contact shields, and shadow shields.

Flat contact shields are made of a combination of vinyl and lead and are placed directly over the gonads of the patient (Fig. 8–9). They are made in various sizes to accommodate the age of the patient. *Shaped contact shields* are cup shaped and designed specifically to protect the gonads of male patients. Because of their shape, they can remain in place more securely, even when the patient must turn to accommodate the examination. *Shadow shields* are mounted to the side of the collimator of the x-ray tube, on a flexible extension arm. They can be manipulated to extend into the path of the beam and cast a shadow on the patient, indicating the area being protected. *Lead rubber blockers* may also be used in some situations.

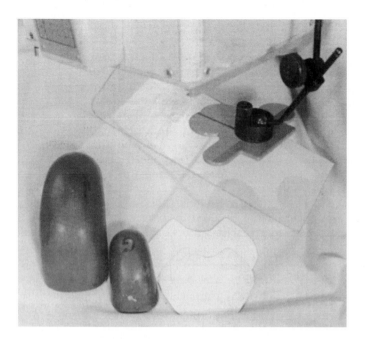

FIGURE 8–9. Gonadal shields (clockwise from top): shadow shield, lead rubber blocker, flat contact shields, shaped shields.

ADDITIONAL METHODS OF PROTECTION

Other factors specific to the production of x-rays can be manipulated with the purpose of minimizing patient exposure. These include beam restriction, film/screen combinations, technical factor selection, and filtration. The radiographer must always restrict the primary beam to the anatomic area of interest, never exceeding the size of the image receptor used to capture the information. This limits the exposure to the area undergoing radiography and does not increase the overall patient dose. Through the use of fast film/screen combinations, a diagnostic image can be produced with less radiation, which minimizes patient exposure. Also, selecting technical factors that use higher kilovoltages increases the probability that Compton interactions occur. This results in less of the energy being directly absorbed by the patient, creating a decrease in patient exposure. When lower kilovoltage techniques are selected, more of that radiation is completely absorbed within the patient, adding to the dose. Finally, using filtration in the path of the x-ray beam absorbs the lower-energy x-rays that only add to the patient's entrance dose. Eliminating their presence in the primary beam does not affect the finished image, since most do not exit the patient to reach the image receptor. Aluminum is the most common material used in filtration. Its atomic number and K-shell binding energies encourage photoelectric absorption of the low-energy x-rays.

Protecting the Radiographer

The same principles of time, distance, and shielding are used to reduce the occupational worker's exposure to radiation. This is done by minimizing the time spent in the room when ionizing radiation is being produced, using the greatest possible distance from the source of exposure, and placing a shield between the worker and the radiation source.

TIME

The radiographer should always spend the least amount of time possible in a room when a source of radiation is active. This risk exists only when exposures are being made: once the exposure is terminated, no radiation remains within the room or the contents of the room. The amount of dose received is directly related to the length of time spent with the source. During fluoroscopy in which radiation is used for imaging dynamic structures, x-rays are emitted for longer periods. Therefore, most units are equipped with 5-minute timers to alert the operator that a period of time has elapsed.

DISTANCE

Distance is the best measure of protection for an occupational worker. The principle of the inverse square law states that the intensity of radiation varies inversely with the square of the distance. Simply put, increasing the distance from the source of the x-ray beam greatly reduces the quantity of radiation that reaches the radiographer (Fig. 8–10). This occurs because the x-rays leaving the tube spread out (diverge) and cover a much larger area, which in turn lessens their intensity. This formula can be used to determine the exact exposure reaching the worker:

$$\frac{\text{new intensity}}{\text{old intensity}} = \frac{(\text{old distance})^2}{(\text{new distance})^2}$$

For example, if the intensity of radiation received by the radiographer was 20 mR at a distance of 1 m from the tube, what would the intensity be at a distance of 2 m from the tube, all other factors remaining the same? Solving for the new intensity, we get:

$$\frac{\text{new intensity}}{20 \text{ mR}} = \frac{(1)^2}{(2)^2}$$

$$\text{new intensity} = \frac{1 \times 20 \text{ mR}}{4} = 5 \text{ mR}$$

Doubling the distance between the radiographer and the source of radiation reduces the exposure by a factor of 4.

A radiographer should not make a practice of holding a patient who cannot cooperate during a radiographic procedure. This places the radiographer closer to the beam and to the patient, who is a source of scatter radiation from Compton interactions. This also increases the time a radiographer is near the source of radiation.

Immobilization devices, such as sandbags or restraint bands, should be used whenever possible. If these are ineffective or unavailable, assistance should be obtained from a nonoccupational worker, such as a nurse, physician, or parent of the patient. The person who assists the patient must wear shielding devices to minimize his or her exposure.

SHIELDING

Shielding must be used by the radiographer whenever time and distance alone cannot satisfactorily protect the worker. Lead is the material used in both fixed protective barriers and accessory devices such as aprons and gloves. Lead aprons and gloves should be worn when it is not possible to take advantage of fixed barriers. They are constructed of lead-impregnated vinyl, having a content between 0.25 and 1.0 mm of lead equivalency. The greater the amount of lead used, the better the protection offered the worker. The greatest drawback to increased lead content is the increase in weight the device possesses. The minimum permissible amount of lead equivalency for aprons used where the peak kilovoltage is 100 is 0.25 mm. Gloves usually possess the same minimum amount.

The shielding garments must be in good condition; cracked aprons and gloves do not successfully attenuate radiation. It is important to store protective apparel properly on specially designed racks, so that cracks do not develop. To determine whether aprons or gloves adequately protect the wearer, they should undergo

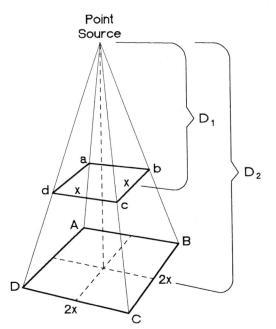

FIGURE 8–10. The inverse square law. The intensity of radiation at a given distance from a point source is inversely proportional to the square of the distance. (Reprinted with permission from Carlton R. Adler A: Principles of Radiographic Imaging: An Art and a Science. Albany, NY, Delmar Publishers, 1992.)

fluoroscopy at least once a year to check for damage.

Fixed protective barriers are part of the radiographic room construction and can be divided into primary and secondary barriers. Primary barriers are those that can be struck by the primary beam exiting the x-ray tube. Secondary barriers are those that can be struck only by secondary, scatter, or leakage radiation. The exact quantity of lead or equivalent thickness of concrete is determined by a diagnostic radiologic physicist, who considers the design and use of the room.

THE PREGNANT STUDENT

Student pregnancy is covered under Nuclear Regulatory Commission (NRC) regulations regarding the declared pregnant worker. Radiologic Sciences programs accredited by the Joint Review Committee on Education in Radiologic Technology must publish and make these regulations known to accepted and enrolled female students. Although there have long been guidelines for exposure to pregnant women, in 1994 the US Nuclear Regulatory Commission became the first regulatory agency to limit the absorbed radiation dose to the unborn child. The dose limit is 0.5 rem (5 mSv) for the declared pregnant woman. In addition, the National Council on Radiation Protection and Measurements (NCRP) recommends that once pregnancy is known, a limit of 0.05 rem (0.5 mSv) per month should apply.

Study of average exposure to radiologic technologists indicates that it is unlikely that exposure to a pregnant woman who is a student would exceed these limits. Consequentially, there is little reason for the pregnant student to decide not to declare her pregnancy or to substantially alter her clinical assignments. It is the responsibility of the pregnant woman to decide what the risk to her fetus may be and to take precautions to avoid excessive radiation exposure. Careful attention to the ALARA concepts of time, distance, and shielding are an important part of this decision.

Due to Supreme Court litigation designed to end sex discrimination against pregnant women in the workplace, American employers may not bar women of childbearing age from jobs because of potential risk to their fetus. Essentially, the ruling upholds the Title VII Civil Rights Act of 1964 as forbidding sex-specific fetal-protection policies. Consequently, the NRC requires that all individuals frequenting any portion of a restricted radiation area be instructed in the risks of radiation exposure to the embryo and fetus. (Restricted areas include diagnostic radiologic rooms, nuclear medicine laboratories, and any other area where ionizing radiation is applied to humans.) These instructions must include the right to declare or not declare pregnancy status. A declared pregnant woman is one who has voluntarily elected to declare her pregnancy. She is not under any regulatory or licensing obligation to do so. If a declaration is made it must be in writing, be dated, and include the estimated month of conception. Acknowledgment of a pregnancy verbally or by visual observation does not meet the requirements of these regulations. Furthermore, the woman has the right to revoke her declaration of pregnancy. Until the proper declaration has been made the total exposure dose limit is 5 rem (50 mSv).

Current recommendations in the literature discourage moving a newly declared pregnant women to an area of lower radiation exposure. This is because reassignments have the potential to increase exposure to others who are not yet aware they are pregnant. However, if students are reassigned to low exposure areas it is necessary to obtain agreement with this practice from all students at the time they begin the educational program. ALARA radiation protection philosophy supports a schedule that evenly distributes exposure risk to all students at a relatively uniform monthly exposures rate to avoid substantial variations among individuals.

NRC regulations require that a personnel monitor be used if the declared pregnant student is likely to receive 10% of the embryo/fetus dose limit. This would be 0.05 rem (0.5 mSv) for the pregnancy or 0.005 rem (0.05 mSv) per month. Regulations require that the film badge (or other approved monitoring device) be worn at the part of the body receiving the highest exposure. No additional monitor is required if the woman has been wearing a personnel monitor at the collar or other location outside a lead apron. However, a single monitor that has been previously worn under a lead apron cannot be moved to the collar or other location. Instead, a second monitor must be worn outside lead aprons while the other monitor is worn in its usual location. This is to avoid abnormal exposure readings from the woman's usual habits.

Radiation Monitoring

Finally, any occupational worker who is regularly exposed to ionizing radiation must be monitored to determine estimated exposure. Any worker who is likely to receive more than one tenth of the recommended dose-equivalent limit should be monitored. Monitors measure the quantity of radiation received, based on conditions in which the radiographer was placed. The most common personnel-monitoring devices are the film badge, thermoluminescent dosimeter, and pocket dosimeter.

FILM BADGES

Film badges are the most popular, least expensive method to monitor personnel exposure (Fig. 8–11). The badge consists of a plastic holder containing different filters and a separate light-tight packet holding two pieces of film having different sensitivity to x-ray. Located on the front of the film packet is the identification information of the person wearing the badge. The film in the holder gets darker in response to the amount and energy of the radiation to which it is exposed. This is analyzed to deter-

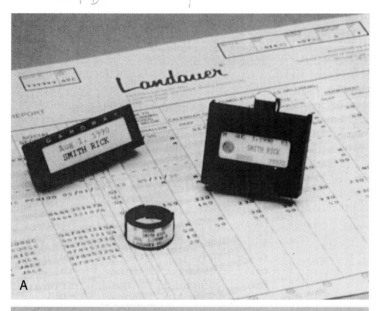

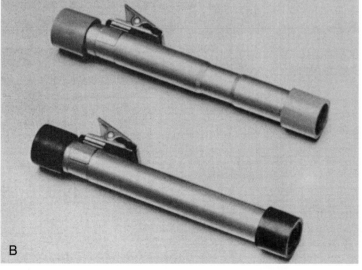

FIGURE 8–11. *A, Left to right,* Typical film badge, thermoluminescent dosimeter ring, and collar badge. *B,* Pocket dosimeters. (Courtesy of Tech/Ops Landauer, Inc.)

mine the occupational worker's exposure. A film badge is sensitive to doses as low as 10 mrem (0.1 mSv) and is usually worn for 1 month. Doses below 10 mrem are not detectable, and are reported as "M" or minimal. The holder should be worn between the collar and waist, on the front of the occupational worker. The main disadvantage to this device is the inability to get an immediate reading of the worker's exposure; the dose can be determined only when the film is processed and analyzed.

THERMOLUMINESCENT DOSIMETERS

A second device to monitor personnel exposure is the thermoluminescent dosimeter (TLD). The TLD consists of a plastic holder containing crystals that absorb a portion of the energy they receive from a radiation exposure. When exposed, the absorbed energy causes the outer valence electrons to be trapped in the forbidden zone, the region immediately past their resting orbit. The number of electrons elevated to this state is directly dependent on the amount of radiation received. When it is time to determine the dose, these crystals are heated so that the trapped electrons return to their original resting state. This results in a release of the extra energy in the form of a light photon. The light is collected and analyzed to determine the quantity of dose received by the TLD.

The crystal most commonly used in TLDs is lithium fluoride. Once the lithium fluoride crystals have been heated (annealed), they can then be reused—something that is not possible with a film badge. The TLD provides readings as low as 5 mrem (0.05 mSv).

POCKET DOSIMETERS

The last device is the pocket dosimeter. It looks like a pen flashlight and is constructed of a central metal electrode surrounded by air, enclosed in a metal holder. The electrode is positively charged, and as the dosimeter is exposed to ionizing radiation, the air in the dosimeter is ionized. Negative ions moving toward the electrode combine with some of the positive charges, neutralizing the electrode. This loss in charge is proportional to the amount of radiation, and a pointer on a scale moves upward relative to the loss in charge. The pocket dosim-

eter is used when an immediate reading of occupational dose is desired. However, it is subject to false readings and does not provide a permanent record.

FIELD SURVEY INSTRUMENTS

Other types of instruments are used to detect the presence of radiation and give the user an indication of the intensity of the source. These are known as field survey instruments. A common instrument used to detect x-radiation, gamma radiation, and beta radiation is the Geiger-Müller counter. It is an ionization chamber constructed of an electrode housed within a chamber. The walls of the chamber are negatively charged, and the electrode is positive. When x-rays pass through the chamber and interact with air, ionization occurs. Free electrons are attracted to the positively charged electrode, where they can be measured. The number of free electrons is directly proportional to the radiation exposure and can be displayed on a special meter that interprets this information and determines the exposure in roentgens or coulombs per kilogram.

Summary

Medical ionizing radiation is a form of electromagnetic radiation capable of penetrating matter and depositing energy as it travels. Although ionizing radiation can interact with matter in five ways, of particular importance to imaging are the photoelectric interaction and Compton interaction. Both contribute to the creation of the diagnostic radiograph, and both contribute to the exposure of the patient and the radiographer to radiation.

The quantities of radiation important in radiography are exposure, absorbed dose, and dose equivalence. The traditional units used to measure these quantities are the roentgen, rad, and rem. The SI units that correspond to the traditional units are coulombs per kilogram, gray, and sievert.

Biologic changes that occur as a result of exposure to radiation begin at the cellular level. The effects depend on what type of cell was struck, how the energy was transferred, the type of radiation, and the sensitivity of the cell. The immediate response of the cell is to repair itself; when this is not possible, other changes begin to take place. These changes have an impact not only on the cells struck but also on all the systems that are composed of those cells. The effects resulting from exposure are either somatic, affecting the individual exposed, or genetic, affecting future generations through changes in germ cells. To minimize these changes, appropriate measures of protection must be used.

To minimize patient exposure, the radiographer must keep in mind all the principles of image production that play a role in patient exposure. Examples of these are kilovoltage, film/screen combinations, collimation, filtration, and repeated exposures. Shields must also be applied to protect the reproductive organs of the patient whenever possible, as long as the examination is not compromised. The radiographer must also protect himself or herself from unnecessary radiation through the use of the cardinal rules of protection: time, distance, and shielding. Finally, a record of the amount of radiation the occupational worker receives or is exposed to can be obtained by using monitoring devices such as film badges, thermoluminescent dosimeters, and pocket dosimeters.

◀R REVIEW QUESTIONS

1 Which of the following is not necessary for x-rays to be produced?
   a) a source of electrons
   b) rapid particle acceleration
   c) a source of protons
   d) instantaneous deceleration

2 For pair production to occur, the energy of the incoming x-ray photon must be at least:
   a) 10 keV
   b) 1.02 keV
   c) 10 MeV
   d) 1.02 MeV

3 The interaction of x-rays with matter that constitutes the greatest hazard to patients in diagnostic radiography is:
   a) photoelectric interaction
   b) Compton interaction
   c) classic coherent scattering
   d) pair production

4 The unit used to measure the amount of ionizing radiation in any medium is the:
   a) rem
   b) rad
   c) roentgen
   d) sievert

5 The maximum accumulated whole-body dose for a 35-year-old occupational worker is:
   a) 85 rem
   b) 5 rem
   c) 35 rem
   d) 0.5 rem

6 According to the law of Bergonie and Tribondeau, the characteristics that determine the sensitivity of a cell to radiation are:
   a) mitotic activity and metabolic function
   b) metabolic function and cell type
   c) mitotic activity and structure and function of the cell
   d) cell type and life span of the cell

7 The intensity of radiation from a radiographic tube was 35 mR at a distance of 2.5 m from the tube. What would the intensity be at a distance of 4 m from the tube, all other factors remaining the same?
   a) 5.5 mR
   b) 55 mR
   c) 14 mR
   d) 90 mR

8 Which of the following is not a component of a film badge?
   a) exposure meter
   b) plastic holder
   c) metal filters
   d) packaged film

9 The type of shielding device that is attached to the side of the collimator on a radiographic tube is a:
   a) flat contact shield
   b) detachable shield
   c) shaped contact shield
   d) shadow shield

10 When ionizing radiation interacts with the suspending medium of the cell, it is termed a:
   a) direct-hit interaction
   b) indirect-hit interaction
   c) target interaction
   d) random interaction

BIBLIOGRAPHY

Bushong C: Radiologic Science for Technologists: Physics, Biology, and Protection. 6th ed. St. Louis, CV Mosby, 1997.

Carlton RC, Adler AM: Principles of Radiographic Imaging: An Art and a Science. 2nd ed. Albany, NY, Delmar Publishers, 1996.

Curry TS, Dowdey JE, Murry RC: Christensen's Introduction to the Physics of Diagnostic Radiology. 4th ed. Philadelphia, Lea & Febiger, 1990.

Dorland's Illustrated Medical Dictionary. 25th ed. Philadelphia, WB Saunders, 1974.

Hall J: Radiobiology for the Radiologist. 4th ed. Philadelphia, JB Lippincott, 1993.

Kane DF, Sims E, Stecker L, et al: The declared pregnant woman in nuclear medicine. J Nucl Med Technol 24(2):83, 1996.

NCRP Report No. 82: SI Units in Radiation Protection and Measurements. Bethesda, MD, National Council on Radiation Protection and Measurements, 1985.

NCRP Report No. 91: Recommendations on Limits for Exposure to Ionizing Radiation. Bethesda, MD, National Council on Radiation Protection and Measurements 1987.

NCRP Report No. 116. Limitation of Exposure to Ionizing Radiation. Bethesda, MD, National Council on Radiation Protection and Measurements, 1993.

Nias AHW: An Introduction to Radiobiology. New York, John Wiley & Sons, 1990.

Selman J: The Fundamentals of X-ray and Radium Physics. 8th ed. Springfield, IL, Charles C Thomas, 1994.

Travis EL: Primer of Medical Radiobiology. 2nd ed. Chicago, Year Book Medical Publishers, 1989.

US Nuclear Regulatory Commission: Standards for Protection Against Radiation. 10 CFR Part 20, Washington, DC: NRC, September 1994.

US Nuclear Regulatory Commission: Instruction Concerning Prenatal Radiation Exposure, Regulatory Guide 8.13, Revision 2, Washington, DC: NRC, December 1987.

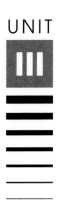
Patient Care

CHAPTER 9

PATIENT INTERACTIONS

C. William Mulkey EdD, RT(R) FASRT, FAERS
Richard R. Carlton, MS, RT(R)(CV), FAERS

Once one learns to cut himself off from his feeling, it is sometimes frightening to realize how difficult it seems to get back in touch with them. This cannot always be done at 5:00 p.m. on schedule, and the student soon learns, like Dr. Jekyll, that the potion doesn't always wear off when it's time to go home.

DAVID REISER AND ANDREA SCHRODER
PATIENT INTERVIEWING: THE HUMAN DIMENSION

OBJECTIVES

On completion of this chapter, the student will be able to:

1 Identify qualities needed to be a caring radiologic technologist.
2 Specify needs that cause people to enter radiologic technology as a profession.
3 Discuss general needs that patients may have according to Maslow's hierarchy of needs.
4 Relate differences between the needs of inpatients and those of outpatients.
5 Explain why patient interaction is important to patients, family, and friends.
6 Analyze effective methods of communication for patients of various ages.
7 Explain appropriate interaction techniques for various types of patients.
8 Discuss considerations of the physical changes of aging for radiologic examinations.
9 Discuss appropriate methods of responding to terminally ill patients.

GLOSSARY

Inpatient: someone who has been admitted to the hospital for diagnostic studies or treatment

Gerontology: pertaining to the study of the aged

Maslow's Hierarchy of Needs: model of human needs developed by Abraham Maslow; it proceeds in five levels: physiologic, safety and security, love and belonging, self-esteem and respect, and self-actualization

Nonverbal Communication: messages sent through methods other than the actual words of speech; for example, tone of voice, speed of speech, and position of the speaker's extremities and torso (body language)

Outpatient: a patient who comes to the hospital for diagnosis or treatment but does not occupy a bed

Palpation: application of light pressure with the fingers

Paralanguage: the music of language; the cadence and rhythm of speech

Verbal Communication: messages sent through spoken words; it can be dramatically shaped by vocabulary, clarity of voice, and even the organization of sentences

Personal Understanding

Radiologic technology is a people-oriented, hands-on profession that requires proficiency in a wide variety of communication techniques. Beginning radiologic technologists must develop effective methods of patient contact early to achieve a successful and enjoyable career.

The importance of interacting effectively with the patient is critical to the radiologic technologist as well as to the patient. These techniques greatly improve the quality of the radiologic images as well as patient care. Obtaining the patient's cooperation is one of the most challenging parts of a radiologic technologist's role. The most seasoned radiologic technologist will have to repeat radiographs if the patient does not understand the procedure or does not cooperate because of poor communication.

The communication skills of the radiologic technologist often determine the patient's opinion of the radiology department. Because hospitals and clinics depend heavily on patients for reimbursement of services, the use of effective interactive skills can make the patient's visit much more pleasant and meaningful and could encourage their return for additional medical care.

Students have needs to satisfy their career ambitions, which often include:

- helping others
- working with people
- making a difference
- thinking critically
- demonstrating creativity
- achieving results

Radiologic technology is capable of fulfilling all these needs and many more. When personal needs are met, it is not unusual to experience increased confidence in technical abilities as well. The patient often perceives this as competence because the external appearance is that of a self-assured individual capable of smoothly carrying out examination procedures.

Maslow's hierarchy of needs provides insight into this type of behavior for all individuals, professionals and patients alike (Fig. 9–1). Maslow suggests that people strive from a basic level of physical needs toward a level of self-actualization. This highest level is characterized by confidence in who one is and what one's goals are in life. Essentially, each level of needs must be satisfied before proceeding to the next level. Radiologic technology students often begin their education at about the third level,

which relates to belonging or affection needs. Once the student has been accepted by instructors, classmates, and staff radiologic technologists, it is important to move toward the fourth level, which addresses self-esteem and respect needs. Many students achieve this level during the second year, once many of the required clinical skills have been mastered. As graduation and the certification examination is successfully completed, level five, the self-actualization level, can begin in a professional context.

As jobs or roles change, it is normal to move up and down the various levels of the hierarchy and to be at different levels in different roles. For example, a new husband may be at the fourth level at work but at the third level in marriage.

Patient Needs

To interact effectively with patients, it is important to understand that patients may be in an altered state of consciousness. They are in an unfamiliar environment where they are no longer in complete control. In addition, they often fear not knowing their exact state of health. It is not unusual for a patient to prefer

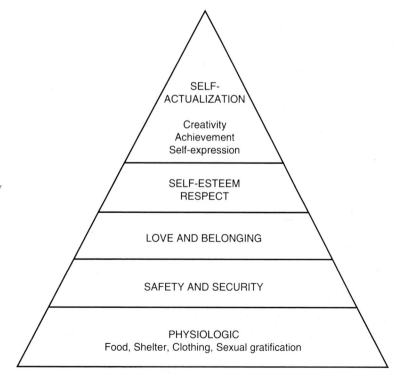

FIGURE 9–1. Maslow's hierarchy of needs.

bad news to uncertainty because at least plans can be made to cope with bad news, whereas uncertainty leaves a person without a means to attempt to control the situation. It is difficult to empathize with these feelings until they have been experienced personally.

Most patients would prefer not to be in the care of a radiologic technologist. Even the kindest and most cooperative patients are simply making the best of a situation they would prefer to avoid. There is a potential for disease or they would not be seeking medical care. It is often patients' fear of what the radiologic technologist will find through the images that causes them to be inconsiderate, arrogant, impatient, rude, or overly talkative, or to exhibit other symptoms as they attempt to cope with their situation.

PATIENT DIGNITY

The patient may arrive for care at the first level of Maslow's hierarchy of needs, which is the physiologic or survival level. Illness may have altered many physiologic functions, which in turn may cause the patient to behave abnormally.

A lack of satisfaction in level one needs can cause a patient to be unable to satisfy the other higher needs. For example, if a patient is very sick, she could lose sleep (level one) over how she will keep her job and maintain her home or belongings (level two). When a patient arrives with a nasogastric (NG) tube in his nose (Fig. 9–2), although he may normally be very friendly and talkative, he may not want to be around other patients with the NG tube in place (level three).

Radiologic technologists have an awesome responsibility when it comes to interacting with patients because of the tremendous power that is held by health professionals over patients. This power is so great that it includes the most basic elements of a person's dignity and self-respect. Inconsiderate abuse of this power may seem to be difficult to avoid because of the nature of the examination procedures. Consequently, special attention is needed to ensure that the power is not abused. For example, it dehumanizes patients when they are required to wear flimsy patient gowns, when they are referred to as the "stomach" or "colon" instead of by name, or when they are placed in proximity to other patients who are more critically ill. It is difficult to maintain self-respect while trying

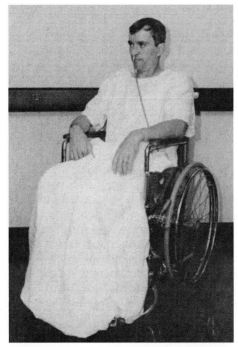

FIGURE 9–2. When patients arrive with a nasogastric tube in the nose, although they may normally be friendly and outgoing, they may prefer to wait in a location where they do not have to face the public.

to get to a toilet before evacuating barium from the bowel, when vomiting, and in other uncomfortable situations.

Top-notch radiologic technologists learn about different types of patients, along with various methods of communication that are effective with each. Two main classifications of patients can be considered: inpatients and outpatients. Each type has typical characteristics that require different approaches and interaction skills on the part of the technologist.

INPATIENTS

An **inpatient** is someone who has been admitted to the hospital for diagnostic studies or treatment. Inpatients often move up and down Maslow's hierarchy before arriving in the care of the radiologic technologist. It is important to gain the patient's confidence even though he or she may be in a somewhat agitated or bewildered state of mind. Previous experiences in the hospital may have shaped the manner in which the patient responds to these initial interactions with the technologist. For example, a patient with severe lower back pain who has been transferred from a bed to a cart by inexperienced nursing staff may be skeptical of a radiologic technologist's assurances of a smooth and careful transfer onto an examination table.

The inpatient may be transported to the radiology department by wheelchair or cart or by walking (ambulating). While in the waiting area of the radiology department, the patient has an opportunity to hear and see many departmental activities. Always be aware that, although you are familiar with the department and may take patients' waiting for granted, the patients are listening and watching everything in anticipation of how they may be treated.

OUTPATIENTS

An **outpatient** is someone who has come to the hospital for diagnosis or treatment but does not occupy a bed. Outpatients arrive in the radiology department with prior expectations. They often expect to be seen immediately on arriving in the department because they have a scheduled appointment. It is difficult to maintain a schedule in any medical setting because of unforeseen circumstances that occur. For example, follow-up films on a previous patient may take longer than expected; a radiologist may require extra projections to be certain of a diagnosis; or patients may become ill, refuse examinations, or be unable to cooperate fully. It is certainly appropriate and important to apologize for delays and to try to keep waiting patients up to date on their status, for example, telling a patient that it will be 20 minutes before he or she can be seen if there are no emergencies. If something unforeseen comes up, it takes no extra time to say, "I'll be with you as soon as I finish one more patient," as you walk by 15 minutes later. Patients greatly appreciate the simple fact that you are aware they are waiting and you perceive their patience. More positive comments are received by hospitals from these types of interactions than for anything else.

Because outpatients often have insurance or government benefits of some type, they may expect priority treatment. As a professional you should provide the same care and attention to all patients regardless of status. This can be especially difficult when a patient is a famous personality, a criminal, or otherwise known.

Interacting With the Patient's Family and Friends

Family and friends of patients who are visiting must also receive attention. Because they spend much time waiting, they tend to critique everything the radiologic technologist does, from appearance to tone of voice to smile (or lack of one). It is important to be courteous to visitors and relatives as well as to the patient. Relatives are justifiably concerned and may ask questions such as whether the technologist sees anything abnormal or whether a fracture is present. It helps to think about how the family and friends feel, or to consider how concerned you would be about a member of your own family.

The same needs function for family and friends as for the patient and technologist. Abnormal or rude behavior may be the result of anxiety, concern, or stress. It is common for the radiologic technologist to be asked for an interpretation of images. Remember that family and friends often listen closely to everything a professional says (Fig. 9–3). Any statements in response to this type of question may be construed as diagnosing, which is practicing medicine and is illegal without a license. The best response is usually to indicate that the findings are available to the referring physician and that only he or she can provide the information.

The radiologic technologist has a responsibil-

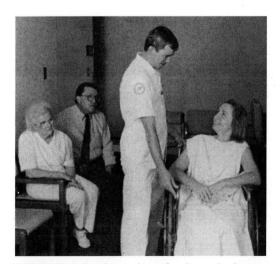

FIGURE 9–3. Family members often listen closely to everything a professional says. It is important to be careful not to attempt to interpret images, because this is diagnosing, which is illegal.

ity to make the patient, the family, and the friends believe they are receiving the best possible care and that they are important and special. A smile and brief explanation of the procedure, with extra attention when delays occur, goes a long way in making everyone feel more relaxed and confident.

Methods of Effective Communication

Attention to the various forms of interaction and communication techniques that have proved effective in improving relationships with patients can produce dramatic results in clinical situations.

VERBAL SKILLS

The methods of **verbal communication** that are used in establishing an open relationship between the health professional and the patient are basic to the quality of the interaction. Vocabulary, clarity of voice, and even the organization of sentences must be at an appropriate level for the patient. For example, discussing units of radiation dose with a Protestant minister is probably not of interest to him or her. Conversely, telling a physics teacher that a chest x-ray dose is similar to a few minutes of sun-tanning is equally inappropriate.

Humor

The value of humor in medical settings is well documented. It is acceptable to use humor to relax and open up conversation, but the radiologic technologist must be extremely careful to avoid cultural slurs and references to age, sex, diseases, and the abilities of health professionals. The fact that many patients use self-depreciating humor about their disabilities or fears as an emotional release must not be construed as permission for the radiographer to joke in a like manner.

NONVERBAL COMMUNICATION

Paralanguage

Paralanguage is the music of language. It produces a sort of **nonverbal communication.**

Patients receive signals about your attitude toward them from the pitch, stress, tone, pauses, speech rate, volume, accent, and quality of your voice. For example, because the mind works faster than the voice, it is common to think of a response when someone who is talking pauses. This knowledge can be used to structure more productive questions. For example, asking a patient, "Exactly where does it hurt most?" may not produce as much information as saying, "You said it hurts a lot around your stomach. Now exactly where would you say the pain is usually greatest?" The second statement gives the patient time to recall what they said and to think more specifically about it before being asked to answer.

Body Language

Patients quickly perceive nonverbal communication such as tone of voice, speed of speech, and the position of the speaker's extremities and torso (body language). Radiographers must be cautious not to give confusing signals to patients by saying one thing and acting in a totally different manner. For example, asking a patient if he or she is comfortable but neglecting to offer a positioning sponge to hold an oblique position may call into question the sincerity, and consequently the trust, of the technologist. Positive nonverbal cues increase the quantity and quality of communication and improve the history. For example, the technologist should look at patients and show interest in their statements. Smiling, responding candidly, and using a friendly tone of voice all work toward this end. Negative nonverbal cues can also be used to improve the history. For example, looking puzzled may prompt the patient to elaborate on exactly how an injury occurred and may provide the radiologist with details on the direction of the force that caused a fracture.

Touch

Three types of touch are commonly used by the radiographer: touching for emotional support, touching for emphasis, and touching for palpation. Few things are more reassuring than a gentle pat on the hand or shoulder as a form of emotional support (Fig. 9–4). Humans respond extremely well to touch, and it is acceptable to use this technique as long as proper social conventions are followed. The use of touch conveys to patients that the technologist

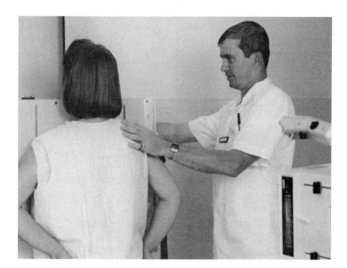

FIGURE 9–4. A gentle touch at the shoulder can be reassuring without being offensive.

is trying to understand, be empathetic, and care about them as people.

Touching for emphasis involves using touch to highlight or to specify instructions or locations. For example, after a posteroanterior chest radiograph has been performed, patients can be instructed to turn their left side toward a chest unit by a gentle touch at the posterior left shoulder accompanied by a similar touch at the anterior right shoulder (Fig. 9–5). For example, after a patient states, "My stomach hurts here," and places a hand on the upper abdomen, the radiographer can elicit further information by asking, "Does it hurt more here or here?" while touching the duodenal and gastric regions.

Palpation is the application of light pressure with the fingers to the body. It is often advisable to palpate to locate various bony landmarks when positioning patients. In a similar fashion it is often useful to use specific palpation to determine a more exact localization during history taking. Effective and precise palpation requires the *gentle* use of fingertips (Fig. 9–6). The use of the palm or several fingers is less precise and in some instances may be painful or even offensive to patients. For example, a 14-year-old girl is usually more comfortable if a male radiographer palpates for the iliac crest with the tip of a finger than if the entire hand is used to feel the hip region.

Professional Appearance

Most programs in radiologic technology have a dress code for students. Although dressing according to a code does not produce a better radiologic technologist, a professional appearance in the medical setting says as much about a person as their technical abilities say about their competence. Professional dress helps the patient feel comfortable and confident in the technologist's abilities. Gaining the patient's confidence and trust is a considerable part of being a competent radiologic technologist.

Physical Presence

Appearance and physical presence go together. Posture is important because it is per-

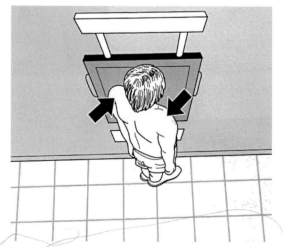

FIGURE 9–5. Touching for emphasis to help a patient turn the left side toward a chest unit. A gentle touch at the posterior left shoulder accompanied by a similar touch at the anterior right shoulder accomplishes the movement quickly and efficiently.

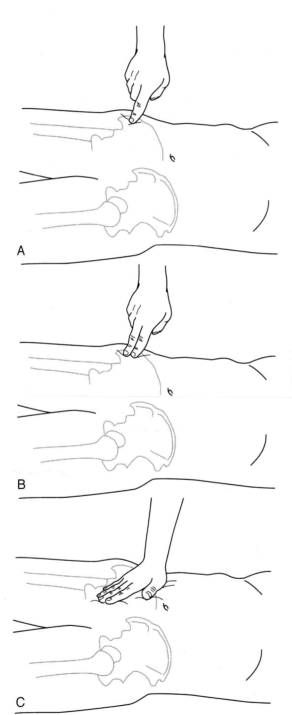

FIGURE 9–6. Proper palpation is accomplished by using fingertips to provide precise and gentle localization information. *A*, Proper use of a single fingertip. *B*, Proper use of several finger. *C*, improper use of the palm.

ceived as relating to confidence and self-esteem. Facial expressions are vital nonverbal cues that give people information on the importance of instructions and questions as well as both positive and negative reinforcement of their actions and statements. For example, confusion and frustration are easily communicated in this manner.

Visual Contact

Eye contact may help ensure that questions, instructions, and other information have been understood. Visual inspection of a patient's condition can be critical when changes such as blood pressure and allergic reactions produce symptoms.

Understanding the Various Types of Patients

Patients in radiology often have unusual conditions in addition to the conditions for which they are undergoing examination. An understanding of the most common special conditions can be valuable in meeting their needs.

SERIOUSLY ILL AND TRAUMATIZED PATIENTS

Not all patients with whom the technologist comes into contact want to talk or are able to cooperate during their examination. A seriously ill or traumatized patient may act differently because of pain, stress, or anxiety. In these instances, it is especially important that the patient hears and understands instructions if at all possible.

First, the technologist should try to communicate with the patient while determining his or her coherence level. This initial communication can provide cues regarding the state of consciousness and coherency of the patient. Some patients may be unable to respond, others may make incoherent statements, and still others may respond coherently but uncooperatively. Inability or unwillingness to communicate can be caused by many factors, including pain, shock, medication, and disorientation.

It is important to work quickly and efficiently while continuing to communicate with the patient even though there is no response. Letting the patient know what is going on during an examination can be reassuring, even when there is no apparent sign of understanding.

Because seriously ill and traumatized patients may not be able to communicate effectively, it becomes especially important to watch for visual indications of changes in vital signs. When patients cannot tell anyone that they are having difficulty breathing, they must rely completely on the technologist to recognize potential problems promptly. Helping someone is a great feeling, but when a seriously ill or injured patient must rely on you, the added responsibility can greatly enhance these feelings.

As a radiologic technologist, you will interact with patients exhibiting a wide variety of impairments. Combining your common sense, empathy, and classroom knowledge will enable you to provide quality radiographs for patients that would otherwise receive suboptimal examinations. Remember that the patient's cooperation is one of the main factors essential to producing quality radiographs.

VISUALLY IMPAIRED PATIENTS

A blind patient, a patient that has decreased vision without glasses, or an optically injured patient needs special attention. The technologist should attempt to gain the patient's confidence as soon as possible by giving clear instructions before the examination, as well as informing him or her at all times of what is occurring. Reassuring the patient through a gentle touch establishes that someone is near if needed.

SPEECH- AND HEARING-IMPAIRED PATIENTS

Patients who are deaf or have impaired hearing also require special attention. For those who can read, the primary means of communication can be writing. The technologist must not insult the patient's intelligence by attempting to simplify terminology. Hearing does not control intelligence.

Pantomime and demonstration work well with hearing-impaired patients. For example, counting to three on your fingers, pinching your nose, and taking a deep breath symbolizes to the patient that you need him or her to hold the breath while you count to three. Patients should return-demonstrate instructions to make sure they understand.

NON–ENGLISH-SPEAKING PATIENTS

Imagine the frustration you would feel if you were in a foreign country where no one understood English. Effective interaction with non–English-speaking patients is greatly enhanced by the use of touch, facial expressions, and pantomime. Nearly all such patients understand basic words such as "yes," "no," and "stop." Everyone appreciates any attempt to speak their language, even if only to say "yes" and "no." Pronunciation and accents are quickly overlooked when good intentions are shown. Most hospitals maintain a list of bilingual employees who are available to help patients and visitors.

MENTALLY IMPAIRED PATIENTS

Working with mentally impaired patients requires a through knowledge of equipment and immobilization techniques as well as interaction skills. Although degrees of mental impairment vary, it is important to use a strong yet reassuring tone of voice with these patients. A continuous conversation while preparing the patient for the examination usually helps to keep the patient calm and aware that the technologist is working with him or her.

SUBSTANCE ABUSERS

Radiologic technologists who work weekends, holidays, and evenings are often involved with patients who are under the influence of drugs or alcohol. These patients may not be totally aware of what they are doing and may need to be restrained from leaving the room, playing with high voltage cables, and so forth.

The best mode of interaction with these patients often includes assessing their capabilities, attempting to establish a means of communication, using technical knowledge, and working efficiently to decrease the total examination time.

Patients who are under the influence of drugs or alcohol may be very relaxed, or they may be hyperactive and irrational. It is important to observe them closely and use immobilization techniques as necessary. If patients are hyperactive and loud, it is obvious that they require close supervision. It is calm and quiet patients who are of greater concern because they may react without warning and fall or otherwise injure themselves.

Some substance abusers respond well to firm directions about what to do, whereas others are best handled by requesting that they return for examination at a later time when the effects have diminished considerably. There will always be patients who simply cannot be examined properly without assistance from other medical personnel. It is often best to wait until the patient becomes more cooperative. Seriously injured patients are seldom uncooperative, especially when they believe their life may be in jeopardy.

Mobile And Surgical Examinations

Many patients who require mobile examination are too sick or injured to be transported to the radiology department for examination. Patients may be comatose and attached to an array of tubes, monitoring lines, ventilators, and other medical equipment. Except in surgery, where the patient is normally incapable of interacting because of anesthesia, it is important to attempt to establish a line of communication with the patient. Begin by calling the patient's name, identifying yourself to the patient, and explaining the procedure. This permits assessment of the patient's condition and level of coherence.

Under no circumstances is it safe to assume that a patient does not comprehend comments that are made within his or her range of hearing. Patients may be cognizant although they appear to be comatose. Several studies have reported instances in which patients in deep anesthesia or even long-term comatose states were able to recall jokes and derogatory comments that were made about them. Both cognizant and incoherent patients are more cooperative if they hear a kind voice of explanation before being touched. Even if the words are not understood, a caring tone of voice and a gentle touch often have a positive effect.

In interacting with the patient's family and friends it is appropriate to introduce yourself, explain the procedure briefly, and explain why they must leave the immediate area during the exposure. There is usually no need to send visitors far, and explaining that the exposure is only a fraction of a second often encourages them to wait nearby while you remove your equipment. Remember that visitors sometimes arrive from distant places at considerable expense and that every moment may be precious with a dying parent or favorite aunt. Visitors appreciate your courtesy and thoughtfulness in taking time with them.

Age as a Factor in Patient Interactions

Age differences between the radiologic technologist and the patient should not be a barrier to effective communication. Nearly everyone has family members and friends of different ages, from grandparents to infants, and interactions with patients should be similar.

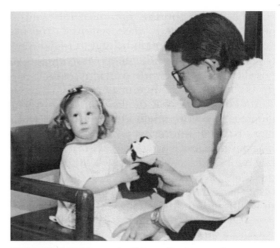

FIGURE 9–7. To stand tall in pediatrics, you have to get down on your knees. Entering the child's environment by squatting to the child's eye level can begin a rewarding relationship.

PEDIATRIC PATIENTS

Pediatric patients always require special attention. The proper method for dealing with young children is summarized by the famous statement of Dr. Armand Brodeur, long-time Chief Radiologist at Cardinal Glennon Children's Hospital in St. Louis: "To stand tall in pediatrics, you have to get down on your knees." In other words, simply getting down to the child's level—physically, in language, and in spirit—establishes a positive relationship. For example, instead of picking a child up and setting him or her on an x-ray table (which is the technologist's environment), it is better to squat at the child's eye level (which is the child's environment) to begin the relationship (Fig. 9–7). The pediatric patient can provide valuable clinical information. For example, a 5-year-old girl may reveal that she has been battered before an examination if she is alone with a friendly and nonthreatening technologist who she believes she can trust.

Children are special patients capable of presenting a challenge to the radiologic technologist's interpersonal skills. A technologist who can effectively and competently perform radiography on the pediatric patient is probably capable of handling any radiographic procedure on any type of patient. Patience, technical knowledge, understanding of the pediatric patient, and the effective use of communication skills

and immobilization devices can assist in obtaining a quality image.

Many hospitals provide soft toys such as stuffed animals for children, and it is a good idea to stock these items in the radiology department. Never try to separate a child from a security object such as a blanket or toy unless absolutely necessary for image quality. Even then, it is important that the object remains within the child's sight and that he or she is assured it will be returned momentarily. If the parents accompany the child, try to sit with the parents in the waiting room while you hold the child and explain the procedure to the parents. This additional time, 2 or 3 minutes, provides the child the opportunity to become familiar with you, your uniform, and the department. Always remember that children must *never* be left alone, even if properly immobilized.

Infants (Birth to 1 Year)

The first communications are through facial expressions, body movements and other nonverbal behaviors, and vocalizations. Very young infants like to be held in a familiar position (observe how the parents are holding the baby or ask what the favorite position is—at the shoulder, lying on the right side, and so forth). In addition, most small infants respond well to being held close with a tight blanket. A steady soothing voice, male or female, also often helps (simply repeating "It's all right; that's okay" usually works).

At about 8 months of age, most infants express definite anxiety when removed from a familiar person. It is often helpful to permit the parents to assist with the entire examination if possible. If separation is necessary, it should be for the minimum amount of time.

At about 12 months of age, children are beginning to develop memories, ideas, and feelings. A child with previous experiences with hospital personnel may rebel at the sight of a laboratory coat or surgical scrub suit. It is amazing how much strength a 1-year-old is capable of mustering when a vivid memory of an injection is triggered.

Toddlers (1 to 3 Years)

Although toddlers may understand simple abstractions, their thinking is basically related to tangible events. They usually cannot take the viewpoint of another (this is why, "See, it doesn't hurt Mommy," is seldom effective), and they cannot understand more than one word for something (it is important to ask a parent what word the child uses for urination, if it will be necessary to ask the child to urinate). Their concept of time is essentially now, and distance is whatever can be seen. Therefore, it is important to speak with simple words that are familiar to children and not to expect them to think about how they will feel in an hour. They are often concerned only with what you are going to do to them right now.

Preschoolers (3 to 5 Years)

Preschool children are not yet able to reason logically or understand cause and effect. Telling a 4-year-old boy that he needs an examination to see if he is sick is meaningless. However, if his arm hurts, he will long remember that he broke it when he fell. Because preschoolers are still very much involved with self-image, this is the age at which children may form an opinion that they are sick because they were bad. They may perceive relationships such as "big," "little," or "first" but cannot understand "next in line." They must see or hear something to understand and must be actively involved to maintain their short attention span. They will not hold still for long, although they can be remarkably cooperative if their trust has been won.

Schoolchildren (6 to 10 Years)

At about age 7, children begin to think logically and to analyze situations. At this point,

children can reflect and develop deeper understandings. With these advancements, children often develop a special fear of bodily injury, disease, separation from loved ones, death, and punishment. Remember that many diagnostic procedures seem like punishment to children, and special attention is warranted to divert their attention from the negative aspects of various examinations. This can often be accomplished by using their capacity for depth of understanding. For example, it is appropriate to help a child rationalize how an intravenous pyelogram helps the doctor find out why it hurts to urinate as a method of diverting attention from the pain of the venipuncture.

Adolescents (10 to 25 Years)

Adolescence is not a well-defined age group, although it begins earlier for girls than boys. The primary consideration in early adolescence focuses on body awareness, and modesty becomes especially important. Persons in this age group usually require special consideration to avoid embarrassment when changing clothes and during examinations. It is appropriate to ask unnecessary personnel to leave a room during these examinations. Same-sex peer groups have a dominant role at this age, and conversation that focuses on friends of the same sex often eases tensions during procedures.

Middle adolescents often are bridging the gap between peer group influence and early sexual relationships. Persons in this age group are often developing their first real independence and often appreciate being treated like adults in conversation, preferences, and consultation about procedures.

Late adolescents are often focusing on mature relationships with both sexes and may be financially independent. They easily relate to adult conversation and should essentially be treated as adults, although their experiences may be limited in some areas.

YOUNG ADULTS (25 TO 45 YEARS)

Young adults are usually entering new roles of responsibility at home and in their work. They often experience problems in handling their multitude of new roles and may neglect one area while they concentrate on another. For example, focusing on child rearing at home may result in neglect of work duties. Conversation and interaction should be on the same level as for other adults.

MIDDLE-AGED PERSONS (45 TO 65 YEARS)

In middle age, most people have found their place in life and tend to be relatively comfortable with their roles and success (or lack of it). When poor health or a threat of poor health occurs, considerable stress and special concern over how to maintain responsibilities, such as keeping a job and providing for a family, may outweigh personal health concerns.

MATURE PERSONS (65 YEARS AND OLDER)

Research shows that most persons 65 years and older do not consider themselves old. They tend to consider themselves middle-aged. Because of this, it is important not to attempt to interact with them as with geriatric patients. Senility is not a natural part of aging, and only 10% of people in this age group demonstrate memory loss. They should be treated as middle-aged persons, with conversation centering on life activities. A much-reprinted saying, "I may be old and wrinkled on the outside but I'm young and vulnerable on the inside," is well worth considering when phrasing statements to this age group.

GERONTOLOGY

Gerontology (geriatrics) is the study of aging and diseases of the elderly. Studies show that the geriatric group will continue to increase in size and importance in American society for many years yet, primarily as a result of improvements in living standards, dietary practices, physical fitness, and medical care. By the mid 1990s there were more than 33 million Americans over 65 years of age, over 12% of the total population, as compared with only 4% in 1900. In addition, the elderly population itself is aging. Between 1960 and 1994, the US population grew by 45% while the over-65 population grew by 100% and the over-85 population grew by almost 275%, to a total of 3 million persons. This has caused significant concern as young workers begin to realize that current retirement

and medical care systems rely on active workers to fund care of the elderly. There is real concern that worldwide economies may not grow sufficiently to fund this increasing burden. As a result, there is now pressure on the medical system to find ways to decrease costs while increasing the efficiency of care for the elderly.

It is inappropriate to refer to all older patients as geriatric. American culture tends to be orientated toward youth, productivity, and a rapid pace. This results in feelings of alienation, which can be made worse by lack of respect. One author points out that although everybody wants to live a long life, hardly anybody wants to be old because the word connotes frailty, narrow-mindedness, incompetence, and loss of attractiveness. Furthermore, the use of words like "senior citizens" or "golden-agers" constitutes prejudice and discrimination and are to be avoided. To minimize these feelings, it is important to treat geriatric patients as mature adults, with all the normal interaction that would be used with healthier or younger patients (Fig. 9–8). Remember not to talk loudly or use childish terms with geriatric patients. At the same time it is also important to accommodate the elderly by the use of gentle handling

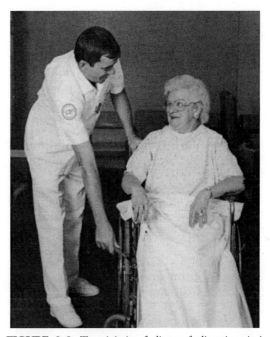

FIGURE 9–8. To minimize feelings of alienation, it is helpful to treat geriatric patients as mature adults, with all the normal interaction that would be used with healthier or younger patients.

and extra time for movements and verbal responses. This is identical to adjustments that must be made for other types of patients, such as a partially paralyzed patient.

Geriatric patients are now being classified as young-old, old-old, and oldest-old in an attempt to differentiate between widely varying conditions that accompany the aging process. Although these can be chronologic classifications, it is more appropriate to classify by functional age. Both classifications are given in Table 9–1. The aging process itself is now divided into primary aging and secondary aging. Primary aging is the gradual and inevitable process of deterioration that begins in childhood and extends through old age. Secondary aging consists of disease, abuse, and disuse, which are often within control of the individual. Some of the changes that occur that are especially important when patients are undergoing radiologic examinations are given in Table 9–2. The cardinal rules when dealing with geriatric patients are patience and respect.

Interacting With the Terminally Ill Patient

It is generally agreed that the primary care of the dying patient falls on the nurse. However, this does not release the radiologic technologist from an obligation to understand the basics of current practices toward terminally ill patients. Because few new radiologic technologists have had experiences with this type of patient, it is important to be prepared personally as well.

Unexpected death is much more complicated but is guided by a principle of trying to meet as many of the patient's requests as possible. Many radiologic technologists eventually experience patient death during radiologic examinations, often as a result of anaphylactic shock. It is always better to call a false emergency code than to wait too long to save a patient. With this guideline followed, it may still become necessary to obtain assistance in working through the personal aspects of having a patient die.

When death is expected because of age or disease, studies show that for most people the crisis is not death, but where and how it will occur. For example, older patients who have adjusted to living at home often are anxious if they are removed from their home before death. However, geriatric patients who have adjusted to living in an institution are much more willing to accept death in the same setting.

Patients who are kept in *closed awareness* are not told of their condition. Many of these patients deduce that they are terminally ill but lack assistance in working through the various stages of acceptance. Even heavily sedated patients may know more than the health care team suspects. Some patients develop *suspicious awareness* in that they watch for clues to their condition but attempt to keep the health care team from knowing exactly how much they understand. A state of *mutual pretense* exists when patient, staff, and family all know but are pretending not to know in hopes of avoiding interpersonal conflicts. A condition of *open awareness* is usually considered to be desirable because it permits everyone to work through the various stages that precede dying.

The stages delineated by Elisabeth Kübler-Ross have been generally regarded as an acceptable sequence of events. *Denial and isolation* may be the initial reactions and should be supported by silence and acceptance of the person without discussing death. *Anger* may occur as a result of the realization that life will be interrupted before everything the person planned has been accomplished, feelings that the person will soon be forgotten, and so forth. Anger is often expressed in terms of complaints about health care, and this may include radiologic services. These complaints should be addressed and special care taken to avoid situations, such as long waits without attention, that will increase the patient's anger.

Some patients experience a *bargaining* stage that focuses on hope and may be based in religion, for example, prayers for small extensions of life to perform good deeds and heal family wounds. It is important to support the patient's beliefs at this time because the hope itself can reduce stress. This stage may be followed by *depression*, which often occurs when remission ends and additional treatments must begin. This is a normal reaction and should be encouraged by giving realistic praise while letting the patient express his or her feelings.

TABLE 9–1. Gerontologic Aging Categories		
	Chronologic	**Functional**
Young-Old	65–74 years	Healthy & active
Old-Old	75–84 years	Transitional
Oldest-Old	85 years and older	Frail & infirm

TABLE 9–2. Physical Changes of Functional Aging

Body System	Physical Change	Considerations for Radiologic Examinations
Nervous	Slowing of psychomotor responses	Give patient time to move.
	Slowing of information processing	Give patient time to think before expecting a response.
	Decreased visual ability	Stand directly in front of patient, hold items to be seen or read at an appropriate distance without moving for a short time and provide extra time for visual adjustments after dramatic changes in light levels.
	Decreased hearing ability	Speak directly to the patient's ear, move closer, or (as a last resort) talk louder.
Respiratory	Decreased cough reflex	Avoid aspiration by giving patient time to swallow when drinking.
Musculoskeletal	Osteoporotic loss of bone mass	Increase sensitivity to patient paranoia about potential falls with potential for permanent loss of mobility.
	Arthritis	Expect decreased joint flexibility.
	Decreased muscle strength	Prepare to provide assistance in moving if needed.
	Atrophied muscle mass	Expect decreased tolerance of positioning requirements and discomfort in placement on hard tabletops.
Cardiovascular	Decreased cardiac efficiency	Avoid orthostatic hypotension by allowing time for blood pressure adjustment when moving a patient from supine to sitting or from sitting to erect position.
	Arteriosclerosis	Avoid chilling discomfort by providing extra blankets and sheets.
Integumentary	Loss of texture and elasticity	Avoid skin lacerations (especially to the backs of hands) by not abrading skin with draw sheets during patient transfers or applying tape to sensitive areas.
Gastrointestinal	Decreased secretions	Expect difficulty when requiring a patient to drink quickly or from a recumbent position.
	Decreased gastrointestinal motility	Expect delays during completion of small bowel studies. (Prepare for long-term patient comfort via extra blankets, pillow under knees, communication of reasons for delays, etc.)
	Decreased sphincter muscle tone	Prepare for potential loss of barium from rectum during lower gastrointestinal examinations. Expect more frequent requests for time or assistance with moving.

Preparatory depression comes with the realization of the inevitability of death and is accompanied by a desire for death as a release from suffering. The most important thing at this time is to permit the behavior. Attempting to cheer the patient may meet the needs of the health care provider but not of the patient. Touch and silence are often construed as acceptance and are appropriate at this time. *Acceptance*, which is considered the final stage, can occur only if enough time is provided and if the patient is helped through the other stages appropriately.

It is characterized by a near-total lack of feelings.

The radiologic technologist also needs to be sure that personal feelings do not override patient concerns when caring for the terminally ill. Most hospitals can offer assistance in dealing with personal feelings about caring for terminally ill patients through their nursing departments. Students should consult with their program directors about assistance or appropriate courses. It is also important not to become hardened in dealing with dying and severely injured patients but to learn to handle feelings appropriately during interactions with the patient, relatives, and friends.

Summary

The importance of interacting effectively with the patient is critical to the radiologic technologist as well as to the patient. Maslow's hierarchy of needs provides insight into the behavior of professionals and patients alike. Maslow's hierarchy proceeds in five levels of needs: physiologic, safety and security, love and belonging, self-esteem and respect, and self-actualization. Great power is held by the technologist, including the most basic elements of a person's dignity and self-respect. Special attention is needed to ensure that the power is not abused.

The inpatient is someone who has been admitted to the hospital for diagnostic studies or treatment. Previous experiences in the hospital may have shaped the manner in which such a patient responds. Outpatients arrive in the radiology department with prior expectations. They often expect to be seen immediately on arriving in the department because they have a scheduled appointment. It is appropriate and important to apologize for delays and to try to keep waiting patients up to date on their status. Family and friends of patients who are visiting must also receive attention.

Attention to the various forms of interaction and communication techniques that have proved effective in improving relationships with patients can produce dramatic results in clinical situations. These include verbal skills (including humor) and nonverbal communications, such as paralanguage, body language, and touch. Touching can be used for emotional support, emphasis, and palpation. Professional appearance, physical presence, and visual contact are also important.

Special consideration and techniques are necessary when dealing with seriously ill and traumatized patients as well as impaired patients. Patients with vision, speech, hearing, and mental impairments; inability to speak English; and substance abuse require extra care. Mobile and surgical examinations also have special techniques for effective communication.

Age is also a special factor in patient interactions. A knowledge of growth and development differences for infants, toddlers, preschoolers, schoolchildren, adolescents, young adults, middle-aged persons, mature persons, and geriatric persons can be useful in clinical practice. The cardinal rules when dealing with geriatric patients are patience and respect.

When death is expected because of age or disease, studies show that for most people the crisis is not death, but where and how it will occur. It is helpful for the radiologic technologist to understand the various stages that many terminally ill patients undergo once they have reached a condition of open awareness about their disease. The Kübler-Ross sequence includes denial and isolation, anger, bargaining, depression, preparatory depression, and acceptance. It is important for the radiologic technologist to personally prepare for dealing with the death of a patient.

◄ R ► R E V I E W Q U E S T I O N S

1 The highest level of Maslow's hierarchy of needs is:
   a) self-actualization
   b) belonging
   c) physiologic
   d) self-esteem

2 The word ambulatory means that the patient:
   a) must be confined to a wheelchair
   b) must be moved by ambulance
   c) can be moved by stretcher
   d) can walk

3 Which of the following would you not want to talk about with a patient?
   a) hobbies
   b) medical chart
   c) ability to walk
   d) weather

4 Questions about the diagnosis of an examination from a patient or visitor are best answered by:
   a) explaining that only a radiologist can read radiographs
   b) providing the best diagnosis available
   c) explaining that the results are not available yet
   d) suggesting that the question is inappropriate

5 Which method is effective in communicating with a patient?
   1. professional appearance
   2. touch

3. pantomime techniques
a) 1 only
b) 1 and 2 only
c) 2 and 3 only
d) 1, 2, and 3

6 When is touching a patient valuable?
a) for emotional support
b) for emphasis
c) for palpation
d) all of the above

7 Which of the following characterize the development of a toddler (1 to 3 years old)?
a) understanding of simple abstractions
b) inability to understand more than one word for something
c) inability to take the viewpoint of another
d) all of the above

8 Of the changes that occur in geriatric patients that are especially important when patients are undergoing radiologic examinations, which of the following may produce patient paranoia about potential falls with potential for permanent loss of mobility?
a) osteoporotic loss of bone mass
b) arthritis
c) decreased muscle strength
d) atrophied muscle mass

9 Which of the following is considered to be the first stage of acceptance of dying for a terminally ill patient?
a) anger
b) frustration
c) denial and isolation
d) shock

10 Which of the following permits the patient to begin to work through the various stages that precede dying?
a) suspicious awareness
b) mutual pretense
c) open awareness
d) all of the above

BIBLIOGRAPHY

Adler R, Towne N: Looking Out/Looking In: Interpersonal Communication. San Francisco, Rinehart Press, 1975.

Freiberg K: Human Development: A Life-Span Approach. 4th ed. Boston, Jones & Bartlett, 1992.

Glaser B, Strauss A: Awareness of Dying. Chicago, Aldine Publishing, 1965.

Gurley LT, Callaway WJ: Introduction to Radiologic Technology. 4th ed. St. Louis, CV Mosby, 1996.

Kübler-Ross E (ed): Death, The Final Stage of Growth. Englewood Cliffs, NJ, Prentice-Hall, 1975.

Maddox J: The Encyclopedia of Aging. New York, Springer, 1987.

Maslow A: Motivation and Personality. 2nd ed. New York, Harper & Row, 1987.

Murray RB, Zentner JP: Nursing Assessment and Health Promotion Strategies Through the Life Span. 4th ed. Englewood Cliffs, NJ, Appleton & Lange, 1989.

Neugarten B, Neugarten DA: The changing meanings of age. Psychology Today 21(5):29, 1987.

Papalia D, Olds SW: Human Development. 6th ed. New York, McGraw-Hill, 1995.

Purtilo R: Health Professional/Patient Interaction. 5th ed. Philadelphia, WB Saunders, 1996.

Torres LS: Basic Medical Techniques and Patient Care for Radiologic Technologists. 5th ed. Philadelphia, JB Lippincott, 1997.

US Bureau of the Census: Growth of America's Oldest-Old Population (Profiles of America's Elderly No. 2). Washington, DC, US Government Printing Office, 1992.

US Bureau of the Census: Sixty-five Plus in America (Current Population Reports, Special Studies, Series P23-178). Washington, DC, US Government Printing Office, 1992.

CHAPTER 10

HISTORY TAKING

Richard R. Carlton, MS, RT(R)(CV), FAERS
Arlene M. Adler, MEd, RT(R), FAERS

When you talk with the patient, you should listen, first for what he wants to tell, secondly for what he does not want to tell, thirdly for what he cannot tell.

L.J. HENDERSON
PHYSICIAN AND PATIENT AS SOCIAL SYSTEMS

The Patient Interview
The Role of the Radiologic
    Technologist
Desirable Qualities of the Interviewer
Data Collection Process
Questioning Skills

**Elements of the Clinical
    History**
Determining the Chief Complaint

The Sacred Seven
    Localization
    Chronology
    Quality
    Severity
    Onset
    Aggravating or Alleviating Factors
    Associated Manifestations

Summary

OBJECTIVES

On completion of this chapter, the student will be able to:

1 Describe the role of the radiologic technologist in taking patient clinical histories.
2 Describe the desirable qualities of a good patient interviewer.
3 Differentiate objective from subjective data.
4 Explain the value of each of the six categories of questions useful in obtaining patient histories.
5 Describe the importance of clarifying the chief complaint.
6 Detail the important elements of each of the Sacred Seven elements of the clinical history.

GLOSSARY

Chief Complaint: primary medical problem as defined by the patient; it is important because it focuses the clinical history toward the single most important issue
Chronology: time element of the history, usu-
ally including the onset, duration, frequency, and course of the symptoms
Clinical History: information available regarding a patient's condition; it is traditionally composed of data on localization, quality, quantity, chronology, setting, aggravating or alleviating factors, and associated manifestations

Leading Question: undesirable method of questioning that provides information that may direct the answer toward a suspected symptom or complaint

Localization: determination of a precise area, usually through gentle palpation or careful wording of questions

Objective: perceptible to the external senses

Quality: description of the character of the symptoms; for example, the color, quantity, and consistency of blood or other body substances; the size or number of lumps or lesions; the frequency of urination or coughing; or the character of pain

Subjective: pertaining to or perceived only by the affected individual; not perceptible to the senses

The Patient Interview

The clinical history describes the information available regarding a patient's condition. To extract as much information as possible during a clinical history, it is important that the event be viewed as an interview with the patient. Because it is often the radiologic technologist's job to obtain the **clinical history,** it is important to learn methods of accomplishing valid patient interviews.

THE ROLE OF THE RADIOLOGIC TECHNOLOGIST

Radiologists usually do not have the opportunity to obtain a clinical history from the patient. Although more complex procedures such as angiography and radiation therapy permit extensive history taking by the radiologist or radiation oncologist, most patients for diagnostic radiography are never examined or interviewed by the radiologist. Because it is one of the most critical and valuable diagnostic tools, good history-taking skills are an essential responsibility of the radiologic technologist.

Few radiologic technologists are aware of the importance of this role as a clinical historian. Unquestionably, it is one of the most valuable opportunities to acquire clinical information that can contribute to the diagnostic process. A radiologist can be instructed to give special attention to the exact anatomic area where pain is focused. For example, stating that a patient has pain in the right hand is less focused than stating the pain is over the anterior aspect of the distal portion of the second metacarpal.

In addition, there is an important role to be played in interacting with the patient. A unique opportunity to actually become part of the healing process presents itself with each new patient. Eric Cassell, a physician noted for his teaching of the art of practicing medicine, relates feeling powerless to help a patient with severe pulmonary edema late one night. While waiting for equipment to arrive, he began to talk calmly, explaining how the water would begin to ease bit by bit until, much to his amazement, that is precisely what happened. By reducing the patient's fear, he had reduced the hypertension and actually eased the pathologic process. Cassell refers to this as the art of healing, and it is directly related to the role of the radiologic technologist when taking a history. Genuine interest in what the patient has to say, attentiveness, and an aura of professional competence can provide patients with a very real sense of caring.

DESIRABLE QUALITIES OF THE INTERVIEWER

Taking a history must be a cooperative event between the patient and the radiologic technologist. Because patients wish to have a medical problem resolved, most want to help with the history. However, sick people may be combative as a symptom of their frustration. In these instances, it often helps to acknowledge the patient's anger as a method of overcoming it. For example, a patient who complains about having already given a history to someone and who then rants about incompetent health professionals will often become an ally if the technologist agrees with the inconvenience and suggests that because the radiologist needs specialized information, the interviewer will be as short as possible and can be taken while getting ready for the x-ray examination.

Carl Rogers identified several qualities that appear to be important in establishing an open dialogue. These include respect, genuineness, and empathy. When patients perceive any of these qualities to be missing, the interview may become more difficult as the good faith between the two persons decreases. Patients need to feel that the information they are providing is important. When they lack these feelings because of intimidation or lack of respect, they may withhold information as unimportant or unworthy of being mentioned. Because physicians are often perceived as busy authority figures by many patients, radiologic technologists can serve a useful role in that they are usually seen as less threatening and easier to talk with than physicians.

The radiologic technologist should maintain a polite and professional demeanor during the interview, especially when introducing himself or herself to the patient, verifying the patient's name (by using Mr. or Ms. instead of first names), and explaining that a history is needed.

Notes should be added to the paperwork (usually the examination request or requisition). Most patients perceive note taking as positive because the technologist is making it clear that the information being given is important enough to be recorded. Additionally, there is little point in acquiring the clinical history if it is not written on the paperwork that will be in front of the radiologist when the images are read.

DATA COLLECTION PROCESS

Good history taking involves the collection of accurate objective and subjective data. **Objective** data are perceptible to the senses, such as signs that can be seen, heard, or felt, and such things as laboratory reports. **Subjective** data pertain to or are perceived by the affected individual only. They include things that involve the patient's emotions and experiences, such as pain and its severity, and are not perceptible to the senses. *Objective data are not necessarily more important than subjective data.* In fact, much has been written on the therapeutic value of the interview itself. Many patients come to see the doctor with a personal agenda of finding a professional to listen to and empathize with a problem, which may or may not have physical manifestations. The technologist must realize that conversation with the patient has great value by itself in addition to the diagnostic information that may be obtained. The art of radiologic technology includes this aspect of patient interaction.

It is important to realize that an objective approach to the collection of subjective data is also necessary. For example, never disregard anything the patient says, *especially* if it does not fit with the opinion you are forming about the patient's symptoms. Disregarding some comments constitutes subjective collection of the data. The diagnostic process can be accelerated considerably by asking patients to define and clarify the words they use. For example, the word *pain* can often provide significant additional information if it can be localized and a chronology established.

QUESTIONING SKILLS

Adult patients are usually experienced in providing medical histories, especially if they have been hospitalized previously. The student can use this to advantage by simply letting the patients tell their stories. Listening instead of asking more questions often provides the necessary information. Better histories result when the following questioning techniques are used:

- Open-ended questions (nondirected, nonleading) let the patient tell the story.
- Facilitation (nod or say "yes," "okay," "go on," etc) encourages elaboration.
- Silence (to give the patient time to remember) facilitates accuracy and elaboration.
- Probing questions (to focus the interview) provide more detail.
- Repetition (rewording) clarifies information.
- Summarization (condensing) verifies accuracy.

All histories should begin with open-ended questions to encourage the patient's spontaneous associations about the clinical problem. For example, "What type of chest problem are you having?" These should be followed with increasingly focused and directed probing questions based on what the patient has already said. For example, "When you breathe deeply, exactly where does it hurt on the left side of your chest?" This technique permits the radiologic technologist to pick up where the patient stops telling the story and provides medically specific information that might not occur to the patient otherwise.

The use of *precise and clear wording* cannot be overemphasized. Words do not always mean the same thing to patients as they do to radiologic technologists. For example, many patients refer to the entire abdomen as the stomach. Therefore, it may be inaccurate to record gastric pain when a patient says the left side of the stomach hurts. If this information is verified by asking the patient to point to the area, it may be discovered that the complaint the patient is actually experiencing is left lower quadrant abdominal distress. The medical terms that are learned in radiologic technology are professional ones and will not be understood by all patients. On the other hand, some patients will understand medical terms, and they should not have their intelligence offended by the use of overly simplified words. For example, there is no need to tell a high school biology teacher that the esophagus is a tube leading to the stomach.

The ability to assess the patient's background can be a difficult skill to develop. Probably the most helpful technique is to begin with a question that provides an opportunity for the patient to respond in a manner that reflects his or her life experience and educational background. For example, when a patient responds to a question about the location of pain with a specific anatomic term, such as *epigastric*, it is a clear signal that medical terminology may be used. Conversely, a response using the word *belly* may indicate lack of knowledge about abdominal organs and should signal the use of simpler terms.

The use of **leading questions** should be avoided whenever possible because they introduce biases into the history. For example, "Does the pain travel down your leg?" may lead the patient to a description of sciatica. Asking, "Does the pain stay deep within your hip or does it move?" provides a more reliable indication.

It is useful to *repeat information* obtained as a part of the histoy for two reasons: to verify that it was perceived correctly by the radiologic technologist and to ensure that the patient has not changed his or her mind.

Elements of the Clinical History (Box 10–1)

DETERMINING THE CHIEF COMPLAINT

Physicians attempt to determine the patient's **chief complaint.** This is a valuable effort because it focuses the history toward the single most important issue. In many cases, the chief complaint is directly related to the first symptom that is discussed. However, there is a danger in becoming too focused on determining a single chief complaint. It is important to permit the patient to add more than a single complaint when it appears that multiple complaints are valid. Ignoring all symptoms except the most predominant can obscure other important clinical information.

THE SACRED SEVEN

The radiologic technologist typically does not need to compile a complete medical history on patients. The physician or the nursing staff who first saw the patient will have completed this job. The technologist's role is to collect a focused history specific to the procedure that is to be performed. Seven elements are recognized for a complete history. These are often referred to as the Sacred Seven. They are:

- Localization
- Chronology
- Quality
- Severity
- Onset
- Aggravating or alleviating factors
- Associated manifestations

Localization

Localization is defining as exact and precise an area as possible for the patient's complaint. It requires the use of carefully worded questions accompanied by proper touching of the patient. By consenting to the procedure, patients give implied consent for the technologist to touch their bodies for both information and for positioning. Remember that the patient can use verbal or nonverbal communication to withdraw this permission at any time. Two types of touch that are commonly used by the technologist in gathering a clinical history are touching for emphasis and touching for palpation.

Touching for emphasis involves using touch to highlight or to specify instructions or specify locations. A history can be clarified by a light touch to specify the region. For example, after a patient states, "My stomach hurts here," and places a hand on the upper abdomen, the radiologic technologist can add information by asking, "Does it hurt more here or here?" while touching the upper left side and then the upper middle region. *Palpation*, or applying the fingers with light pressure, can also be useful in history taking. For example, palpating the olecranon process of the elbow can assist the patient in the localization of pain within that region.

BOX 10-1

Sample Patient History Guide

REVIEW THE CHIEF COMPLAINT

Indications for this examination
    Localization
    Chronology
    Quality
    Severity
    Onset
    Aggravating or alleviating factors
    Associated manifestations
    Has there been any trauma?
    Has there been any previous surgery?

DEPENDING ON THE CHIEF COMPLAINT

Skeletal system
    Pain location
    Injury location
    Injury chronology
Central nervous system
    Pain
    Unconsciousness or lethargy
    Bleeding location
    Vision
    Vertigo
    Convulsions
Respiratory system
    Cough

Dyspnea
Hemoptysis
Infection
Pain location
Pain duration
Gastrointestinal and genitourinary systems
    Pain location
    Gastric
        Nausea
        Vomiting
    Bowel
        Constipation
        Diarrhea
        Stool description
        Date of last bowel movement
    Urinary
        Known allergies and contrast media
            reactions
        Blood pressure
        Hematuria
        Blood urea nitrates
        Creatinine
        Burning
        Frequency

Sometimes localization is not possible because of the nature of the problem. For example, a radiating pain may also be a deep pain that the patient cannot localize. When this occurs, the radiologist should be informed that the pain is not localized. This description tells the radiologist that attempts were made to confine the complaint to a specific region. The term *nonlocalized* then becomes valuable clinical information.

Chronology

The **chronology** is the time element of the history. The *duration* since onset, *frequency*, and *course* of the symptoms should be established. This information should be described in seconds, minutes, hours, days, weeks, or months. For example, the onset of a chest problem may have been several weeks prior to the examination, the duration of coughing may average 10 to 15 seconds, the frequency may be several times per hour, and the course may reveal that it is worse during the night and in the morning. Radiologists may derive important diagnostic clues from a good chronology. For example, a stress fracture may first be visualized 10 to 20 days after the onset of symptoms.

Students should avoid giving dates or days as a chronology. For example, reporting that an injury occurred last Thursday or on July 14th requires that the radiologist find a calendar to determine how much time elapsed between the trauma and the examination.

Quality

The **quality** describes the character of the symptoms. Examples include the color and consistency of body fluids, the presence of clots or sores, the size of lumps or lesions, the type of cough, and the character of pain.

When pain is involved, it must be described carefully. This description should include either the word *acute*, meaning having a sudden onset, or *chronic*, meaning having a prolonged course. It should also include more specific descriptors such as *burning*, *throbbing*, *dull*, *sharp*, *cutting*, *aching*, *prickling*, *radiating*, *pressure*, and *crushing*. Again, the patient's understanding of medical terms is important. For example, a patient may describe acute pain as *sharp* or *recent*. Gaining this additional information often requires the use of focused, probing questions, such as, "When did the pain begin?"

Severity

The severity of a condition describes the intensity, the quantity, or the extensiveness of the problem. Examples are the intensity of pain, the number of lesions or lumps, and the extent of a burn. A patient may say that there is a light burning sensation versus a very intense burning sensation.

Onset

Describing the onset of the complaint involves the patient's explaining what he or she was doing when the illness or condition began. A review of the onset can help to determine whether there were predictable events that preceded the recurrence of a symptom. For example, a patient might have had a series of mild headaches before a convulsion.

Aggravating or Alleviating Factors

The circumstances that produce the problem or intensify it should be well defined, including anything that aggravates, alleviates, or otherwise modifies it. For example, heartburn may occur only after a full meal or a stressful day on the job and may be aggravated by certain foods and alleviated by assuming a right anterior oblique position with the head elevated slightly.

Associated Manifestations

It may be necessary to determine whether there are other symptoms that accompany the chief complaint. This is necessary to determine whether all of the symptoms relate to the chief complaint or are related to a separate condition. For example, the patient may describe gastrointestinal symptoms as a part of, or separate from, a cardiac condition.

Summary

The radiologic technologist who sees himself or herself as a clinical historian realizes the value of this service. Understanding the fine art of accomplishing patient interviews can often assist in gaining better insight and information that can add significantly to the radiologist's ability to diagnose.

Good history taking involves the collection of accurate objective and subjective data. Objective data are perceptible to the senses. Subjective data pertain to or are perceived by the affected individual only.

Better histories result using such techniques as open-ended questions, facilitation, silence, probing questions, repetition, and summarization.

Physicians need to attempt to determine the patient's chief complaint. This is a valuable effort because it focuses the history toward the single most important issue. There are seven elements that are recognized for a complete history. These are often referred to as the Sacred Seven and are localization, chronology, quality, severity, onset, aggravating or alleviating factors, and associated manifestations.

◀R REVIEW QUESTIONS

1 Which of the following is undesirable for conducting a clinical history interview?
   a. clarifying terminology
   b. asking open-ended questions
   c. asking vague questions
   d. repeating information

2 Which of the following includes a description of the color, quantity, and consistency of blood or other body substances?
   a. localization
   b. chronology
   c. quality
   d. occurrence

3 Which of the following is the determination of a precise area, usually

through gentle palpation or careful wording of questions?
a. localization
b. chronology
c. quality
d. occurrence

4 Which of the following is/are usually included as part of the chronology of a clinical history?
a. onset
b. duration
c. frequency
d. all of the above

5 Which of the following includes the tone of voice, speed of speech, and the position of the speaker's extremities and torso?
a. nonverbal communication
b. palpation
c. quality
d. facilitation

6 What term describes the primary medical problem as defined by the patient?
a. chief complaint
b. palpation
c. onset
d. nonverbal communication

7 Which of the following describes an undesirable method of questioning that provides information that may direct the answer toward a suspected symptom or complaint?
a. facilitation
b. palpation
c. nonverbal communication
d. leading question

8 Which of the following is/are part of the Sacred Seven elements of the patient clinical history?
a. localization
b. aggravating factors
c. quality
d. all of the above

9 Which of the following is/are desirable methods of conducting a clinical history interview?

a. positive nonverbal communication
b. defining and specifying terms
c. subjectiveness
d. a and b

10 Which term describes gentle touching to determine the precise location of a symptom or complaint?
a. nonverbal communication
b. palpation
c. quality
d. facilitation

BIBLIOGRAPHY

Bates RC: The Fine Art of Understanding Patients. Oradell, NJ, Medical Economics Book Division, 1972.

Billings JA, Stoeckle J: The Clinical Encounter: A Guide to the Medical Interview and Case Presentation. Chicago, Year Book Medical Publishers, 1989.

Cassell E: Talking With Patients, Vol. 1: Theory of Doctor-Patient Communication. Cambridge, MA, MIT Press, 1985.

Cassell E: Talking With Patients, Vol. 2: Clinical Technique. Cambridge, MA, MIT Press, 1985.

Cassell E: The Healer's Art: A New Approach to the Doctor-Patient Relationship. Philadelphia, JB Lippincott, 1976.

Carlton R: Radiographers as clinical historians. RT Image 4(29):16–17, 1991.

Carlton R, Adler AM: Repeating radiographs: Setting imaging standards. Postgraduate Advances in Radiologic Technology. Berryville, VA, Forum Medicum, 1989.

Carnevali DL, Mitchell PH, Woods NF, Tanner CA: Diagnostic Reasoning in Nursing. Philadelphia, JB Lippincott, 1984.

Coulehan JL, Block MR: The Medical Interview: A Primer for Students of the Art. Philadelphia, FA Davis, 1987.

Enelow A, Swisher S: Interviewing and Patient Care. New York, Oxford University Press, 1972.

Engel G, Morgan W Jr: Interviewing the Patient. Philadelphia, WB Saunders, 1973.

Feinstein A: Clinical Judgment. Baltimore, Williams & Wilkins, 1967.

Hillman R, et al: Clinical Skills: Interviewing, History Taking, and Physical Diagnosis. New York, McGraw-Hill, 1981.

Levinson D: A Guide to the Clinical Interview. Philadelphia, WB Saunders, 1987.

Prior JA, Silberstein JS, Stang JM: Physical Diagnosis: The History and Examination of the Patient. St. Louis, CV Mosby, 1981.

Purtilo R: Health Professional and Patient Interaction. 4th ed. Philadelphia, WB Saunders, 1990.

CHAPTER 11

TRANSFER TECHNIQUES

Jan Bruckner, PhD, PT

At no time in the day is the patient in more peril than when being transferred from bed to wheelchair. More injuries of consequence occur to patients, and health care personnel serving them, during transfer than at any other time.

MARILYN RANTZ AND DONALD COURTAIL
LIFTING, MOVING, AND TRANSFERRING PATIENTS, 1977

Body Mechanics
Base of Support
Center of Gravity
White and Red Muscles

Principles of Lifting

Wheelchair Transfers
Standby Assist Transfer
Assisted Standing Pivot Transfer

Two-Person Lift
Hydraulic Lift Techniques

Cart Transfers

Positioning

Summary

OBJECTIVES

On completion of this chapter, the student will be able to:

1 Define the terms associated with body mechanics.
2 Describe the cause, signs, symptoms, and treatment of orthostatic hypotension.
3 Describe the basic principles of proper lifting and transfer techniques.
4 Describe four types of wheelchair-to-bed transfers.
5 Describe a standard cart transfer procedure.
6 Identify five standard patient positions.

GLOSSARY

Base of Support: foundation on which a body rests or stands; when a person is standing, the feet and the space between them define the base of support

Biomechanics: study of the laws of physics, specifically the laws of mechanics, as they apply to living bodies at rest and in motion

Center of Gravity: hypothetical point around which all mass appears to be concentrated

Mobility Muscles: muscles that are found in the four extremities and that are designed for movement; examples include biceps femoris, biceps brachii, and gastrocnemius

Orthostatic Hypotension: drop in blood pressure when a person stands up quickly from a sitting or supine position

Stability Muscles: muscles that support the torso and are designed to provide postural stability; examples include latissimus dorsi, the abdominal group, and erector spinae

Body Mechanics

The use of proper lifting and transfer techniques is crucial to job safety. Radiologic technologists who use these techniques can reduce their injuries and minimize low back pain. Low back pain causes major disability in adults aged 45 years and younger and results in major activity limitations in people aged 45 to 64 years. The annual cost of this disability to Americans has recently been estimated at $14 billion. Much of this pain, suffering, and expense could be avoided if health professionals would learn and use basic principles of body mechanics.

Biomechanics is a branch of science that applies the laws of physics, specifically the action of forces on bodies at rest or in motion, to living creatures. For example, by studying biomechanics, one can gain a better understanding of how people walk, what the best ways are to exercise, and how to develop greater athletic skills. Studies in biomechanics also yield insights into the mechanisms of injury. From these studies, researchers discover how people sustain injuries, what can be done to prevent injuries, and how to promote fitness.

An understanding of the basic aspects of biomechanics can help prevent back injury while promoting safe and effective patient transfers. Fundamental to good patient transfer techniques are the concepts of base of support, center of gravity, white muscles, and red muscles.

BASE OF SUPPORT

The **base of support** is the foundation on which a body rests. When a person is standing, the feet and the space between the feet constitute that person's base of support (Fig. 11–1A). Standing with the feet wide apart enlarges the base of support (Fig. 11–1B). Standing on one foot provides the person with a narrow base of support (Fig. 11–1C). Narrow bases of support characterize unstable and mobile systems.

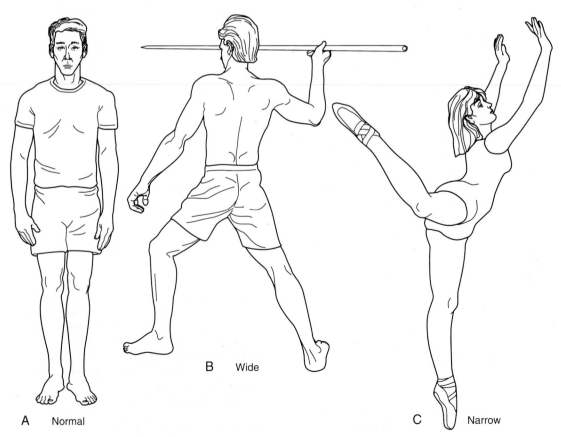

A Normal   B Wide   C Narrow

FIGURE 11–1. Variations in base of support: *A*, normal; *B*, wide; *C*, narrow.

Wide bases of support characterize stable systems. When transferring a patient, the health professional needs to establish as stable a base of support as possible. Standing with feet apart to increase the base of support improves stability.

CENTER OF GRAVITY

A second concept of importance is **center of gravity,** a hypothetical point at which all the mass appears to be concentrated (Fig. 11–2). The force of gravity appears to act on the entire body from this specific point. In humans aligned in the anatomic position, the center of gravity is at approximately sacral level two (S2) with slight variations between men and women. Stability can be achieved when a body's center of gravity is over its base of support (Fig. 11–3*A*). Instability results when the center of gravity moves beyond the boundaries of the base (Fig. 11–3*B*). For safe, stable lifting, the center of gravity must always be over the base of support.

WHITE AND RED MUSCLES

The body contains muscles that are designed for mobility and other muscles that are designed for stability. **Mobility muscles** are found in the limbs. Typically, these muscles have long white tendons and cross two or more joints. Examples include the biceps muscles, which flex the elbow, and the hamstring muscle, which flexes the knee (Fig. 11–4). **Stability muscles** are found in the torso. Typically, stability muscles are large expanses of red muscle that provide postural support. Examples include latissimus dorsi of the back and rectus abdominis of the anterior abdomen. For effective transfers, technologists should use white mobility muscles for lifting and red postural muscles for support. Lifting should be done by bending and straightening the knees. The back should be kept straight or in a position of slightly increased lumbar lordosis.

Principles of Lifting

The best way to perform a transfer is to let the patient do as much of the work as possible (Box 11–1). Before attempting a transfer, always ask patients whether they can do the transfer independently. Often, patients can transfer on

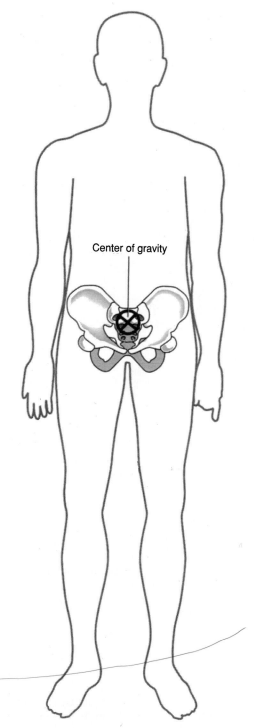

FIGURE 11–2. The center of gravity for most people is located at approximately S2.

their own or with minimal assistance. If assistance is required, let the patient help. This approach minimizes the trauma to the patient and

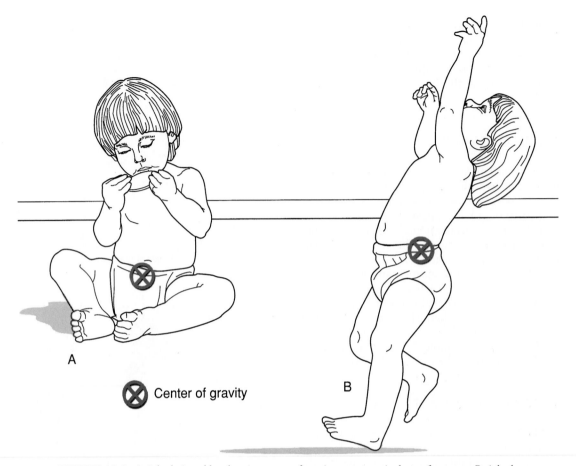

FIGURE 11–3. *A*, A body is stable when its center of gravity rests over its base of support. *B*, A body is unstable when its center of gravity is not over its base of support.

avoids stress on the technologist. In addition, this approach enhances rapport and mutual respect between the patient and the technologist.

Patients may be unsure whether they need assistance. It is not unusual for patients to believe that they are capable of transferring themselves when they are not. Before executing the transfer, check the patient's chart. Verify whether the patient has a restricted weight-bearing status. Be especially protective of patients with diagnoses such as lower extremity or pelvic girdle fracture; any disease or disorder that results in painful, inflamed, or unstable joints; or any weakened or debilitated condition. If any of these conditions appear, it is important to be especially gentle in handling the patient. Offer assistance as required. Always inform the patient of what you are going to do and how you intend to proceed. For example, tell the patient you are going to assist him or her in standing, turning toward the wheelchair, and

sitting gently. It is difficult for a patient to help you if he or she is uncertain of exactly what you are doing. Execute the transfer slowly enough for the patient to feel secure.

Safe, effective transfers rely on proper body mechanics. When lifting a patient, the person performing the transfer should stand with feet apart to increase the base of support. The patient's center of gravity (S2) should be held close to the transferrer's center of gravity (S2). This positioning provides the best mechanical advantage for lifting. Some patients may be wearing bathrobes or hospital gowns. Loose clothing inhibits one's ability to hold a patient securely. One solution is to place a transfer belt around the patient's waist. Transfer belts are usually made of webbing or muslin and can provide a good grip with minimal trauma to the patient. It is a good practice to take a transfer belt when planning to perform transfers. When lifting patients, it is important to *keep the back stationary*

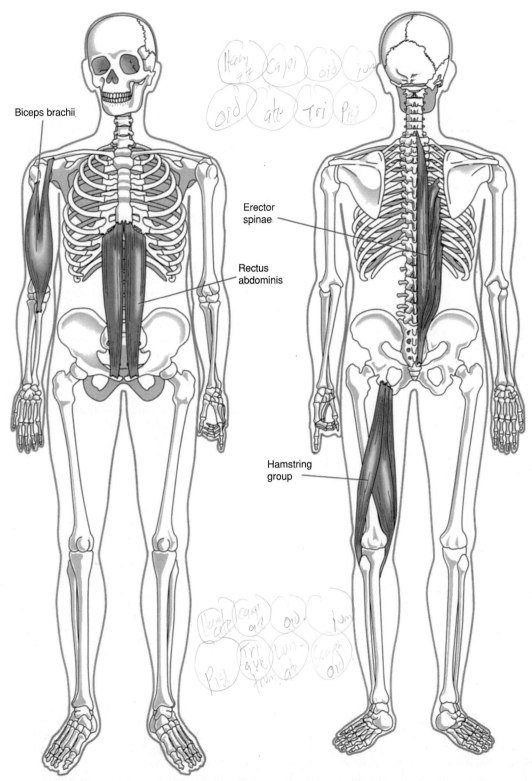

Biceps brachii

Erector
spinae

Rectus
abdominis

Hamstring
group

FIGURE 11–4. Mobility muscles include the biceps brachii and the hamstring group. Postural muscles include the rectus abdominis and the erector spinae muscles.

BOX 11–1

Principles for Safe Transfers

- Let the patient do as much of the transfer as possible.
- Check chart for precautions, such as weight-bearing status and joint disease, before executing the transfer to minimize patient discomfort and harm.
- Use a wide base of support for your stability.
- Hold the patient's center of gravity close to your own center of gravity for a better mechanical advantage.
- Hold the patient with a transfer belt around the patient's waist to minimize stress on the patient's shoulder girdle.
- Lift the patient with your legs. Avoid back bending.
- Avoid trunk twisting during transfer.
- Never lift more than you can. Ask for assistance when needed.
- Watch the patient for signs of orthostatic hypotension and take precautions to minimize its effects.

and do all of the lifting with the legs. It is important to avoid twisting. After the patient is standing, help him or her to pivot around to a bed or x-ray table and to sit down.

Technologists should be aware of **orthostatic hypotension,** the drop in blood pressure that occurs when a person stands up. A slight drop in blood pressure occurs normally when any person rises quickly from a recumbent to an upright position. This condition becomes more serious when patients have been in bed for long periods and have a debilitated status. These weakened patients tend to have blood vessels with decreased vasomotor tone and other problems in their circulatory systems. As a result, circulation and blood pressure may be affected. Rising too quickly can deprive patients of oxygen-rich blood to the brain. Symptoms of orthostatic hypotension include dizziness, fainting, blurred vision, and slurred speech.

To minimize the severity of orthostatic hypotension, have the patient stand slowly. Encourage the patient to talk during the transfer by asking simple questions—for example, "How

are you feeling?" or "Can you turn toward the bed now?" Slowing or slurring of speech may be indicative of decreased blood flow to the brain. If symptoms do occur, it is important to slow down the speed of the transfer; ask the patient to take slow, deep breaths; and provide additional assistance in the execution of the transfer. If patients report symptoms when returning to a wheelchair, let them pause for a few moments until they feel better. *Do not send symptomatic patients on their way* and risk having them faint on the way to their rooms.

Wheelchair Transfers

Four types of wheelchair transfers are used by radiologic technologists: standby assist, assisted standing pivot, two-person lift, and hydraulic lift. Begin by determining whether the patient has a strong side and a weak side or if both sides are equal. Unilateral problems such as a fracture, a lower extremity amputation, or a stroke determine which way the patient is transferred. Check the patient's chart, ask the patient, and inquire of staff about transfer precautions such as restricted weight-bearing status, debilitated state, or arthritic conditions. This is valuable information. If the patient has a strong side and a weak side, *always position the patient so that he or she is transferring toward the strong side.*

STANDBY ASSIST TRANSFER

Some patients have the ability to transfer from a wheelchair to a table on their own. Position the wheelchair at a 45-degree angle to the table (Fig. 11–5). Talk to the patient before he or she moves to determine how much, if any, assistance is required. Divide the transfer into single-step components and talk the patient through each step. Give the following commands to the patient to provide verbal assistance for a wheelchair-to-table transfer:

1 "Move the wheelchair footrests out of the way."
2 "Be sure that the wheelchair is locked."
3 "Sit on the edge of the wheelchair seat."
4 "Push down on the arms of the chair to assist in rising."
5 "Stand up slowly."
6 "Reach out and hold onto the table with the hand closest to the table."

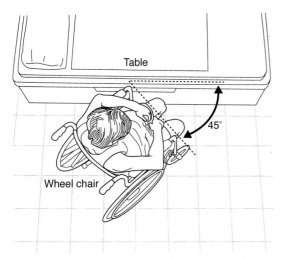

FIGURE 11–5. Angle the wheelchair to be 45 degrees from the table.

7 "Turn slowly until you feel the table behind you."

8 "Hold onto the table with both hands."

9 "Sit down."

If the table is too high for the patient to sit comfortably, after step 6, give the patient a footstool. Provide assistance as needed for the patient to step up on the stool and sit on the table.

ASSISTED STANDING PIVOT TRANSFER

For patients who cannot transfer independently, a standing pivot technique is used. Position the wheelchair at a 45-degree angle to the table with the patient's stronger side closest to the table. If the patient has on loose-fitting clothes, place a transfer belt around the patient's waist (Fig. 11–6A). It is important to have a secure grip on the patient without traumatizing any of the patient's joints. Execute the following steps one at a time:

1 Move the wheelchair footrests out of the way.

2 Be sure that the wheelchair is locked.

3 Have the patient sit on the edge of the wheelchair seat (Fig. 11–6B). Provide assistance as needed.

4 Have the patient push down on the arms of the wheelchair to assist in rising (Fig. 11–6C).

5 Bend at the knees, keeping your back straight, and grasp the transfer belt with both hands. The patient's feet and knees must be blocked to provide stability, especially for paraplegic and hemiplegic patients who are partially paralyzed and may not be able to move or feel sensation in a lower extremity. This is accomplished by placing one foot outside the patient's foot while the knee is placed at the medial (inside) surface of the patient's knee (Fig. 11–6D).

6 As the patient rises to a standing position, rise also by straightening your knees (Fig. 11–6E).

7 When the patient is standing, ask, "Are you feeling all right?" If the patient reports any feelings of dizziness or exhibits any of the other signs of orthostatic hypotension, let him or her stand for a moment until recovered.

8 When the patient is ready, both of you pivot toward the table until the patient can feel the table against the back of the thighs (Fig. 11–6F).

9 Ask the patient to support himself or herself on the table with both hands and to sit down (Fig. 11–6G).

10 Help the patient to sit by gradually lowering him or her to the table. Be sure that your back remains straight and that the lowering occurs from the knees.

TWO-PERSON LIFT

Some patients cannot bear weight on their lower extremities and must be lifted onto the table. If the patient is lightweight, a two-person lift can be executed. The stronger person should lift the patient's torso while the other person lifts the patient's feet. The person lifting the patient's torso is usually in charge of the transfer and directs the other person's actions.

Prepare for the transfer by verbally planning out the procedure. This verbal planning enables a coordinated effort among the transferrers and the patient. Verbal planning also allows for troubleshooting before the execution of the transfer.

Before the patient is moved, lock the wheelchair, remove the armrests, and swing away or remove the legrests. The patient is asked to cross his or her arms over the chest. The transferrer stands behind the patient, reaches under the patient's axillae, and grasps the patient's crossed forearms. The other person should

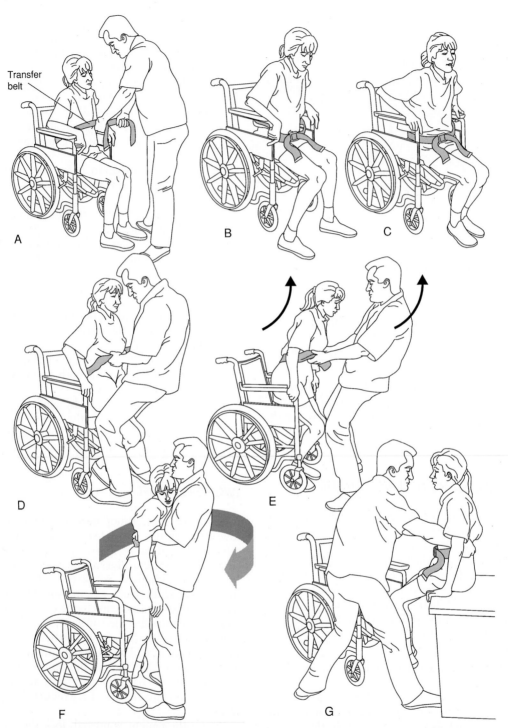

Transfer belt

A

B

C

D

E

F

G

FIGURE 11–6. An assisted standing/pivot transfer is used when transferring a patient from a wheelchair to a table. *A*, Use a transfer belt to hold the patient securely. *B*, Have the patient sit on the edge of the wheelchair seat. Provide assistance as needed. *C*, Have the patient push down on the arms of the wheelchair to assist in rising. *D*, Bend at the knees, keeping the back straight, and grasp the transfer belt with both hands. *E*, As the patient rises to standing, rise also by straightening your knees. *F*, When the patient is ready, pivot toward the table until the patient can feel the table against the back of the thighs. *G*, Ask the patient to hold onto the table with both hands and to slowly sit down.

squat in front of the patient and cradle the patient's thighs in one hand and the calves in the other hand (Fig. 11–7A). At the command of the transferrer, the patient is lifted to clear the wheelchair and moved as a unit to the desired place (Fig. 11–7B).

HYDRAULIC LIFT TECHNIQUES

Some patients are too heavy to lift manually and require a hydraulic lift. Before attempting to lift a patient with this particular piece of equipment, practice to become familiar with it.

Most hydraulic lifts have several basic features. To facilitate moving, they often have four caster wheels but no wheel locks. The lift's base of support can be widened or narrowed by means of a lever. Most lifts have two handles for steering, a manual pump for raising the support arm, a release valve for lowering the support arm, and a spreader bar for the sling attachment (Fig. 11–8). Identify these features and learn their operation before attempting to use the lift.

For patients who need to be transferred using a hydraulic lift, prior arrangement should be made with the nursing staff to have these patients arrive in the radiology department sitting in a wheelchair on a transfer sling. If the patient arrives without a sling, assistance should be requested. It is better to send a patient back to the ward to return sitting on a sling than to risk injury to the patient, the transferrer, or both by attempting transfer without using one.

The sling attaches to the spreader bar by hooks and chains. The chains have a short segment for attachment to the sling back and a longer segment for attachment to the sling seat. Adjust the chain length according to the size of the patient. Hook the chains to the sling from the inside out (Fig. 11–9A). This minimizes the risk of a patient being injured by the hooks.

Check that the release valve is closed and that the patient is positioned comfortably in the sling. Gently begin to raise the patient (Fig. 11–9B). When the patient has cleared the wheelchair seat, the wheelchair can be removed and the patient can be positioned on the table. Manual assistance may be required to position the patient's legs appropriately.

To lower the patient, open the release valve and gently lower the patient. Guard the patient's head from contact with the spreader bar. Remove the chains with care; they have a tendency to swing and must be steadied to avoid patient injury. After the patient has achieved a safe, stable position, the lift can be removed.

Cart Transfers

Many patients are transported by cart (also called a stretcher or gurney). To move a patient from a cart onto a radiographic table, position the cart alongside the table on the patient's strong or less affected side. The cart must be as close to the table as possible and then secured. Simply depressing wheel locks may not be sufficient to keep a cart from moving. It is often necessary to place sandbags or other devices on the floor to block the wheels satisfactorily.

If the patient can assist with the transfer, all that may be required is stabilization of the cart and support for the involved body part. For example, a patient may move his or her body if a leg in a cast is supported during the transfer. If the patient cannot assist, a moving device should be used. If no moving devices are available, three people can be used for a cart-to-table transfer.

There are numerous commercially manufactured moving devices. Some are smooth, thin sheets of plastic, others are composed of canvas or plastic over small rollers, but all are designed to be used as aids during cart-to-table transfers. The patient is rolled away from the table while the moving device is placed to the midpoint of the back. Then the patient is returned to a supine position so that he or she is halfway onto the moving device. The draw sheet is then used to slowly move the patient onto the table (Fig. 11–10). If necessary, the patient may be rolled to remove the moving device.

A second type of moving device is a low-friction polyester sheet that enables health practitioners to slide rather than lift their patients during transfers. The Arjo Company manufactures such products under the names of Maxi-Slide, MaxiTube, and MaxiTransfer. A patient must be placed on a double thickness of this fabric and then glided from one place to another. The top layer moves with the patient so the patient's skin is protected from abrasions. Since the patient is pushed or pulled into position rather than lifted, each transfer requires less effort and fewer personnel.

To perform a lateral transfer from, for example, a gurney to a radiographic table, two sheets are needed. One sheet must be directly under

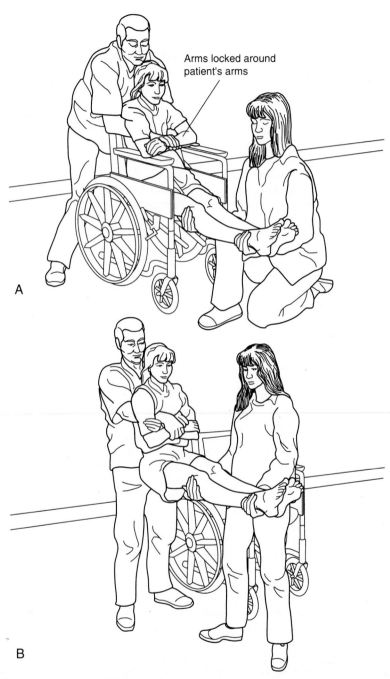

Arms locked around
patient's arms

A

B

FIGURE 11–7. A two-person lift. *A*, The first person asks the patient to cross his or her arms over the chest. The person making the transfer stands behind the patient, reaches under the patient's axillae, and grasps the patient's crossed forearms. The assistant squats in front of the patient and cradles the patient's thighs in one hand and the patient's calves in the other. *B*, At the command of the person supporting the patient's upper body, the patient is lifted to clear the wheelchair and moved as a unit to the desired place.

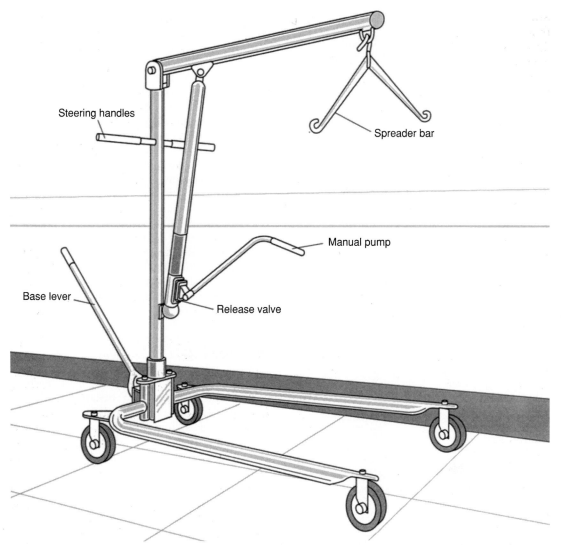

FIGURE 11–8. Hydraulic lifts often have four caster wheels but no wheel locks. The lift's base of support can be widened or narrowed by means of a lever. The lift has two handles for steering, a manual pump for raising the support arm, a release valve for lowering the support arm, and a spreader bar for the sling attachment.

the patient and the second sheet must be under the first sheet to serve as a track on which the patient will slide. If the patient arrives without a transfer sheet, one can be easily placed under the patient. Roll the patient to one side, place a double-thickness of the sheeting under the patient and then roll the patient on top of the transfer sheets.

For the actual lateral transfer, both transfer surfaces must be side to side, as close to each other as possible, and at the same height. The wheels of the gurney must be locked so the two surfaces can not separate during the transfer.

The transfer sheets have handles. Two technologists, one at the patient's head and chest and a second at the patient's pelvis and legs, can grasp the top sheet and slide the patient laterally into the desired position.

To perform a cart-to-table transfer without a moving device, begin by rolling up the draw sheet on both sides of the patient (Fig. 11–11A). If the draw sheet is not completely under the patient, it must be properly positioned before the transfer. This transfer cannot be accomplished without a draw sheet. The person directing the transfer should support the patient's head and

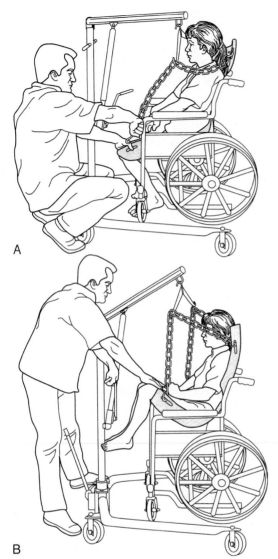

A

B

FIGURE 11–9. A hydraulic lift transfer. *A*, The chains have a short segment for attachment to the sling back and a longer segment for attachment to the sling seat. Adjust the chain length according to the patient's size. Hook the chains to the sling from the inside out. This minimizes the risk of a patient's being injured by the hooks. *B*, Check that the release valve is closed and that the patient is positioned comfortably in the sling. Gently begin to raise the patient.

upper body from the far side of the radiographic table. Another person should support the patient's pelvic girdle from the cart side. A third person should support the patient's legs from the table side. The patient's arms should be crossed over the chest to avoid injury or interfering with a smooth transfer (Fig. 11–11*B*).

The person supporting the pelvic girdle stands on the opposite side of the cart and

makes sure that the cart does not move away from the table during the transfer. The person in charge, at the patient's head, gives the commands and directs the transfer. On command, everyone grasps the rolled-up draw sheet and slowly pulls the patient to the edge of the cart. Depending on the length of their reach, the assistants may need to reposition themselves in anticipation of moving the patient from the cart onto the table. When everyone is ready, the person in charge again issues the command and the patient is slowly lifted and pulled onto the table.

The transfer without a moving device is difficult. Because there is potential for strain and injury to the persons performing the maneuver, it is generally not recommended for most patients, especially those who are heavy or who have serious injuries. It is never recommended that the transferrers attempt to kneel or stand on the radiographic table to perform this type of transfer.

Positioning

To examine the desired body part, patients need to be moved into a variety of different positions. In general, the patient needs to be transferred as a single unit; placed on the table in a safe, secure position; and then moved segmentally into the desired body position. Before executing the move, talk through the steps to prepare the patient and any assistants. Let the patient assist as much as possible. To minimize trauma and discomfort for the patient, take an extra moment to make sure that the patient is ready to make the move. Try to roll the patient toward you. Provide positioning sponges to support the patient comfortably in the desired position. The proper terms for the most common positions are given in Figure 11–12. All radiologic technologists should become familiar with both the positions and appropriate methods to assist patients to achieve them.

Summary

To execute safe, efficient patient transfers with minimal stress and discomfort for health professionals and patients, the radiologic technologist must maintain a wide base of support, hold patients close to the center of gravity, avoid trunk twisting, keep the back stable, lift from the knees, and let the patients assist as much as possible. Prepare both patients and the assis-

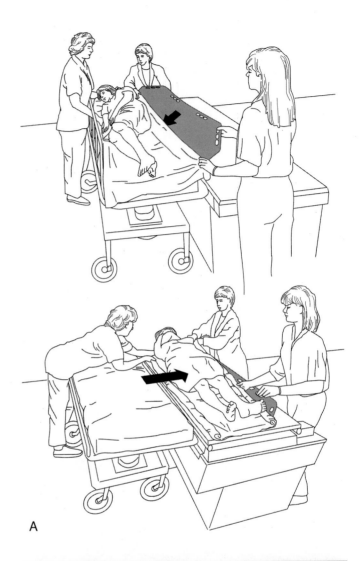

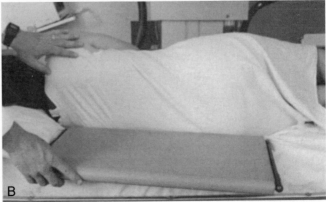

A

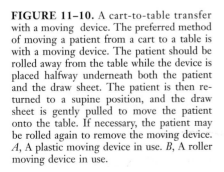

B

FIGURE 11–10. A cart-to-table transfer with a moving device. The preferred method of moving a patient from a cart to a table is with a moving device. The patient should be rolled away from the table while the device is placed halfway underneath both the patient and the draw sheet. The patient is then returned to a supine position, and the draw sheet is gently pulled to move the patient onto the table. If necessary, the patient may be rolled again to remove the moving device. *A,* A plastic moving device in use. *B,* A roller moving device in use.

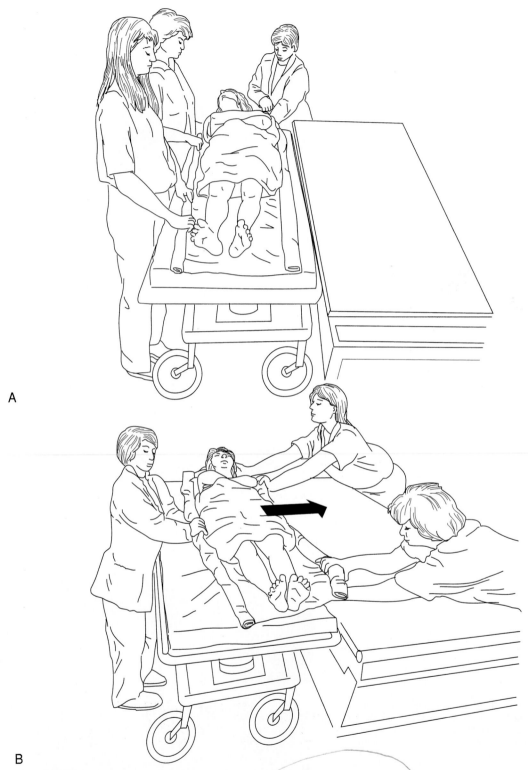

FIGURE 11–11. A cart-to-table transfer without a moving device. *A*, Begin by rolling up the draw sheet on both sides of the patient. *B*, The person directing the transfer supports the patient's head and upper body from the far side of the radiographic table. An assistant supports the patient's pelvic girdle from the cart side. A second assistant supports the patient's legs from the table side. The patient's arms can be crossed over the chest to avoid injury or getting in the way.

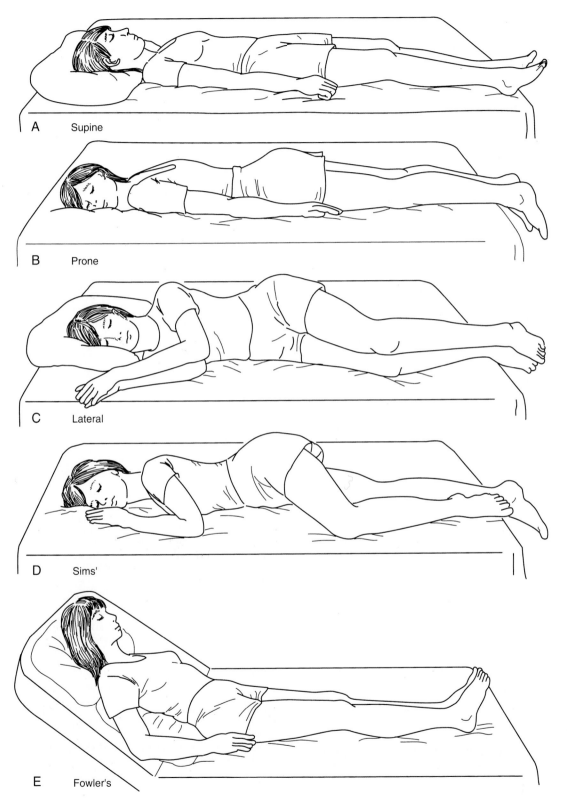

A Supine

B Prone

C Lateral

D Sims'

E Fowler's

FIGURE 11–12. Patient positioning.

tants for transfers by verbally planning out and rehearsing the procedures. Take the time to be gentle and safe, and to move slowly. These extra moments could prevent a serious injury.

◀R REVIEW QUESTIONS

1 Which of the following is the foundation on which a body rests?
a) center of gravity
b) base of support
c) orthostatic hypotension
d) biomechanics

2 What term is used to describe the drop in blood pressure some patients experience when they stand up quickly?
a) center of gravity
b) base of support
c) orthostatic hypotension
d) a and b

3 Where is the human center of gravity located?
a) at the center of the diaphragm
b) within 1 to 2 inches of the umbilicus
c) midway between the hip joints
d) at approximately sacral level two

4 Which of the following transfers can be used to move a patient from a wheelchair to an examination table?
a) pivot
b) assisted standing
c) standby assist
d) all of the above

5 Toward which side should all transfers be initiated?
a) the left
b) the right
c) the patient's weak side
d) the patient's strong side

6 What causes patients to feel lightheaded, queasy, or faint when they stand up quickly from a sitting or supine position?
a) increased respiration from the effort of standing
b) decreased blood pressure
c) increased body temperature
d) increased pulse rate

7 What term describes the hypothetical point around which all mass appears to be concentrated?
a) center of gravity
b) base of support
c) orthostatic hypotension
d) a and b

8 If a patient arrives in a wheelchair and on a sling, which type of transfer is indicated?
a) hydraulic lift
b) pivot
c) standby assist
d) cart to table by means of a moving device

9 How can the base of support be increased?
a) standing on one toe
b) standing on one foot
c) standing with the legs farther apart
d) bending the knees with the feet together

10 What is the minimum number of persons to use for a cart-to-table transfer when no moving devices are available?
a) one
b) two
c) three
d) four

BIBLIOGRAPHY

Delitto RS, Rose SJ, Apts DW: Electromyographic analysis of two techniques for squat lifting. Physical Ther 67:1329–1334, 1987.

Ehrlich RA, McCloskey E: Patient Care in Radiography. 3rd ed. St. Louis, CV Mosby, 1989.

Hollis M, Davis PR: Safer Lifting for Patient Care. Oxford, UK, Blackwell Scientific Publications, 1981.

Kelsey JL, White AA, Pastides H, et al: The impact of musculoskeletal disorders on the population of the United States. J Bone Joint Surg [Am] 61:959–963, 1979.

Minor MA, Minor SD: Patient Care Skills. 3rd ed. Norwalk, CT, Appleton & Lange, 1995.

Norkin CC, Levangie PK: Biomechanics. In Norkin and Levangie (eds): Joint Structure and Function: A Comprehensive Analysis. Philadelphia, FA Davis, 1983.

Rantz MF, Corntial D: Lifting, Moving and Transferring Patients: A Manual. 2nd ed. St. Louis, CV Mosby, 1981.

Smidt GL: Biomechanics and physical therapy: a perspective. Physical Ther 64:1807–1808, 1984.

Sullivan MS: Back support mechanisms during manual lifting. Physical Ther 69:38–45, 1989.

Torres L: Basic Medical Techniques and Patient Care for Radiologic Technologists. 4th ed. Philadelphia, JB Lippincott, 1993.

White AA, Gordon SL: Synopsis: Workshop on idiopathic low back pain. Spine 7:141–149, 1982.

CHAPTER 12

IMMOBILIZATION TECHNIQUES

Dennis Spragg, MS Ed, RT(R)

Uncooperative behavior can be viewed as active resistance, a defensive action which serves to preserve self-esteem and ward off the invasiveness of intervention . . . . Resistance is therefore a sign of strength; . . . the therapeutic solution is not to confront resistance, but to honor it.

HELEN BURR, 1987

OBJECTIVES

On completion of this chapter, the student will be able to:

1 Demonstrate a range of immobilization techniques.
2 Explain the importance of quality communication with the patient.
3 Describe reduction of patient radiation exposure by using proper immobilization methods.
4 Apply immobilization techniques in routine situations.
5 Use immobilization devices effectively.
6 Describe trauma immobilization techniques as they pertain to specific anatomic involvement.
7 Explain the importance of establishing rapport with pediatric patients.
8 Use various methods of pediatric immobilization.
9 Describe appropriate application of immobilization techniques pertinent to geriatric patients.

GLOSSARY

Ambulatory: able to walk

Anteroposterior: direction of x-ray beam from front to back

Artifact: substance or structure not naturally present but of which an authentic image appears on a radiograph

Axial Projection: any projection not at right angles to the long axis of an anatomic structure

Empathy: recognition of and entering into the feelings of another person

Flexion: act of bending or condition of being bent

Geriatric: pertaining to the treatment of the aged

Homogeneous: of a uniform quality throughout

Immobilization: act of rendering immovable

Neonate: newborn infant

Pediatric: pertaining to that branch of medicine that treats children

Plantar Surface: sole of the foot

Rapport: relation of harmony and accord between two persons

Restraint: hindrance of an action (movement)

Trauma: wound or injury

Scope of Immobilization Techniques

When discussing **immobilization** techniques, it is important to understand the effect of motion and positioning inaccuracy on the diagnostic quality of the procedure. One of the many factors that affect diagnostic quality is motion. When attempting to photograph a fast-moving object (a sprinter or a race car, for example), there is a a good possibility that the image on the developed film will appear streaked or blurry because of the motion of the object photographed.

The same phenomenon occurs when radiographing a wiggly 3-year-old patient's chest or the shaking hand of a badly injured accident victim. The movement of the toddler or the shaking hand results in a blurred image and greatly reduces the radiologist's ability to make a diagnosis. The important fact is that the motion of the subject does not have to be considerable or exaggerated to affect the procedure. Even the slightest movement may seriously compromise the radiograph.

Another important factor that affects diagnostic information is inaccuracy when positioning the patient during an examination. Many positions for procedures require exact degrees of rotation of the patient or body part. Use of positioning aids such as sponges or supports enables the radiologic technologist to more accurately position the patient. At the same time, this support of the patient significantly lessens the possibility of motion.

A thorough knowledge of the various methods that may be used to reduce the possibility of motion and to ensure positioning accuracy is therefore extremely important when studying the art and practice of radiologic technology.

SIMPLE VERSUS INVOLVED IMMOBILIZATION TECHNIQUES

On first encountering the term *immobilization*, it might be easy for a new radiologic technology student to envision a patient hog-tied and bound to an x-ray table (Fig. 12–1). While some forms of immobilization techniques are somewhat intricate, it is important to understand that immobilization techniques cover a wide range of applications from minimal to highly sophisticated.

The simplest techniques involve the use of a positioning sponge to support the anatomic area of interest or gently laying a sandbag across a patient's forearm to minimize shaking due to patient anxiety. More complex techniques might involve completely wrapping an infant or small child in a sheet (often referred to as a mummy wrap) or securing an accident victim to a backboard to facilitate transport of the patient to the emergency department and to minimize the possibility of more severe complications such as spinal cord damage during the transport process. In the latter case, the radiologic technologist has not applied the immobilization device but must recognize the importance of the device and be able to use it to the best advantage.

RADIATION PROTECTION

The underlying concept of a conscientious, professional radiologic technologist is the ability to produce the most diagnostic film possible with the least amount of radiation to the patient and others. If there is movement by the patient, either voluntary or involuntary, the radiographs

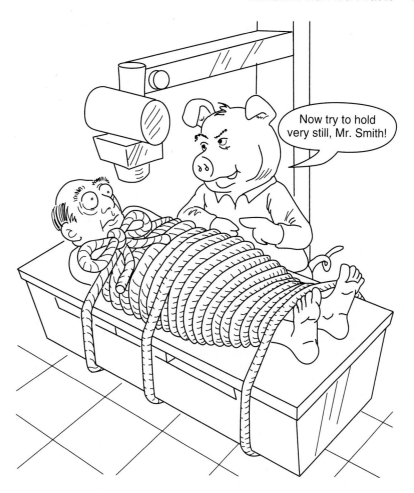

FIGURE 12–1.

may be of less than optimal quality. Voluntary movement can be controlled by the patient and most often occurs as a result of inadequate communication by the technologist. Involuntary movement is the result of many contributing factors (eg, examination room temperature, medication, posttraumatic shock) and cannot be controlled by the patient. The importance of performing the procedure correctly the first time is obvious.

COMMUNICATION

Various physical **restraints** may be used to reduce the possibility of motion, but perhaps one of the most effective means of reducing motion on the part of the patient is also one of the most simple and, unfortunately, one of the most overlooked. The method is communication.

The art of communication is a skill that is often used ineffectively. Ineffective or unskillful communication can occur at all levels: between radiologist and radiologic technologist, from one technologist to another, clinical instructor to student, department manager to secretary, technologist to patient and so forth. Keeping in mind the objective of reducing repeated procedures and radiation exposure, it may well be that the most important communication that goes on in a hospital department takes place between the technologist and patient.

Often the patient is capable of cooperation and would be more than willing to facilitate the examination if he or she were simply informed of what was going to happen and apprised of the importance of cooperation in producing an accurate diagnosis. A key component to effective communication with the patient is the establishment of rapport.

Rapport is a relation of harmony and accord between two persons, as between patient and physician. This harmony and relationship building should begin as soon as the technologist comes into contact with the patient. It begins as the radiologic technologist introduces himself or herself to the patient and continues throughout the history taking process. During this history taking, the technologist has the opportunity to display empathy, respect, and concern for the patient as a person, as well as to ascertain the clinical facts behind the examination. Once the radiologic technologist has established rapport with the patient, the patient becomes more comfortable, a sense of trust and confidence is established, and the patient is better able to focus on the explanation of what will occur during the examination.

While a good explanation of the examination is important and will better enable the patient to cooperate, the explanation generally need not be highly technical or filled with professional jargon. A simple explanation in lay terms with stress on the importance of cooperation on the part of the patient is usually all that is needed. Care must be taken, however, that in simplifying the explanation, the patient is not insulted by underestimation of his or her intelligence. A proper assessment of the patient's replies and questions allows the technologist to explain the examination at a level appropriate to each patient. The explanation should emphasize that cooperation on the part of the patient will make the examination proceed much more quickly and result in the highest possible diagnostic information. It is important to keep the explanation simple but make sure the patient understands that his or her cooperation is essential.

The radiologic technologist will not always be able to communicate effectively in a verbal sense, as in the case of a very young child or someone who is highly stressed because of the nature of his or her injury or condition. If the technologist is truly genuine in his or her **empathy** for the patient, communication of a more subtle nature will occur. For example, a newborn infant often senses and responds positively to warmth, gentle holding, a soft calm voice, and a sense of security.

Routine Applications

Although some immobilization methods may seem mundane to the experienced technologist, their dedicated use results in fewer repeated procedures as a result of patient motion.

POSITIONING SPONGES

One of the most common methods of reducing patient motion is the use of positioning sponges. These sponges come in a variety of shapes and sizes and are designed to support the patient or the anatomic area of interest by reducing physical strain on the patient from having to hold a position that might otherwise be difficult to achieve (Fig. 12–2). Positioning sponges also allow for more accuracy in positioning by supporting the patient or anatomic area of interest in the correct position and relation to the film. The use of positioning sponges is limited only by the creativity of the technologist.

VELCRO STRAPS

Although often not considered a form of restraint, Velcro straps can be effective as restraining or positioning devices. A good example of the use of straps is provided by an upright lateral chest position (Fig. 12–3). It is important for the patient to stand for a chest examination if at all possible. While capable of standing, a patient who has not been regularly **ambulatory** for a time may be unsteady when standing at the upright cassette holder. Placing Velcro straps across the patient's arms and hips helps the patient to hold still and also provides a sense of security. Holding the arms up out of the way on a lateral chest position raises the center of balance and can cause slight swaying even in the most steady subject.

Velcro straps may also be used in immobilizing only the area of interest during the procedure. For example, an **axial projection** of the calcaneus requires extreme dorsiflexion of the ankle to produce an optimally diagnostic radiograph (Fig. 12–4). The use of the strap beneath the **plantar surface** of the foot allows the patient to maintain the extreme **flexion** required and at the same time reduces the possibility of motion that may result from maintaining an uncomfortable position.

Velcro straps can serve as a safety precaution when performing a procedure on a patient who is not completely cognizant, such as those who are heavily medicated or intoxicated, or who have diminished mental capacities. This type of patient should never be left unattended; the straps serve only to facilitate in protecting the patient from injury. With straps in place, sudden

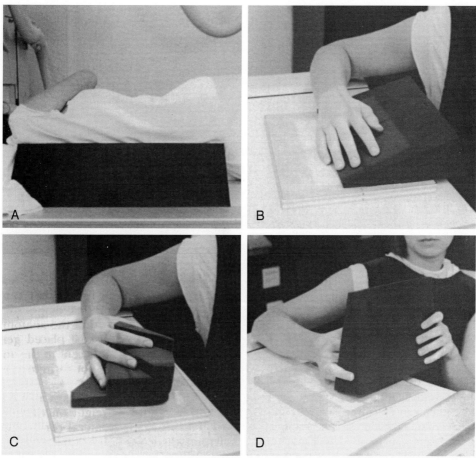

FIGURE 12–2. *A,* Patient positioned with sponge for oblique lumbar spine radiograph. *B,* Hand in oblique position on sponge. *C,* Hand in fan lateral position on sponge. *D,* Fourth finger in lateral position using sponge.

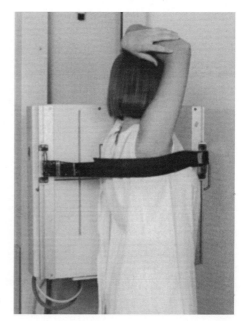

FIGURE 12–3. Patient positioned for lateral upright chest radiograph with straps in place.

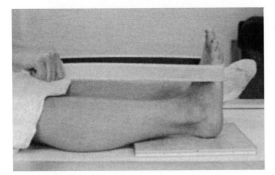

FIGURE 12–4. Patient positioned for axial calcaneus radiograph using strap.

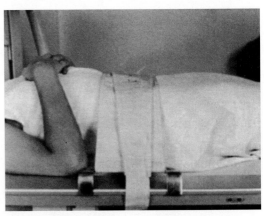

FIGURE 12–5. Patient supine on table with Velcro straps in place.

or unexpected movement by the patient would not result in injury to the patient and would allow the attendant to respond to the situation.

COMPRESSION BANDS

Compression bands are designed to be attached to the sides of a table and removed. They apply controlled, gentle pressure on the abdomen, which can enhance diagnostic information in certain procedures. For example, a compression band can be used to cause more **homogeneous** tissue density in the abdomen of a patient undergoing a small bowel examination who is unable to lie prone. Compression bands

can be used in much the same way as Velcro straps, although their use may be somewhat more limited because they must be attached to the table (Fig. 12–5).

When performing some abdominal examinations, it may be desirable to have the patient standing erect. In instances in which a patient is too weak to stand unassisted, compression bands across the patient's chest, hips, and knees allow the table to be placed in a semierect position while securely supporting the patient during the procedure (Fig. 12–6). Compression bands, like Velcro straps, can also be used when

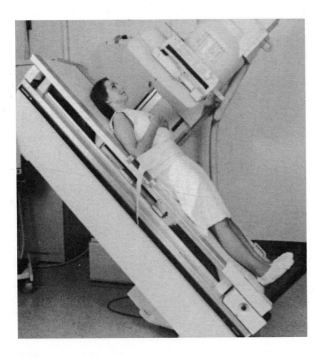

FIGURE 12–6. Table in semierect position with compression band over patient. If more support is needed, additional bands may be applied to the chest, hips, and knees.

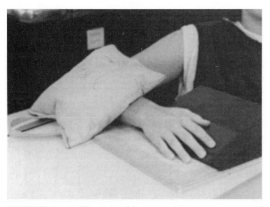

FIGURE 12–7. Hand in oblique position on sponge with sandbag across forearm.

examining a patient who is not completely cognizant.

SANDBAGS

Sandbags are useful positioning and immobilization devices and can be used in a variety of ways. By themselves or in combination with positioning sponges, sandbags are extremely helpful in reducing voluntary motion (Figs. 12–7 and 12–8). Sandbags, unlike radiolucent positioning sponges, are radiopaque (ie, radiation does not pass through easily). As a result, they cannot be placed in such a way that diagnostic information is obscured within the anatomic area of interest. They must be placed gently on or against the areas adjacent to the anatomic area of interest so as not to injure or cause further damage.

A common use of sandbags as positioning aids is for placing weight on the shoulders when performing a lateral cervical spine or acromio-

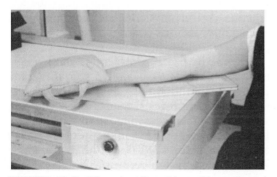

FIGURE 12–8. Elbow in AP position with sandbag on palm.

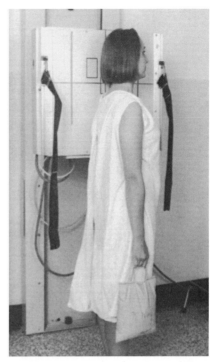

FIGURE 12–9. Patient in erect lateral cervical position with sandbags.

clavicular joints examination. It is important to lower the shoulders as much as possible for this projection, and having the patient hold heavy sandbags in each hand causes the shoulders to be pulled lower (Fig. 12–9).

Here again, as in the case of positioning sponges, the variety of uses for sandbags is limited only by the technologist's imagination.

HEAD CLAMPS

Head clamps can be attached to radiographic imaging devices (eg, radiographic table or upright cassette holder) and are designed strictly for use in positioning various projections of the skull. When applied safely and appropriately, head clamps serve more as a positioning aid than as an immobilization device. A patient so desiring can easily pull away from the head clamps. Head clamps serve more as a reminder to the patient of the importance of remaining as still as possible, and they ensure the reduction of voluntary movement on the part of the patient (Fig. 12–10).

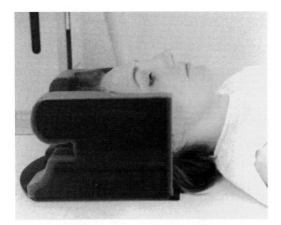

FIGURE 12–10. Patient positioned for AP skull radiograph with head clamps in place.

Special Applications

Immobilization techniques often are required for nonroutine situations, and patients and the technologist must be adept in their use. These special applications include trauma, pediatric, and geriatric patients.

TRAUMA APPLICATIONS

Methods for safely and expeditiously performing examinations on badly traumatized patients involve entirely different concepts. Immobilization is one of the most critical considerations when working with seriously injured patients. In these instances, the technologist is faced with immobilization devices that have already been applied to the **trauma** victim by the emergency medical team to stabilize the area of injury and to facilitate safe transport to the trauma center. The technologist must be familiar with the various types of traction and immobilization techniques and devices used by emergency medical personnel. This familiarity must include knowledge of which devices are radiolucent, which must be left in place for initial examinations, and when these devices can safely be removed for more detailed procedures.

In many situations, the technologist must consider performing the initial examination with immobilization devices left in place. In fact, more often than not, there is no choice but to perform the procedure in this manner. Fortunately, manufacturers of emergency traction devices are designing equipment to use radiolucent materials whenever possible. This permits initial studies to result in more diagnostic information without endangering the accident victim by necessitating the removal of immobilization devices.

In most instances, initial images can and should be produced without removal of immobilization devices. Only after the initial radiographs are read by a radiologist or an attending physician and approval has been given should the technologist remove the immobilization device for a more complete examination.

Immobilization devices should be removed gently while maintaining patient comfort and safety by immobilizing the injured area above and below the device. Positioning sponges should be placed to support the anatomic area of interest. Depending on condition, the patient may be moved or rolled slightly to facilitate removal of the device. If help is available, it is always safer and easier for the patient if two people, working together, remove immobilization devices.

Spinal Trauma

Probably the most common spinal trauma traction device encountered by a technologist is the cervical collar. This device is designed to place traction on the cervical spine to prevent further life-threatening movement in this vital area. The lateral position is the most important when performing a cervical trauma examination. It is essential in evaluating cervical trauma. After evaluating this radiograph, the attending physician or neurosurgeon can determine the next step in treatment. Other projections can be produced with the cervical collar in place, but the most critical diagnostic information is obtained from the lateral position (Fig. 12–11). In all instances, the cervical collar must be left in place until a physician has seen the initial radiographs and has approved removal of the collar.

The backboard or spineboard is another spinal immobilization device often seen in trauma situations. Although the backboard is mentioned here under spinal trauma considerations, its uses are by no means limited to spinal injury. It is used to immobilize and support the victim's entire body. A backboard may be used if there is involvement of the thoracic or lumbar spine. Additional trauma situations in which the backboard is used include injuries to the pelvis, hips,

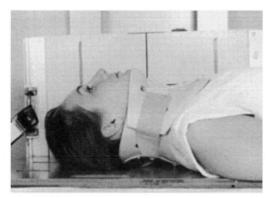

FIGURE 12–11. Patient positioned for recumbent lateral cervical spine radiograph with cervical collar in place.

and lower extremities or when there are multiple injuries in addition to spinal trauma.

Most backboards are made from radiolucent materials (eg, wood or plastic), making radiography of patients relatively easy. With assistance, one end of the backboard can be lifted and a cassette placed under the area of interest beneath the board (Fig. 12–12). All **anteroposterior** (AP) projections from head to toe can be accomplished in this manner.

Another advantageous way of using the backboard is to transport a stable trauma patient to

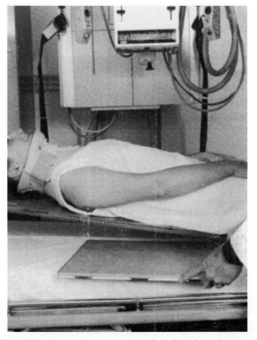

FIGURE 12–12. Patient on backboard with grid cassette placed under backboard for AP lumbar spine radiograph.

the radiology department for the initial examination. It is much easier and more comfortable to move the patient onto the table by sliding the entire backboard onto the examination table. Once the initial radiographs have been evaluated by a radiologist, the backboard can be moved from under the patient for further projections. Conversely, if the findings indicate the presence of fracture or other traumatic involvement, the patient can be safely moved back onto a stretcher for transport to surgery, the emergency department, or the appropriate treatment area.

Head Trauma

The technologist will encounter trauma immobilization devices applied to other areas of interest besides the spine. Many times it is necessary to examine the skull of a patient wearing a cervical collar or similar immobilization device. Because of the presence of the cervical collar, a radiographer must become versatile in the production of skull radiographs. Instead of being able to rotate and tilt the head or flex and extend the neck to position the patient correctly, the radiographer must be able to manipulate the radiographic equipment to compensate for the patient's lack of mobility (Fig. 12–13). The cervical collar often cannot be removed for more difficult skull projections until after approval by a physician.

Extremity Trauma

Other anatomic areas of interest that may involve the use of traction devices are the extremities, particularly the lower extremities. In these cases, the traction devices are in the form of splints, most often inflation or traction splints.

An inflation or air splint is simply an inflatable plastic cuff that is slipped over the affected limb and inflated to provide stability for transport by the emergency team (Fig. 12–14). These splints are readily radiolucent, and routine radiography can usually be achieved with little discomfort or danger to the patient. An exception would be if there are multiple injuries that complicate the procedures.

Traction splints are designed for use on the lower extremities. They exert a steady force on the affected limb by applying pressure against the pelvis and groin area (Fig. 12–15). Although traction splints often contain radiopaque mate-

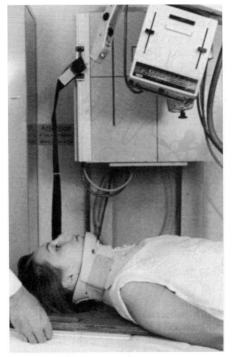

FIGURE 12–13. Patient on backboard positioned for acanthioparietal projection with cervical collar in place.

rials, satisfactory initial radiographs can be obtained with the splint in place. Most splints designed for use on the upper extremities are made from radiolucent materials and do not present any great obstacles for the procurement of diagnostic radiographs.

An antishock garment might also be occasionally encountered. The antishock garment is a pair of inflatable trousers applied to the victim. This device is used in instances in which there is trauma to the abdomen, pelvis, or lower extremities and internal hemorrhaging is sus-

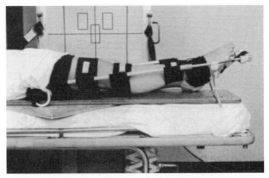

FIGURE 12–15. Traction splint on lower leg.

pected. Once the antishock garment is in place around the patient, the garment is inflated to slow the rate of hemorrhage. It is sometimes necessary to perform radiography on these patients for pelvic or other fractures with the garment in place. Because the trousers are radiolucent, they should be left in place while the examination is being performed (Fig. 12–16).

PEDIATRIC APPLICATIONS

Special problems are encountered when performing radiographic examinations on **pediatric** patients. While there are many methods and devices available to facilitate pediatric radiography, perhaps the most overlooked aspect of positioning and immobilizing children is communication and the establishment of rapport. Often, children as young as 3 or 4 years old can be convinced to hold still without immobilization when communication is well done. This rapport is established with kindness, patience, honesty, and understanding. Although this may not be difficult to convey under normal circumstances, an entirely different situation arises

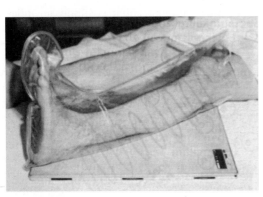

FIGURE 12–14. Inflation (air) splint on lower leg.

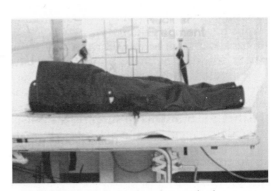

FIGURE 12–16. Patient wearing antishock garment.

within the context of a busy radiographic department with a child who is injured or sick. Kindness, patience, honesty, and understanding are best conveyed to children literally on their level by dropping to one knee to talk with the children face to face. To quote Armand Brodeur, former chief radiologist at Cardinal Glennon Children's Hospital in St. Louis, "To stand tall in pediatric radiology, you have to get down on your knees." A diagnostic examination will be obtained much more quickly if a little time is spent in establishing rapport with the child. Speak in a calm, soothing voice, perhaps while offering a toy to the child. Often young children respond well to making a game of having their "picture taken" or seeing how long they can hold still. Allow the child time to explore the new surroundings and ask questions. Threats and force must be avoided at all times, with restraints being applied gently.

Another preliminary consideration for pediatric radiography is how to handle parents while the examination is being performed. Two schools of thought exist for whether to allow the parents to accompany the child into the radiographic room. Often departmental policy has been established addressing this issue, but there can always be exceptions because of extenuating circumstances. Some parents are understanding and extremely helpful when allowed to accompany their child to the radiographic room.

As is often the case, when departmental policy or the situation calls for parents to be present during the examination, it is imperative that the radiographer give the parents a crash course in the importance of cooperation and understanding. It is difficult for parents to be objective when they observe their child being placed in a pediatric immobilization device. Although a child who is confined in an upright chest immobilization device or strapped to a restraint board may look uncomfortable, the parent must be made to understand that the technique or device used for immobilization is the safest and surest way to produce optimal diagnostic radiographs with a minimal amount of discomfort and radiation exposure to the child.

Pediatric positioning and immobilization are more appropriate for **neonates** and small children. If well done and genuine, rapport and communication should be all that is necessary for older children. The radiographer must determine what methods are required according to the situation.

Sheet Restraints

One of the most effective, simple, inexpensive, and reliable methods of restraining or immobilizing a child is mummification. While this method can be used on children 4 or 5 years old, it is more beneficial for children who are still too young to understand cooperation. Basically, the child is wrapped in a sheet, which effectively limits the movement of the extremities and also gives the technique its name (Fig. 12–17). There are many ways to use sheets or blankets for immobilizing infants and small children, and other mummification variations exist. Again, the technologist is limited only by imagination.

Commercial Restraints

Commercial restraints usually take one of two forms: upright restraint devices and restraint boards. One of the most common and useful upright restraint devices is the Pigg-O-Stat (Fig. 12–18). This device is made of radiolucent materials and can be useful for upright chest and abdominal radiographic examinations. It is large enough to accommodate children up to about 3 years of age. Once secured, the patient can be rotated 360 degrees to demonstrate various oblique and lateral positions. Examinations are facilitated by a built-in, adjustable lead shield for gonadal protection, respiration phase indicators, and left and right markers. Because the Pigg-O-Stat is made of clear plastic, patient movement is easily observable during exposures. It holds the child securely and safely and greatly reduces the need for repeated exposures or the necessity of having someone hold the patient. One disadvantage of the device is possible **artifacts** caused by the plastic sides, which can overlap the anatomic area of interest.

Another type of commercial restraint device occasionally used in radiology departments is the restraint board (sometimes called a circumcision board). Even though several variations of restraint boards exist, all consist basically of a contour-fitting pad, mold, or sponge with attached Velcro straps for securing the patient (Fig. 12–19). The restraint board is a good way to immobilize an infant or small child when radiographic studies of the abdomen are desirable. Like the upright restraint device, these restraint boards allow the child to be safely and securely immobilized while eliminating the need for someone to hold the child.

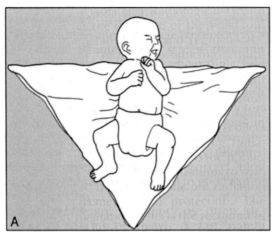

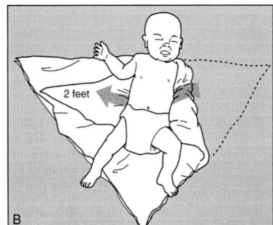

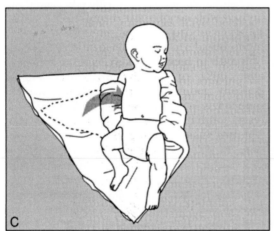

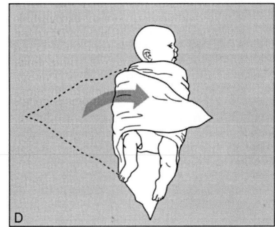

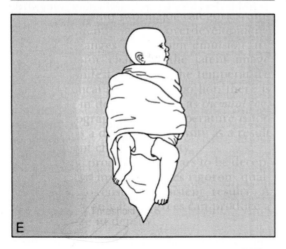

FIGURE 12–17. Sheet restraint (mummification technique) sequence. *A*, The child is placed in the center of a triangular folded sheet as shown so that the shoulders are just above the top fold. *B*, The left corner of the sheet is brought over the left arm and under the body so that about 2 ft of the sheet extends beyond the right side of the body. Make sure the child is not lying on the left arm. *C*, Tuck the 2 ft of sheet over the right arm and under the body. Again make sure the child is not lying on the arm. *D*, Bring the remaining sheet over the body. *E*, Tuck the sheet securely under the left side of the body. Remember that this technique restrains most movement but is not satisfactory as a complete immobilization procedure. Restraint bands are still required and the child should not be left alone, even long enough to make a radiographic exposure.

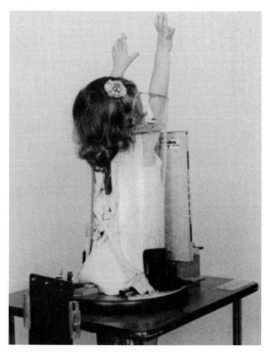

FIGURE 12–18. Patient positioned in Pigg-O-Stat for PA chest radiograph.

A modification of the Velcro strap restraint board is the Octastop board (Fig. 12–20). Octagonal metal frames are attached to the end of the board, and the child is restrained on the board with Velcro straps around the limbs and across the torso and head. The patient can then be rotated 360 degrees into eight different positions (Fig. 12–21). The disadvantage of the regular restraint board and the octagonal framed

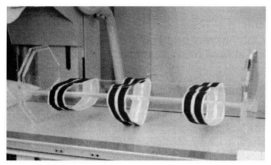

FIGURE 12–20. Octastop restraint board.

version is size. Only infants and small children up to 1 year old should be immobilized with these devices.

Noncommercial Restraints

A clever means of immobilizing the hands, fingers, feet, and toes of young patients is the use of a radiolucent Plexiglas paddle (Fig. 12–22). Little people have a tendency to wiggle fingers and toes. Applying gentle pressure to the affected area of interest aids the child in holding still while at the same time allowing the production of a diagnostic radiograph of the entire subject with one exposure.

One other immobilization technique worthy of consideration is the use of Velcro straps and tape. Velcro straps may be used in pediatric situations in much the same way as for adult applications. Because children are curious, they tend to be easily distracted by the new surroundings of a radiographic room with all its new information. With their attention wander-

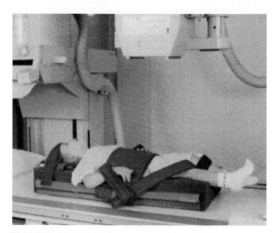

FIGURE 12–19. Pediatric patient in a Velcro strap restraint board.

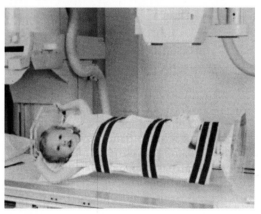

FIGURE 12–21. Child on Octastop restraint board in oblique position.

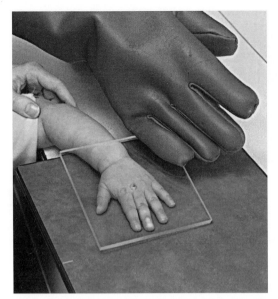

FIGURE 12–22. Positioning for pediatric PA hand radiograph using Plexiglas paddle.

ing from one new wonder to another, even the best rapport and communication may not be able to entirely overcome a slight bit of motion as the child continues to investigate the surroundings during the examination. Using Velcro straps for a 5- or 6-year-old during an upright chest examination not only keeps the patient more still but also serves as a reminder to the child that he or she should hold still.

Tape is also sometimes employed when immobilizing pediatric patients. Tape should be used more as a reminder to the patient to hold still than as an absolute restraining device. The radiographer should keep in mind that the skin of infants and young children is much more tender and sensitive than that of an adult. Caution should be taken when using tape to restrain so as not to abrade the skin of the child. When tape is used, it should be twisted where it comes in contact with the skin so that the nonadhesive side is in contact with the skin (Fig. 12–23A). Another technique to protect the skin is to place a gauze pad between the skin and the tape (Fig. 12–23B).

A stockinette is also an invaluable pediatric immobilization device. A stockinette is stretchable cotton fabric in the shape of a sleeve that is pulled over a fractured extremity before a plaster cast is applied. Its purpose is to prevent chafing and irritation of the skin while the limb is in the cast. It comes in a roll and can be cut to any length. A stockinette is effective as a restraint when pulled over the upper or lower extremities of a child and secured with tape. This is a good technique for immobilizing the upper limbs above and behind the child's head (Fig. 12–24).

Pediatric radiography is an art in itself, and it is a special radiographer who is its master. Conversely, radiography of a patient who is at the other extreme of age also requires a skillful and professional radiographer.

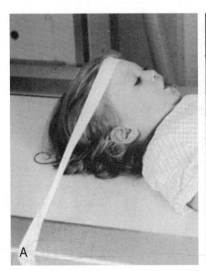
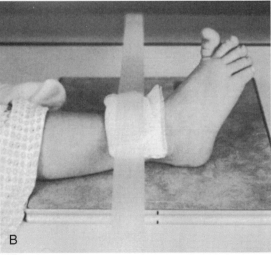

FIGURE 12–23. *A*, Patient positioned for AP skull radiograph with tape twisted across forehead. *B*, Gauze pad between skin and tape for an AP ankle radiograph.

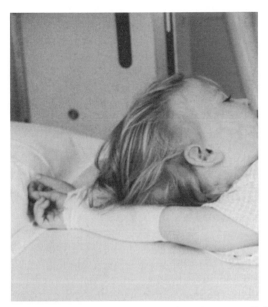

FIGURE 12–24. Pediatric patient with stockinette applied to upper extremities.

GERIATRIC APPLICATIONS

Radiographic studies on **geriatric** patients can be difficult, but the radiographer can make the examination go much more smoothly if a few considerations are kept in mind. The first of these considerations is security.

Often, one of the greatest concerns of an older person is fear of falling. A natural part of the aging process is loss of mobility, agility, and sense of balance. What would be considered a minor fall for a younger person may often have catastrophic results for an elderly person. Therefore, in addition to communication and rapport, the radiographer must take extra care to make a geriatric patient feel secure. This always includes patience in allowing for extra time during the examination so that the geriatric patient does not feel rushed or hurried. Using an extra assistant or two to help move the older patient onto the radiographic table can increase the patient's feeling of security. Always take extra care not to make the geriatric patient feel disoriented by rushing through the examination or by quickly moving from one radiographic position to another. This will allow the geriatric patient to feel more relaxed and better able to concentrate on holding still, thus reducing the need for repeated exposures.

An often overlooked consideration of geriatric radiography that goes along with security is

keeping the patient warm. Elderly persons tend to become chilled easily. That fact along with the necessity of wearing thin hospital gowns and robes can add to the difficulty of a geriatric radiographic examination. If the patient is cold and concentrating on trying to keep warm, he or she will be less likely to be able to cooperate by maintaining a radiographic position. If the elderly patient is going to be in the department for a long time or is undergoing a lengthy examination such as an excretory urogram, which requires an extended time on the radiographic table, the radiographer should cover the patient or offer extra blankets between radiographic exposures.

A third factor that can interfere with an older patient's ability to cooperate and maintain position is comfort, and this too must be considered during the radiographic examination. Just as security and warmth are part of patient comfort, consideration must be given to how long the geriatric patient must lie on the radiographic table. Radiographic tables are hard and cold. Many elderly patients are thin and more conscious of the hardness of the table. To enable the geriatric patient to more easily and fully cooperate, a radiolucent pad should be placed on the table before the examination (Fig. 12–25). A radiographic examination that might take 20 to 30 minutes can seem like an eternity on an unpadded radiographic table. Additionally, a sponge or radiolucent pad beneath the patient's knees can greatly reduce strain on the patient's back and increase the patient's ability to cooper-

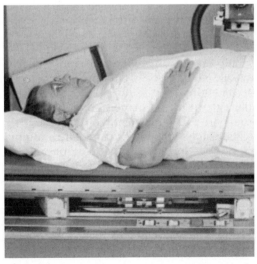

FIGURE 12–25. Geriatric patient on radiolucent pad.

ate during the examination. A disadvantage of using a pad is the possibility for slight artifact production or loss of radiographic detail because of increased object-to-film distance. In some instances, this might be objectionable to a radiologist.

While the previously mentioned aspects of security, warmth, and comfort should be considered for all patients, these elements are of extra importance for geriatric patients and can greatly reduce the amount of stress to the patient and radiographer during a radiographic examination if extra emphasis is placed on them.

Summary

Although patient immobilization is only one of many factors in the production of a successful radiographic study, awareness of the various elements to be considered in immobilization techniques must be a part of the radiographer's professional repertoire.

Before learning the various methods of immobilization and restraint that are pertinent to radiographic studies, the radiographer must first understand that immobilization techniques are used to eliminate or minimize movement by the patient and to enhance the proper positioning of the anatomic area of interest. Appropriate use of immobilization or restraint techniques can greatly reduce the negative effects of movement or improper positioning on the diagnostic quality of the finished radiograph.

The skill that may be the single most important technique in patient immobilization and the one that must be developed by all radiographers is high-quality communication. Quality communication allows the patient to become an active participant and assistant in the radiographic examination, thus accelerating the examination and reducing the need for repeated exposures. Two key essentials for effective communication are explanation and establishment of rapport with the patient.

The range of immobilization techniques runs from simple involvement, such as the use of a positioning sponge or sandbag to reduce patient motion, to rather involved techniques, such as sheet restraints in pediatric radiographic studies or making decisions about removal of traction splints in trauma situations. Within this range are a significant number of different immobilization techniques and considerations for their use. The radiographer should be familiar with all of these applications and be able to adapt them to fit each radiographic situation and patient condition.

Some of the more commonly used routine immobilization methods are positioning sponges, Velcro straps, compression bands, sandbags, and head clamps. There are many ways to use these sundry methods of immobilization, and their use is limited only by the creativity of the radiographer.

Because immobilization is one of the most critical aspects of trauma radiography, the radiographer should be familiar with numerous trauma immobilization devices, methods for producing diagnostic radiographs with these devices in place, and when it is appropriate to remove these devices for further radiographic studies. Some of these trauma immobilization devices are cervical collars, backboards, air splints, traction splints, and antishock garments.

One area of radiography that often requires the use of immobilization methods is pediatric radiography. Perhaps the most effective method of immobilization is establishing rapport with the young patient. Methods for pediatric immobilization with which the radiographer should be acquainted are sheet restraints, upright and board restraint devices, radiolucent paddles, stockinettes, and the correct use of tape.

Although radiographic examination of geriatric patients can be difficult, certain considerations can greatly facilitate these studies. In addition to communication, rapport, and respect, key considerations for successful geriatric radiography are security, warmth, and comfort.

Familiarity with various immobilization techniques is one aspect of the art of radiography that enables the radiographer to attain the highest levels of professional standards—that is, the production of optimal diagnostic quality images with the least amount of radiation exposure to patient, radiographer, and ancillary personnel.

◀R REVIEW QUESTIONS

1 Voluntary motion is under the control of the:
   a) technologist
   b) patient
   c) radiologist
   d) student

2 The most important communication that occurs in a radiology department takes place between the radiographer and the:

a) administrator
b) patient
c) radiologist
d) student

3 A key component to effective communication with a patient is:
a) establishing rapport
b) assessing the patient's physical condition
c) introducing the patient to the radiologist
d) giving a detailed, technical explanation of the examination

4 What is the most commonly used immobilization device?
a) sheet restraint
b) cervical collar
c) positioning sponge
d) Velcro straps

5 Which of the following might be used to immobilize a patient for an upright lateral chest radiograph?
a) sandbags
b) Velcro straps
c) head clamps
d) positioning sponge

6 Which of the following is an example of a spinal trauma immobilization device?
a) air splint
b) antishock garment
c) traction splint
d) backboard

7 When is it permissible to remove a cervical collar?
a) before the initial radiographic examination
b) after a radiographer reads the radiograph and approves removal
c) after a radiologist reads the radiograph and approves removal
d) after a paramedic reads the radiograph and approves removal

8 Which of the following devices might be encountered by a radiographer when hemorrhaging is suspected as a result of pelvic trauma?
a) air splint
b) compression band
c) antishock garment
d) traction splint

9 What is an important initial consideration for pediatric radiography?
a) what method of sheet restraint to use
b) which position to radiograph first
c) the proper use of tape
d) establishment of rapport with the patient

10 One of the greatest fears of a geriatric patient is:
a) falling
b) not being able to hear the radiographer
c) having to lie on a radiolucent pad
d) getting lost on the way to the radiology department

BIBLIOGRAPHY

Ballinger P: Merrill's Atlas of Radiographic Positions and Radiologic Procedures. 7th ed. St. Louis, Mosby-Year Book, 1991.

Bontrager K, Anthony B: Textbook of Radiographic Positioning and Related Anatomy. 3rd ed. St. Louis, CV Mosby, 1993.

Campbell J: Basic Trauma Life Support. 2nd ed. Englewood Cliffs, NJ, Prentice-Hall, 1988.

Darling D: Radiography of Infants and Children. 3rd ed. Springfield, IL, Charles C Thomas, 1979.

Ehrlich R, Givens E: Patient Care in Radiography. 4th ed. St. Louis, CV Mosby, 1993.

Gurley L, Callaway W: Introduction to Radiologic Technology, 4th ed. St. Louis, CV Mosby, 1996.

Torres L: Basic Medical Techniques and Patient Care for Radiologic Technologist. 5th ed. Philadelphia, JB Lippincott, 1997.

Wilmot DM, Sharko GA: Pediatric Imaging for the Technologist. New York, Springer-Verlag, 1987.

CHAPTER 13

VITAL SIGNS AND OXYGEN

Cheryl Oprisko, JD, RRT
Denise E. Moore, BS, RT(R)

Life is only known as the complex of many functions, and health as the integrity of these functions, each in itself and in harmony.

PETER LATHAM
GENERAL REMARKS ON THE PRACTICE OF MEDICINE

OBJECTIVES

On completion of this chapter, the student will be able to:

1 Discuss the significance of homeostasis.
2 Explain the mechanisms that adapt and maintain homeostasis.
3 Discuss the significance of each of the four vital signs: temperature, respiration, pulse, and blood pressure.
4 Identify the normal range for each of the vital signs.
5 Explain the implication of abnormal vital signs.
6 Describe how vital signs are assessed.
7 Explain the indications for administering oxygen therapy.
8 Identify high-flow and low-flow oxygen delivery devices.

9 Explain why caution must be used in performing radiographic procedures on patients receiving oxygen therapy.

10 Describe the use and radiographic appearance of various chest tubes and lines.

GLOSSARY

Apnea: cessation of spontaneous ventilation

Atelectasis: absence of gas from part or the whole of the lungs, due to failure of expansion or reabsorption of gas from the alveoli

Body Temperature: a measurement of the degree of heat of the deep tissues of the human body.

Bradycardia: slowness of the heart beat, as evidenced by slowing of the pulse rate to less than 60 beats per minute

Bradypnea: abnormal slowness of breathing

Diaphoresis: profuse sweating

Diastolic: pertaining to dilatation, or period of dilatation, of the heart, especially of the ventricles

Dyspnea: difficult or labored breathing

Febrile: pertaining to or characterized by fever

Homeostasis: a constancy in the internal environment of the body, naturally maintained by adaptive responses that promote healthy survival

Hypertension: persistently high arterial blood pressure

Hyperthermia: abnormally high body temperature, especially that induced for therapeutic purposes

Hypotension: abnormally low blood pressure; seen in shock but not necessarily indicative of shock

Hypothermia: low body temperature

Hypoxemia: decreased oxygen tension (concentration) in the blood

Hypoxia: the reduction of oxygen supply to the tissue

Intubation: insertion of a tubular device into a canal, hollow organ, or cavity

Pleural Effusion: increased amounts of fluid within the pleural cavity, usually due to inflammation

Pneumothorax: the presence of air or gas in the pleural cavity

Pulse Oximeter: photoelectric device for determining the oxygen saturation of the blood

Sphygmomanometer: instrument for measuring blood pressure

Systolic: pertaining to contraction, or period of contraction, of the heart, especially that of the ventricles

Tachycardia: rapidity of the heart action, usually defined as a heart rate greater than 100 beats per minute

Tachypnea: abnormal rapidity of breathing

Ventilation: the mechanical movement of air into and out of the lungs

Vital Signs as an Indication of the Patient's Homeostasis Status

Homeostasis is a relative constancy in the internal environment of the body, naturally maintained by adaptive responses that promote healthy survival. The primary mechanisms that function to maintain homeostasis are the heart beat, blood pressure, body temperature, respiratory rate, and electrolyte balance. These adaptive response mechanisms are continuously interacting with and adjusting to changes originating within or outside the body, to maintain the constant internal environment identified as homeostasis. Every health care professional should have a fundamental comprehension of the mechanisms that function to maintain homeostasis. For example, vital signs are primary mechanisms that are able to adapt to responses, within or outside of the body, to maintain homeostasis. Collectively, the vital signs are body temperature, pulse rate, blood pressure, and respiratory rate. In addition, assessment of the patient's mental alertness (sensorium) is often reported along with the vital signs.

The vital signs, which can be obtained quickly in the clinical setting, are an objective noninvasive evaluation of the patient's immediate condition or response to therapy. Most notably, vital signs provide important information because they may reveal the first clue of adverse reactions to treatment. Improvement in a patient's vital signs is strong evidence that a given treatment is having a positive effect. For example, a decrease in the patient's heart rate and respiratory rate, toward normal, after oxygen therapy suggests a beneficial effect.

Body Temperature

DESCRIPTION

Body temperature is a measurement of the degree of heat of the deep tissues of the human body. The normal mean body temperature is about 37°C (98.6°F), with a daily variation of 0.5–1.0°C (1–2°F). Because humans are warm-blooded animals, the cells of the human body function best within a narrow range of temperature variations. Body temperature must maintain a relatively constant level despite extremes in environmental temperatures. *Thermoregulation* is the term used to describe the body's maintenance of heat production and heat loss. The hypothalamus plays an important role in regulating heat loss and can initiate peripheral vasodilatation and sweating (**diaphoresis**) to dissipate body heat. Likewise, the respiratory system also plays an important role by removing excess heat via ventilation. The hypothalamus also plays an important role in the preservation of heat by initiating shivering (to generate heat) and vasoconstriction (to conserve heat).

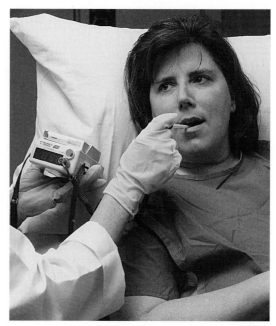

FIGURE 13–1. The most common method for measuring body temperature is the oral route, the thermometer being placed under the tongue.

MEASUREMENT

Four routes are commonly used to measure body temperature: oral, axillary, tympanic, and rectal. Oral measurements are obtained by placing a thermometer under the tongue. Depending on the type of thermometer used, electronic or glass bulb, the thermometer stays in place for 20 seconds to 3 minutes until a stable reading is obtained. Oral temperature readings are the most common method of determining the body temperature of an adult or a cooperative child (Fig. 13–1).

Axillary temperatures are obtained by placing the thermometer high between the upper arm and the torso. This method, used for children and infants, is notoriously inaccurate and time-consuming. The thermometer must remain in place 5 to 10 minutes to obtain a stable reading. The shortcomings make this technique almost useless.

Tympanic and rectal temperatures are the preferred readings for infants as well as for adults when oral temperatures are not feasible. Tympanic temperatures are obtained by placing an electronic thermometer in the ear. A stable reading is displayed within 3 seconds. To obtain rectal temperatures, the bulb of a rectal thermometer is lubricated and placed in the rectum of the patient for 2.5 to 5 minutes.

Body temperature readings may be measured in either degrees Fahrenheit (°F) or degrees Celsius (°C). Oral temperature readings in healthy adults and children are within the narrow range of 97.7° to 99.5°F (36.5° to 37.5°C) (Table 13–1). Axillary temperatures register slightly lower and rectal temperatures register approximately 1°F higher than oral readings.

SIGNIFICANCE OF ABNORMALITIES

When the oral temperature is higher than 99.5°F, a fever exists (**hyperthermia**). A patient

TABLE 13–1. **Normal Vital Signs**	
Sign	**Range**
Temperature	97.7°–99.5°F (36.5°–37.5°C)
Respirations	
Adult	12–20 breaths per minute
Child	20–30 breaths per minute
Pulse	
Adult	60–100 beats per minute
Child	70–120 beats per minute
Blood pressure	
Systolic	95–140 mm Hg
Diastolic	60–90 mm Hg

with a fever is said to be **febrile.** When the body temperature falls outside the normal range, for example with an illness or head injury, the metabolic rate changes accordingly, and the demands on the cardiopulmonary system also change. For example, when the body temperature increases, the metabolic rate also increases, resulting in more O_2 consumption and CO_2 production at the cellular level. As the metabolic rate increases, the cardiopulmonary system must work harder to meet the additional cellular demands, by providing more O_2 and eliminating CO_2. As a result of increased body temperature, an increase in cellular metabolism occurs; therefore, any event that increases cellular metabolism also increases body temperature.

Conversely, when the patient's temperature falls below the normal range, **hypothermia** is said to be present. While not common, hypothermia may be present in patients exposed to cold environmental temperatures and in those with trauma to the hypothalamus. Also, medically induced hypothermia is used during heart surgery to decrease the metabolic demands, therefore decreasing the demand on the cardiopulmonary system.

Fevers are common with viral and bacterial infections as a natural response of the human body to increase cellular activity to combat the invading organism. Likewise, a patient may become febrile for a day or two after a surgical procedure as the body responds to initiate healing. Prolonged fever in these patients is evidence of postoperative infection. The culprit is often an infection in the wound, lungs, or urinary tract. Patients suffering from a myocardial infarction might also be febrile because of increased cellular activity. Hyperthermia may also be a result of injury to the temperature-regulating center of the hypothalamus, causing it to set the thermostat at a higher level. This may occur as a result of a cerebrovascular accident, cerebral edema (swelling), or tumor.

Despite the increased body temperature in some disease states, cellular function is optimal within only a narrow temperature range. Prolonged hyperthermia can lead to serious complications and resultant cellular damage. Patients suffering from hyperthermia may become confused, dizzy, and even comatose. Conversely, hypothermia may be medically induced or may be the consequence of accidental exposure. Medically induced hypothermia is an attempt to therapeutically decrease the body's need for oxygen. Because temperature is an easily obtained indicator of the presence of disease, it is routinely followed as a yardstick of response to therapy for many conditions.

Respiratory Rate

DESCRIPTION

While assessing a patient's respiratory rate, the health care professional obtains a general impression of the respiratory system functioning. The respiratory system is responsible for delivering oxygen from the environment to the tissues and eliminating carbon dioxide from the tissues to the environment. The cells of the body require a constant supply of oxygen for cellular metabolism. As a result of cellular metabolism, the waste product carbon dioxide is produced. Unless oxygen is continually supplied and carbon dioxide is continually eliminated, death will occur. Consequently, failure of the respiratory system is a life-threatening event.

MEASUREMENT

The major muscle of **ventilation** is the diaphragm. During inspiration, the diaphragm contracts, moving downward in the abdominal cavity and pushing the abdominal contents outward. The downward movement of the diaphragm causes an expansion of the chest cavity, and air rushes into the lungs. Expiration is achieved by simple relaxation of the diaphragm. As the diaphragm relaxes, it returns to its original position at the floor of the chest cavity. This action causes the pressure of air in the lungs to increase. Subsequently, air flows out of the lungs, escaping to the environment (Fig. 13–2).

In a healthy adult, a single respiration consists of an inspiratory phase and an expiratory phase. Because the diaphragm is responsible for the movement of air in and out of the lungs, respirations are often counted by observing the movement of the abdomen. A respiratory rate may also be obtained by observing the rise (inspiration) and fall (expiration) of the chest. However, abdominal and chest wall movement may be difficult to detect by observation alone. This is particularly true with patients who are breathing shallowly. In this case, a hand may be placed on the patient's abdomen or chest to assist in assessing each respiration. However, it is best to obtain a patient's respiratory rate with-

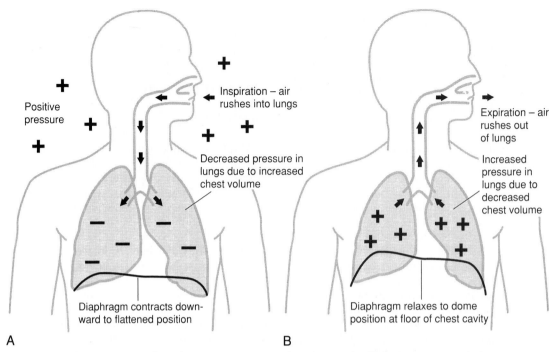

Positive pressure

Inspiration – air rushes into lungs

Decreased pressure in lungs due to increased chest volume

Diaphragm contracts downward to flattened position

Expiration – air rushes out of lungs

Increased pressure in lungs due to decreased chest volume

Diaphragm relaxes to dome position at floor of chest cavity

A

B

FIGURE 13–2. Normal ventilation. *A,* During normal inspiration, the diaphragm contracts, causing an expansion of the chest cavity. This expansion decreases the pressure in the lungs to below the atmospheric pressure; consequently, air rushes into the lungs. *B,* During normal expiration, the diaphragm relaxes, returning to its original position at the floor of the chest cavity and causing a decrease in the volume of the chest cavity. The decrease in chest cavity volume increases the pressure of air in the lungs to above atmospheric pressure, so that air flows out of the lungs.

out the patient's knowledge. This is true because patients aware that their respirations are being monitored often alter their breathing rate and pattern. Therefore, after obtaining a pulse rate, many health care professionals leave their hand on the patient's wrist and count the respiratory rate, while the patient assumes a pulse rate is still being assessed.

In the healthy adult, normal respirations are silent and effortless, automatically occurring at regular intervals. Respiratory rates are measured as the number of breaths per minute with the normal range at rest of 12 to 20 breaths per minute (see Table 13–1). Children under the age of 10 have slightly increased rates, averaging between 20 and 30 breaths per minute. Newborn respiratory rate averages between 30 and 60 breaths per minute. Since respiratory rates are increased in children, it is important to count respirations for a minimum of 1 minute to obtain an accurate measurement. Also, while counting respirations, the health care professional assesses the depth (shallow, normal, or deep) and pattern (regular or irregular) of venti-

lation. Therefore, by assessing the rate, depth, and pattern, an overall impression of the respiratory system may be obtained.

SIGNIFICANCE OF ABNORMALITIES

Any deviation from normal indicates a change in the status of the respiratory system. If cellular metabolism increases, the demand for oxygen increases, as does the production of carbon dioxide. The respiratory system responds by increasing the respiratory rate to deliver additional oxygen to the blood. Likewise, with increasing respiratory rates more CO_2 will be exhaled by the lungs. **Tachypnea** is the term used to describe respiratory rates greater than 20 breaths per minute. Common causes of tachypnea include exercise, fevers, anxiety, pain, infection, heart failure, chest trauma, decreased oxygen in the blood, and central nervous system disease.

Bradypnea is the term used to describe a decrease in respiratory rate. Bradypnea occurs much less frequently than tachypnea. Bradypnea results from depression of the respiratory center of the brain common with drug overdoses, head trauma, and hypothermia. **Dyspnea** is a common term used to describe difficult breathing. **Apnea** is the term used to identify the absence of spontaneous ventilation; it is an ominous sign.

Pulse

DESCRIPTION

The cardiovascular system is a closed fluid system composed of a pump (the heart) and many blood vessels. When the left ventricle of the heart contracts, blood is pumped out of the heart into the aorta and throughout the arteries of the body. The function of the cardiovascular system is to transport oxygenated blood from the lungs to the cells of the body and to return unoxygenated blood back to the heart and lungs to become reoxygenated. Also, the cardiovascular system transports CO_2 from the cells to the lungs for removal.

As previously stated, the cells of the human body require a constant supply of oxygen to function. Therefore, any impairment to the cardiovascular system will result in decreased oxygen to the cells and injury. Further, if the heart stops beating, death is imminent.

MEASUREMENT

Under normal conditions, the pulse can be palpated at superficially located arteries. Three common sites are the radial artery, on the thumb side of the wrist; the brachial artery, in the antecubital fossa of adults and upper arm of infants; and the carotid artery in the neck (Fig. 13–3). Femoral pulses often are palpated during cardiac arrest, but this site is not routinely used to obtain pulse rates. Since the pulse rate reflects the rapidity of each heart contraction, pulse rates may also be obtained by listening to the chest with a stethoscope for each heart beat. Pulses obtained in this manner are called *apical* pulses (Fig. 13–4).

Pulse rates are recorded in number of beats per minute. It is important to count the pulse rate for 1 minute for an accurate measurement. Resting pulse rates in the normal adult have a variation of 60 to 100 beats per minute (see

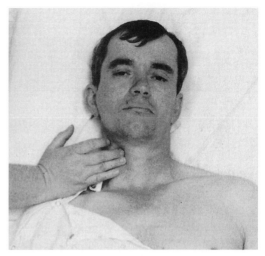

FIGURE 13–3. One of the common sites for measuring pulse is the carotid artery in the neck.

Table 13–1). A normal pulse for children under the age of 10 is anywhere between 70 and 120 beats per minute.

In critical care settings, patients' arterial oxygen saturation (SaO_2), respiratory rate, and pulse rate are continuously monitored. An example of devices that can provide continuous monitoring are electrocardiograms, arterial lines, and pulse oximeters. Electrocardiograms continually monitor the patient's pulse rate and rhythm. Electrodes placed on the patient's chest monitor the electrical activity of the heart and transform

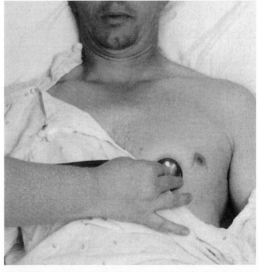

FIGURE 13–4. Apical pulses can be obtained by listening to the chest with a stethoscope.

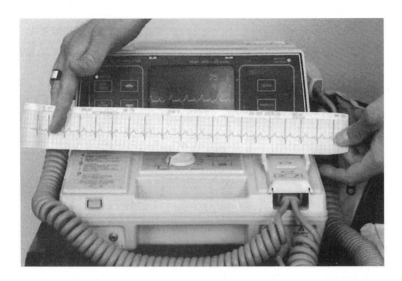

FIGURE 13–5. Electrodes placed on the patient's chest transform the electrical activity into pulse rate values and wave forms visible on a monitor.

that electrical activity to pulse rate values and wave forms visible on a monitor (Fig. 13–5).

An arterial line is a catheter inserted into an artery. The catheter is connected to a pressure transducer that is attached to a monitor. A continual measurement of the patient's heart rate and blood pressure is visible on the monitor.

A **pulse oximeter** is a noninvasive device used to provide ongoing assessment of the hemoglobin oxygen saturation of arterial blood. It displays the pulse rate as well. A light-emitting probe is placed on the finger, foot, toe, earlobe, temple, nose, or forehead of a patient. Arterial oxygen saturation and pulse rate are determined by measuring absorption of selected wavelengths of light by the circulating blood. The oximeter converts the light intensity information into oxygen saturation and pulse rate values (Fig. 13–6).

Several factors may affect the accuracy of electronic devices used to monitor pulse rates. Patient movement may give rise to inaccurate readings. Misplaced or loose electrodes, lines, or probes also yield inaccurate values. Low blood pressure and nail polish are common causes of pulse oximetry inaccuracies. However, when the factors or situations that limit the device's precision are corrected, these monitoring instruments provide reliable, continual, and rapid assessment of patients.

SIGNIFICANCE OF ABNORMALITIES

Because the cardiovascular system is responsible for delivering oxygenated blood to the cells, when cellular demand for oxygen increases, the heart responds by sending more blood to the

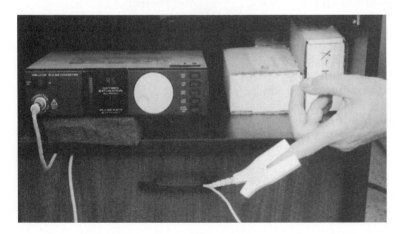

FIGURE 13–6. A pulse oximeter can be used to display a patient's pulse and oxygen saturation.

tissues. The heart accomplishes this by increasing the number or force of each contraction. When heart contractions, and therefore pulse rates, increase by more than 20 beats per minute in the resting adult or reach a rate greater than 100 beats per minute, the patient is said to be experiencing **tachycardia.** Exercise, fever, anemia, respiratory disorders, congestive heart failure, hypoxemia, and shock may all cause a patient to become tachycardic because of the increased cellular demands for oxygen. Pain, anger, fear, anxiety, and medications may also induce tachycardia, but the stimulus is through the nervous system, not an increased demand for oxygen.

Bradycardia refers to a decrease in heart rate. While pain may initially cause tachycardia, unrelieved severe pain may in fact lead to bradycardia and subsequent heart problems or failure. Also, bradycardia may be seen in hypothermia and in physically fit athletes.

If no pulse can be felt at the wrist, or in the event that cardiac arrest is suspected, the pulse should be assessed at the carotid artery for a full 5 seconds while emergency help is summoned.

If pulse irregularities are accompanied by patient complaints of palpitations, dizziness, or feeling faint, a physician should be notified, since these irregularities can be life threatening.

Blood Pressure

DESCRIPTION

Blood pressure is a measure of the force exerted by blood on the arterial walls during contraction and relaxation of the heart. An analogy can be made to water being pumped through a hose. A constant pressure is exerted on the inner surface of the hose by the water. When pumping occurs, the pressure increases as more water is added to the system, causing the water to flow. A similar situation exists in the human body. The pump is the heart, arterial blood vessels are analogous to the hose, and the fluid component is blood instead of water. A constant pressure is still exerted on the arterial vessels by the blood when the heart is relaxed. This pressure is called the **diastolic** pressure. During a contraction of the heart, blood is ejected from the left ventricle into the arterial blood vessels, creating an increase in pressure. The peak pressure present during contraction of the heart is known as the **systolic** pressure.

MEASUREMENT

Blood pressure readings are obtained with the use of a **sphygmomanometer** and stethoscope. The cuff of the sphygmomanometer is placed on the upper arm midway between the elbow and shoulder. Inflation of the cuff above the patient's systolic pressure stops blood flow to the arm by collapsing the brachial artery. With the stethoscope placed over the brachial artery in the antecubital fossa of the elbow, the cuff of the sphygmomanometer is slowly deflated. When cuff pressure no longer exceeds the internal pressure of blood in the brachial artery, blood flow returns and can be heard through the stethoscope. The first sound of blood flow is the systolic pressure. When the sound of blood flowing through the arm can no longer be heard, the diastolic pressure is reached (Fig. 13–7). Blood pressures are recorded in millimeters of mercury (mm Hg) with systolic measurements recorded over diastolic measurements (systolic/diastolic).

Normal blood pressure readings in the healthy adult range from systolic pressure of 95 to 140 mm Hg and diastolic pressure of 60 to 90 mm Hg (see Table 13–1). Pressures are most often recorded with the patient in a sitting position and the arm at about the level of the heart. Variations of these conditions may cause some difference in blood pressure readings.

SIGNIFICANCE OF ABNORMALITIES

The persistent elevation of blood pressure above 140/90 mm Hg is known as **hypertension.** Hypertension is common, but patients are usually unaware of its existence because there are no symptoms. Hypertension causes a significant increase on the workload of the heart. Extreme elevations in the blood pressure can damage the brain within minutes. More moderate degrees of hypertension can cause damage to the heart, brain, kidneys, lungs, and other organ systems. In addition to various disease states, stress, medications, obesity, and smoking can contribute to hypertension. The incidence of hypertension is higher in men than in women, and it is twice as common in black people as in white.

Hypotension is identified by a blood pressure of less than 95/60 mm Hg. In a healthy adult without any accompanying symptoms, hypotension presents no cause for alarm. A hypo-

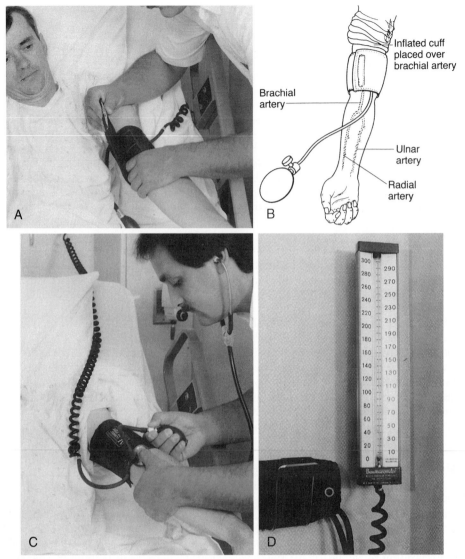

FIGURE 13–7. Blood pressure is obtained by use of a sphygmomanometer and a stethoscope. *A*, The cuff of the sphygmomanometer is placed on the upper arm midway between the elbow and shoulder and is then inflated. *B*, Proper placement of the cuff. *C*, The stethoscope is placed over the brachial artery. Gradually release the cuff pressure and listen for pulse changes through the stethoscope. *D*, A sphygmomanometer gauge. (*B* reprinted with permission from Craig M: Introduction to Ultrasonography and Patient Care. Philadelphia, WB Saunders, 1992.)

tensive patient complaining of dizziness, confusion, or blurred vision may have an inadequate circulating blood volume, and further evaluation needs to be initiated immediately. A patient in shock from severe bleeding, burns, vomiting, diarrhea, trauma, or heat exhaustion is hypotensive as a result of a decrease in total blood volume. These individuals require immediate care.

Oxygen Therapy

The moment-to-moment sustenance of human life depends on a single external substance. This substance is so important that its absence in the environment causes irreversible damage to the brain in approximately 6 minutes. In its absence, production of cellular metabolism is grossly inadequate, and death ultimately occurs.

This substance is, of course, oxygen, which is essential to each of the billions of cells making up the human body. Oxygen is a colorless, tasteless, and odorless gas that plays a critical role in efficient cellular metabolism. Oxygen is not flammable, but it does support combustion. Oxygen constitutes 21% of atmospheric gases.

The need for oxygen becomes critical to patients when the internal environment of the body is not consistent. Normally, 21% of oxygen maintains homeostasis. However, when oxygenation levels become low, the metabolic rate is compromised and the patient's homeostasis is altered. Accordingly, the patient's cardiopulmonary system has to adapt to **hypoxemia** to maintain homeostasis. Approximately one third of all patients in acute care settings have oxygen therapy of some type. The overall goal of oxygen therapy is to maintain adequate tissue oxygenation while minimizing cardiopulmonary work.

INDICATIONS FOR OXYGEN THERAPY

The primary clinical indications for oxygen administration are to correct hypoxemia or suspected tissue hypoxia; to prevent or minimize the increased cardiopulmonary workload (increased heart rate, blood pressure, and respiratory rate). Tissue **hypoxia** is a term used to describe the inadequate amount of oxygen at the cellular (tissue) level. The tissues most sensitive to hypoxia are the brain, heart, lungs, and liver. When hypoxia is present, the metabolic rate of the body is compromised, resulting in altered homeostasis.

To compensate for hypoxia, respiratory rates, depth of breathing, blood pressure, and heart rates increase. A hypoxic patient feels short of breath and has to work harder to breathe, thereby allowing the body's adaptive response mechanisms to function to maintain homeostasis. At this time, oxygen therapy is administered to alleviate the cardiopulmonary work. As a result, blood pressure, heart rate, and respiratory rate and depth return toward normal.

OXYGEN AS A DRUG

Oxygen is listed in the *U.S. Pharmacopeia* and is defined as being a drug in the Federal Food, Drug, and Cosmetic Act of 1962. Like any drug, oxygen has both good and bad biologic effects.

As such, the minimum dose should always be given to obtain the desired result, and no more. Oxygen, therefore, must be prescribed by a physician. In terms of dosage and depending on equipment, oxygen usually is ordered either in liters per minute or as a concentration. When a concentration is prescribed, it may be either a percentage, such as 24%, or a fractional concentration (FIO_2), such as 0.24. Once the desired result is achieved, the dosage is maintained and the patient's response is continually monitored.

Oxygen Devices

The radiologic technologist will encounter a variety of devices used to deliver oxygen. Most of these devices in no way hamper the technologist's ability to perform radiologic procedures, although sometimes repositioning of the devices is necessary to avoid artifacts on the film. If the oxygen device must be repositioned, it is the responsibility of the technologist to ascertain that any tubing leading to the device is not kinked or disconnected and that the device is properly repositioned on the patient at the conclusion of the radiologic procedure. *Under no circumstances should an oxygen device be completely removed from the patient for the purpose of taking a radiograph without the consent or supervision of a physician or attending nurse.*

Oxygen devices are divided into low-flow and high-flow delivery systems. A high-flow device, sometimes referred to as a fixed-performance device, supplies a consistent oxygen concentration for the patient and provides his or her entire inspiratory volume. The inspired concentration of oxygen does not change with altered breathing patterns. For example, if a patient exhibits a variable respiratory rate and has irregularly increasing and decreasing inspiratory volumes, the high-flow device supplies an exact oxygen concentration, no matter how much the patient's breathing fluctuates. A low-flow, or variable-performance, device does not supply a consistent oxygen concentration because it is incapable of providing all the gas required for patient inspiration. Because the device provides only part of the inspired gas, the delivered oxygen is diluted with room air. Consequently, the percentage of oxygen that a patient receives may fluctuate with a change in depth of respiration, respiratory rate, or breathing pattern.

NASAL CANNULA

The most common device used to deliver low concentrations of oxygen is the nasal cannula (Fig. 13–8). The nasal cannula delivers oxygen through short prongs inserted into the nares. Because the patient inhales oxygen from the cannula as well as room air, this is classified as a low-flow device. Usually, oxygen flow rates of 1 to 4 L/min are used, delivering approximately 24% to 36%. Flow rates over 6 L/min should not be used, since high flow rates can dry out the nasal mucosa and cause severe sinus pain. The nasal cannula is well tolerated by the patient because talking, eating, and sleeping are not hindered.

MASKS

Various kinds of masks, including simple, nonrebreathing, aerosol, and air-entrainment are used for oxygen therapy. A mask is generally not tolerated as well as a nasal cannula. Masks can be hot, and because they are made of plastic, they tend to stick to the patient's face. Masks need to be removed while eating. They muffle speech, and frequently the head strap does not fit well around the patient's head. Therefore, masks often become dislodged during sleep. Masks also increase the risk of aspiration in the patient who vomits. Despite these disadvantages, masks provide an effective way to deliver accurate as well as high concentrations of oxygen.

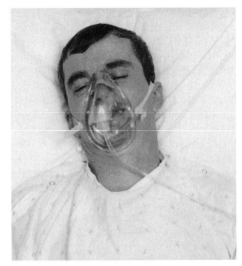

FIGURE 13–9. Simple oxygen mask.

Simple oxygen masks, low-flow devices, cover the patient's nose and mouth (Fig. 13–9). They require oxygen flow rates of higher than 5 L/min to prevent an accumulation of carbon dioxide. They are capable of delivering 35% to 60% oxygen, depending on the oxygen flow rate and the respiratory pattern of the patient. Although not commonly used, simple masks are convenient for short-term oxygen therapy.

A nonrebreathing mask may be used to deliver a higher percentage of oxygen (Fig. 13–10). These disposable units are constructed with one-way valves, preventing exhaled air from being rebreathed and ensuring that only oxygen from the device is inhaled. A partial rebreathing mask is similar to a nonrebreathing mask, but it does not contain the valve. Nonrebreathing masks have bags attached to them known as *reservoirs*. These reservoirs fill with oxygen. Because of the small volume of the reservoir, the partial rebreathing mask and nonrebreathing mask may not necessarily meet the total inspiratory demands of a patient exhibiting variable respiratory rates or variable inspiratory volumes. The masks should always be maintained with a liter flow high enough to keep the reservoir bag inflated. Theoretically, a high liter flow and a tight seal against the face should provide 100% oxygen. However, clinically these devices may deliver as little as 60% or as much as 90% oxygen, depending on how tightly the mask is affixed to the face.

Aerosol masks are commonly used when both high oxygen concentrations and humidity are

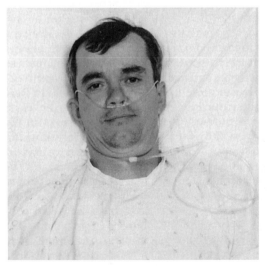

FIGURE 13–8. Nasal cannula.

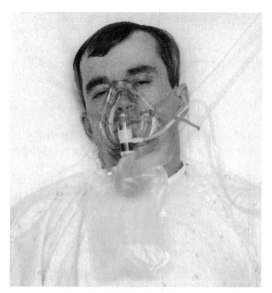

FIGURE 13–10. Nonrebreathing mask. (A partial rebreathing mask looks similar to this.)

needed (Fig. 13–11). Because therapeutic gases are extremely drying to the respiratory mucosa, the mask is attached to a bottle of sterile distilled water via corrugated tubing. To prevent carbon dioxide accumulation under the mask, the oxygen should never be adjusted to less than 6 L/min. Aerosol masks can deliver FIO_2 values of 21% to 100%.

The air-entrainment mask, a high-flow device, is constructed to provide an accurate concentration of oxygen to the patient by propelling a high velocity of source oxygen through a narrowed opening near the mask (Fig. 13–12). This results in room air being drawn into the mask. The source oxygen, along with the entrained room air, provides a flow of gas that is capable of meeting the total need of the inspiratory capacity of the patient. Therefore, it is essential for the purpose of maintaining accurate oxygen concentrations that the set liter flow not be altered. Air-entrainment masks provide consistent concentrations of oxygen, even though the patient's respiratory pattern may change. Depending on the manufacturer, air-entrainment masks generally can provide consistent FIO_2 values at 24%, 28%, 35%, 40%, and 50%.

In the patient's hospital room, these oxygen devices are usually attached to a wall outlet through which oxygen is piped. However, many times a patient who requires oxygen must be transported to the radiographic examination room. This is accomplished by attaching the tubing from the oxygen device to a portable oxygen cylinder that has two regulator valves (Fig. 13–13). One of the valves controls the pressure and indicates how full the cylinder is, and the other valve indicates the rate of oxygen flow, in liters, to the patient. Although oxygen cylinders and regulators are extremely durable, they should be secured during transport and

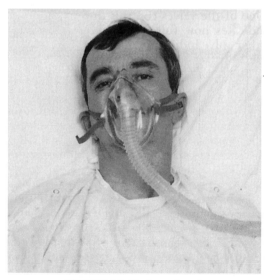

FIGURE 13–11. Aerosol mask.

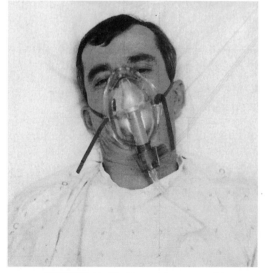

FIGURE 13–12. Air-entrainment mask.

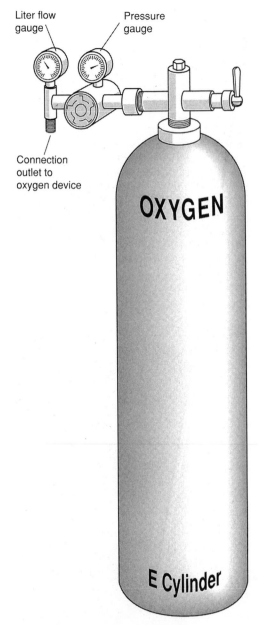

Liter flow gauge

Pressure gauge

Connection outlet to oxygen device

OXYGEN

E Cylinder

FIGURE 13–13. Typical portable oxygen cylinder.

use to prevent them from falling and possibly developing cracks or leaks.

TENT AND OXYHOOD

Pediatric patients requiring oxygen therapy and additional humidity can be found either in oxygen tents or in oxyhoods. An oxygen tent covers the child's bed. It is difficult to control the oxygen concentration in a tent, since frequent openings necessary for child care allow oxygen to escape. Because oxygen supports combustion, care should be exercised and machines that are likely to produce sparks should not be used in the vicinity of oxygen tents or free-flowing oxygen. Therefore, the technologist is responsible for ascertaining that the mobile x-ray unit is safe for use in combustible situations.

Oxyhoods are generally used on very small babies. The oxyhood consists of a disposable or permanent plastic box that fits over the infant's head (Fig. 13–14). Oxygen concentrations between 21% and 100% can be delivered in an oxyhood.

VENTILATORS

When the cardiopulmonary system of a patient is unable to supply adequate oxygen to the tissue, a patient may have an artificial airway inserted into the trachea, which is then connected to a mechanical ventilator (Fig. 13–15). The ventilator delivers a controlled respiratory rate, preset inspiratory volume, and consistent FIO_2. Frequently, a radiograph of the patient's chest is required to determine whether the artificial airway is in the proper place (Fig. 13–16). The attending nurse or respiratory care practitioner must be informed before the initiation of any radiologic procedure, because it is important that care be taken not to dislodge the artificial airway when positioning the patient or when adjusting the ventilator tubing. The radiographer must also be aware that proper head position is critical, since flexing or extending the head may adversely influence artificial airway placement.

If a mobile procedure is to be performed on a mechanically ventilated patient, the radiographer must carefully observe the rise and fall of the patient's chest to determine full inspiration or full expiration.

Audio and visual alarms on the ventilator monitor the patient's response. Occasionally, the alarms sound when the patient is repositioned. *These alarms should not be silenced or altered on the ventilator.* The nursing staff or respiratory care practitioners should assist the technologist in positioning the patient, thereby preventing accidental disconnection and patient endangerment.

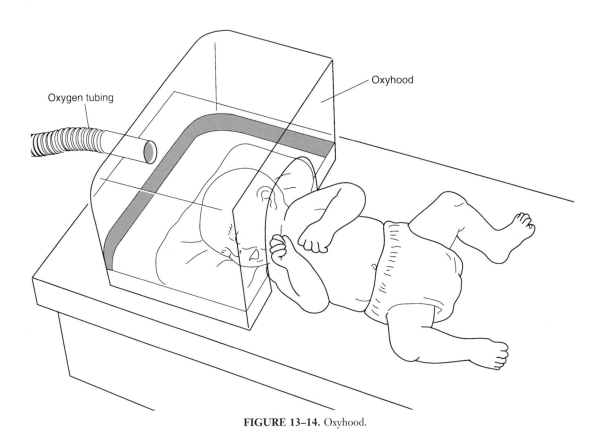

Oxygen tubing

Oxyhood

FIGURE 13–14. Oxyhood.

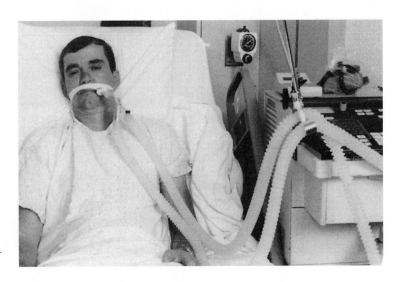

FIGURE 13–15. Mechanical ventilator.

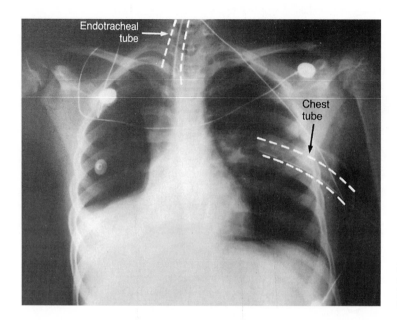

FIGURE 13–16. Chest radiograph of an 8-year-old girl demonstrating a properly placed endotracheal tube and a chest tube.

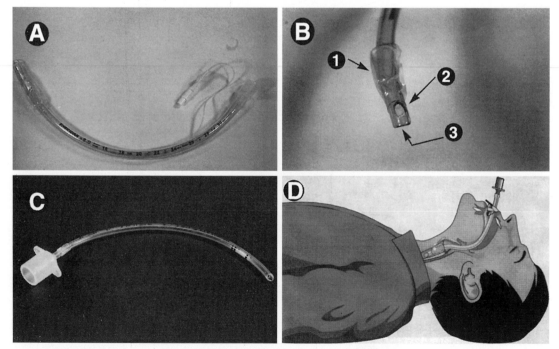

FIGURE 13–17. *A*, Adult endotracheal tube. *B*, Distal end of endotracheal tube with cuff deflated (1); side hole (2); and end hole (3). *C*, Pediatric endotracheal tube; note the absence of cuff. *D*, Patient intubated with an endotracheal tube. (From Moore DE: ET, CV, VAD, PA, Swan: What's It All About? Semin Radiol Technol 5(2):49, 1997. *D* originally from LifeART Collection Images; copyright 1989–1997 by TechPool Studios, Inc, Cleveland, OH.)

Chest Tubes and Lines*

Provided they are informed, radiographers can play an important role in the early detection of problems associated with malpositioned lines. As experts in radiographic quality, radiographers have a clear responsibility in this area that is separate from the issue of interpretation of images. Without any expectation of the radiographer to interpret the image from a pathologic diagnostic standpoint, when malpositioning is suspected, alerting the appropriate authority (eg, radiologist or attending physician) is both appropriate and beneficial to the patient.

ENDOTRACHEAL TUBES

Endotracheal tubes are used to manage a variety of respiratory complications (Fig. 13–17). Indications for use include: (1) a need for mechanical ventilation or oxygen delivery due to inadequate ventilation (breathing), inadequate arterial oxygenation, severe airway obstruction, shock, and parenchymal diseases that impair gas exchange; (2) upper airway obstruction; (3) pending gastric acid reflux or aspiration; and (4) provisions for tracheobronchial toilet (lavage).

Tracheal **intubation** is accomplished most often using a translaryngeal approach via the mouth or nose, but in certain cases, the use of a tracheostomy is necessary (Fig. 13–18). Other than during emergency situations and when administering anesthesia, the nasotracheal approach is preferred. Formerly, cuff structure and its pressure often damaged the tracheal mucosa, especially during long-term care; thus, in extended care settings, tracheostomies were often substituted. Today, endotracheal cuffs are softer and exert lower pressure on tracheal tissues and as such are more compatible with long-term use.

Once an endotracheal tube is inserted, placement of the tube is confirmed by chest radiography and is assessed periodically thereafter. Properly positioned tubes will show the distal tip 1 to 2 inches (3–5 cm) superior to the tracheal bifurcation (Fig. 13–19). The cuff is inflated with air and is positioned at midtrachea; however, the cuff is not radiographically apparent. The most common example of malpositioning involves intubation of the right main

*This section is extracted from Moore DE: ET, CV, VAD, PA, Swan: What's It All About? Semin Radiol Technol 5(2):49, 1997. Reprinted with permission.

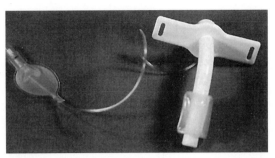

FIGURE 13–18. Tracheostomy tube. (From Moore DE: ET, CV, VAD, PA, Swan: What's It All About? Semin Radiol Technol 5(2):49, 1997.)

stem bronchus because it originates at the trachea at a lesser angle compared with the left main bronchus. Complications may include overventilation of the right lung and potential airway obstruction of the left. When the tip of the tube slides into the right main bronchus, it is possible for its shaft to occlude the left main bronchus, causing severe **atelectasis** of the left lung (Fig. 13–20).

Occasionally, endobronchial tubes are used to provide ventilation to one lung, as in the case of pneumonectomy, or to use two mechanical ventilators, one for each lung. Endobronchial tubes are designed so that the tip is inserted in one of the main stem bronchi. In such cases, the tip will locate in either the right or left system. Once inserted properly, two cuffs are inflated to anchor the endobronchial tube in

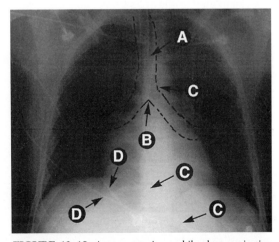

FIGURE 13–19. Anteroposterior mobile chest projection showing trachea (*dotted line*) with endotracheal tube (A) positioned approximately 2 inches superior to the carina (B); nasogastric tube (C); cardiac monitor leads/electrodes (D). (From Moore DE: ET, CV, VAD, PA, Swan: What's It All About? Semin Radiol Technol 5(2):49, 1997.)

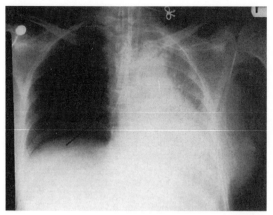

FIGURE 13–20. Intubation of right main stem bronchus with complete occlusion of the left bronchus causing left lung atelectasis. (From Moore DE: ET, CV, VAD, PA, Swan: What's It All About? Semin Radiol Technol 5(2):49, 1997.)

THORACOSTOMY TUBES

Thoracostomy (intrapleural) tubes, more commonly called chest tubes (Fig. 13–22), are used to drain the intrapleural space and the mediastinum (Fig. 13–23). Fluid or air accumulation, or both, in either space will have deleterious effects and may be life threatening, depending on volume.

The pleural cavity is a potential space in which parietal and visceral pleurae meet. A minimal amount of serous fluid exists to provide a lubricant for ease of movement between the two pleural layers during breathing. Negative pressure in the intrapleural space provides a suction-type mechanism between the lung and thorax that facilitates lung expansion. When fluids or air accumulate in the space, negative

position, one at the bronchial end and one in the trachea. When dual ventilation is used, a side hole in the endobronchial tube is positioned adjacent to the nonintubated bronchus to facilitate ventilation to the contralateral lung.

Radiographic demonstration of complications associated with tracheal intubation and mechanical ventilation include the following:

1 Bronchial intubation, most often involving the right main stem bronchus (Fig. 13–21)
2 Erosion of the tracheal mucosa due to cuff trauma causing subcutaneous or mediastinal emphysema
3 Pneumothorax

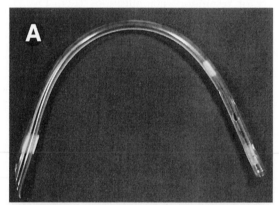

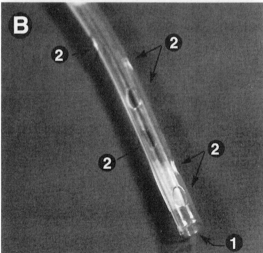

FIGURE 13–22. *A*, Thoracostomy tube. *B*, Thoracostomy tube: end hole (1) and side holes (2). (From Moore DE: ET, CV, VAD, PA, Swan: What's It All About? Semin Radiol Technol 5(2):49, 1997.)

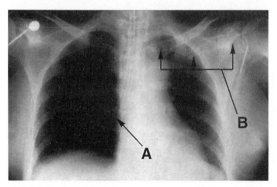

FIGURE 13–21. Distal tip of endotracheal tube in right main bronchus (A); central venous catheter in the left subclavian vein (B). (From Moore DE: ET, CV, VAD, PA, Swan: What's It All About? Semin Radiol Technol 5(2):49, 1997.)

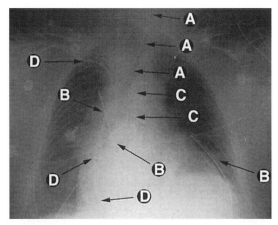

FIGURE 13–23. Postoperative cardiac surgery AP mobile chest projection showing endotracheal tube (A) approximately 2 inches superior to the carina; two chest tubes (B); mediastinal drain (C); pulmonary arterial catheter passing through the right atrium and ventricle (D) (tip in pulmonary artery not visible). Note cardiac monitor wires and electrodes. (From Moore DE: ET, CV, VAD, PA, Swan: What's It All About? Semin Radiol Technol 5(2):49, 1997.)

pressure is lowered or lost and the lung fails to fully expand. If pressure falls too low, the lung will collapse.

Thoracostomy tubes are inserted through the chest wall to re-establish negative intrapleural pressure in cases of **pneumothorax,** hemothorax, **pleural effusion,** and empyema. In addition to chest tubes, mediastinal drains (usually small chest tubes) are used after cardiac surgery to drain residual blood from the mediastinum. Postoperative blood accumulation around the pericardium can cause cardiac tamponade, which is a life-threatening event.

Insertion sites for thoracostomy vary depending on the intrapleural substances to be removed. In the case of hemothorax and pleural effusions, fluids flow with gravity and tend to accumulate near the lung base. Typical insertion sites in these instances are the fifth to six intercostal space, laterally at the midaxillary line. Tubes may also be inserted as high as the fourth and as low as the eighth rib. In cases of pneumothoraces, air will rise to the upper pleural spaces, requiring higher insertion sites in the apical region. Generally, the second to third intercostal space at the midclavicular line is preferred.

Pleural fluid accumulation becomes apparent radiographically when enough fluid is present to show costophrenic blunting. Once radiographically apparent, the angles typically show medial displacement. Costophrenic fluids may approach 300 mL or more before becoming radiographically evident on posteroanterior or anteroposterior chest projections, but as little as 150 mL of fluid may be visible on lateral decubitus views. Supine filming may obscure visualization of pleural fluids and should be avoided when possible.

Causes of pneumothorax include break in the continuity of the visceral pleura (rupture of an emphysematous bleb, fractured rib, central venous line insertion error), penetration of the external chest wall seen in trauma, or in rare instances, a gas-producing microorganism (empyema). When air accumulates in the intrapleural space, creating a loss of negative pressure, the lungs cannot fully expand, creating a space between the lung edge and the costal border.

Radiographically, pneumothoraces are shown when the increased density of the collapsed lung is contrasted with a lateral radiolucency that is absent of lung markings (Fig. 13–24). During inspiration, the lung expands laterally and meets the lateral rib edge, rendering small pneumothoraces that are difficult to detect. Therefore, pneumothoraces are best shown by expiratory posteroanterior or anteroposterior projections of the chest. Lateral decubitus filming with the ipsilateral side up may also be useful.

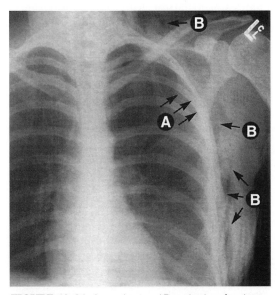

FIGURE 13–24. An expiratory, AP projection showing an approximate 10% pneumothorax on the left (A); also note moderate subcutaneous emphysema in the left chest wall extending up to the neck (B). (From Moore DE: ET, CV, VAD, PA, Swan: What's It All About? Semin Radiol Technol 5(2):49, 1997.)

After thoracostomy, sutures are applied to anchor the tube so patients can move with caution. Radiographic studies require erect or semierect filming whenever possible, and care must be exercised to avoid dislodging the tube. Partially dislodged tubes, leaks at the insertion site, and extracostal insertions may lead to subcutaneous emphysema (Fig. 13–24).

Various degrees of pneumothoraces exist. Small pneumothoraces are typically classified as simple and spontaneous, usually caused by a ruptured bleb, and may resorb naturally. Secondary pneumothoraces are complications of parenchymal disease or may be caused iatrogenically during central venous catheter insertion. Because of coexisting conditions and the fact that these patients are already in a compromised state, secondary pneumothoraces require chest tube evacuation of the pleural cavity.

Tension pneumothorax is a dramatic event that requires aggressive care. In these cases, air continues to enter the pleural cavity either through a valve-like opening in the external chest wall (trauma) or similar opening in the visceral pleura, whereby air continues to enter the pleural space but cannot escape. Pressure increases on the ipsilateral side causing a shift of the mediastinum toward the opposite side and producing a life-threatening event.

Tension pneumothorax may occur during mechanical ventilation. Rupture of the visceral pleura allows air to enter the pleural space without escape. Immediate aspiration of the intrapleural air relieves pressures and is standard treatment for tension pneumothorax.

CENTRAL VENOUS LINES

Central venous (CV) lines are catheters that are inserted into a large vein. They have a multitude of uses and descriptive terms. Initially, CV lines were developed to administer chemotherapeutic drugs and parenteral nutrition. Today they may also be used to administer a variety of drugs, manage fluid volume, serve as a conduit for blood analysis and transfusions, and monitor cardiac pressures.

Known commonly as central venous catheters and venous access devices, venous lines are also named by the developer. One of the first modern CV lines was developed by Broviac and later enlarged by Hickman. Leonard and Groshong catheters are also widely used. Groshong catheters have a unique rounded, closed-end tip with

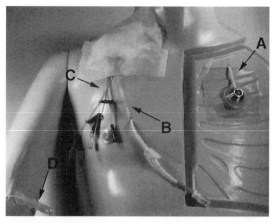

FIGURE 13–25. Various central venous catheters inserted in a model. Subcutaneously implanted port (A); tunneled catheter into subclavian vein (B); triple-lumen subclavian line (C); peripheral catheter in the antecubital area (D). (From Moore DE: ET, CV, VAD, PA, Swan: What's It All About? Semin Radiol Technol 5(2):49, 1997.)

a three-way valve mechanism that reduces the risk of blood loss and air embolism during withdrawals and infusions.

Catheters generally vary by size and composition and are available in single, double, and multiple lumens for short- and long-term care use. They are available as percutaneous catheters (subclavian insertion catheter), totally implanted access ports (Infusa Port, Port-a-Cath, Mediport), peripherally inserted central catheters (peripherally inserted central catheter lines) (Fig. 13–25), and externally tunneled catheters (Broviac, Hickman, Groshong) (Fig. 13–26). Implantable ports are desired when access is

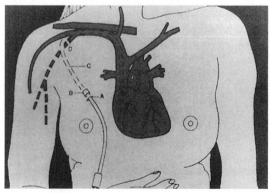

FIGURE 13–26. Tunneled catheter. Subcutaneous insertion site (A); catheter cuff (B); subcutaneous tunnel (C); subclavian insertion site (D). (From Infuse-a-Cath: Central Venous Catheter Nursing Manual. Beverly, MA, Strato Medical Corp, 1992.)

required intermittently over a long period of time.

Regardless of the style used, the goal is to position the catheter tip in a central vein. The preferred location is the superior vena cava, approximately 2 to 3 cm above the right atrial junction (Fig. 13–27). Superior vena caval placement is preferred because of its size. Infusions of intravenous fluids are much less caustic in central veins than in smaller, peripheral veins.

The most common insertion site for central venous catheters is the subclavian vein (see Fig. 13–27A). Other common sites include the internal jugular (Fig. 13–27D) and femoral veins. Recent technologic advancements in catheters

and safer insertion techniques now provide the opportunity to access the subclavian vein from a peripheral approach. When percutaneous subclavian and internal jugular approaches are contraindicated, the antecubital area may be accessed for line insertion. Ports used in conjunction with peripherally inserted central catheters are smaller than those used in a subcutaneous pocket in the thorax but functionally are identical.

Pulmonary arterial (PA) lines are commonly called Swan-Ganz catheters, so named for the developers of the catheter. PA lines are specialized, single, or multilumen CV lines that incorporate a small electrode at the distal end used

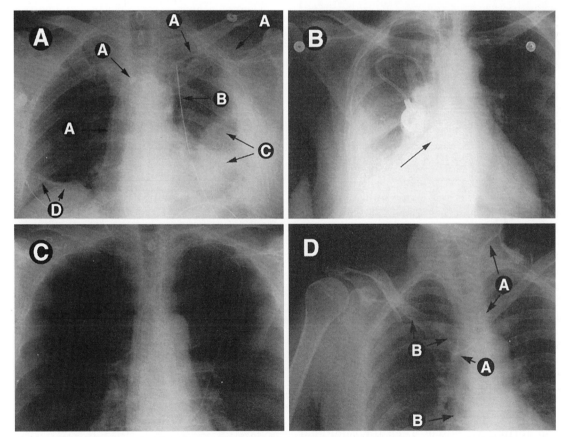

FIGURE 13–27. *A,* AP projection of the chest shows a subclavian catheter inserted from the left side and advanced to the superior vena cava (A); a thoracostomy tube (B) with moderate pleural infiltration in the left lung (C) and with some atelectasis noted in the right lung base (D). *B,* Implanted central venous port with its tip in the superior vena cava. The catheter does not cross midline when advanced from the right side. *C,* Groshong catheter subcutaneously tunneled into the left subclavian vein and advanced to the superior vena cava. *D,* Two central venous catheters are seen. A catheter is inserted into the internal jugular vein with its tip positioned in the proximal portion of the superior vena cava (A). A tunneled catheter is inserted from the right subclavian vein with its tip positioned lower in the superior vena cava (B). (From Moore DE: ET, CV, VAD, PA, Swan: What's It All About? Semin Radiol Technol 5(2):49, 1997.)

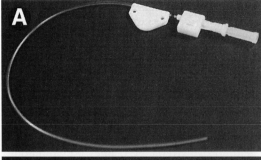

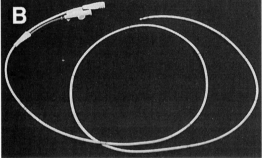

FIGURE 13–28. *A,* Single lumen central venous catheter. *B,* Single lumen pulmonary arterial catheter. Note the distal tip with a deflated balloon and electrode. During pressure measurement, the balloon in inflated, drifting the catheter into a small pulmonary artery where it wedges. The electrode at the tip of the catheter measures pulmonary pressure. (From Moore DE: ET, CV, VAD, PA, Swan: What's It All About? Semin Radiol Technol 5(2):49, 1997.)

PA-wedged pressure is indicative of left atrial pressure, which in turn is indicative of left ventricular pressure.

Other than PA lines, no central catheter should appear beyond the superior vena cava. In the case of PA lines, the distal tip will locate in one of the two pulmonary arteries (Fig. 13–29). During pressure recordings, the balloon floats and wedges in a small arterial branch. Balloon wedging is synchronized with the cardiac monitor and lasts momentarily to avoid potential ischemia and infarction of the lung. Pressure tracings are generated by the cardiac monitor during the wedge procedure. Once the measurement is complete, the balloon is deflated and blood flow beyond the catheter tip is resumed (Fig. 13–30).

Central venous access devices can improve and extend quality of life for many patients, but the potential for complications demands the attention of all members of the health care team. Reported incidence of CV complications vary, but those related to health care worker management of CV lines approach 55%. Managerial complications include catheter dislodgment and occlusions due to the accumulation of blood clots or drug precipitates. Catheter flushing procedures conducted by nursing staff

to monitor pulmonary arterial pressures (Fig. 13–28).

Pulmonary arterial lines are used to estimate left ventricular end-diastolic pressure. Access to the left ventricle requires an arterial approach, and because catheter placement in the left ventricle has major physiologic consequences, the safest way to assess left heart pressure is to extrapolate its value by monitoring right heart and pulmonary pressures. Cardiopulmonary circulation is a continuous network of vascular structures interconnected by valves. Some valves are open while others are simultaneously closed. When atrioventricular valves (tricuspid and bicuspid) are open, semilunar valves (pulmonary and aortic) are closed; when the semilunar valves open, the atrioventricular valves close.

Pulmonary arterial catheters have a balloon located at the distal end, and during pressure monitoring it is inflated, allowing the catheter tip to float and wedge in a small pulmonary artery. During this interval, the electrode, at the most distal end of the catheter, measures pulmonary arterial (wedged capillary) pressures.

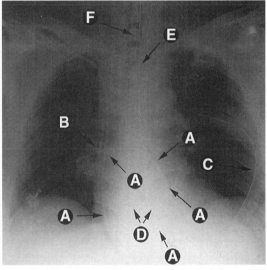

FIGURE 13–29. Postoperative AP chest projection showing several lines: pulmonary arterial catheter with the tip in the right pulmonary artery (A); a second central venous line seen in the superior vena cava (B); thoracostomy tube in the right lung (C); mediastinal drains (D); nasogastric tube in the esophagus (E); and endotracheal tube (F). (From Moore DE: ET, CV, VAD, PA, Swan: What's It All About? Semin Radiol Technol 5(2):49, 1997.)

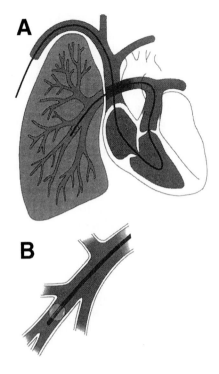

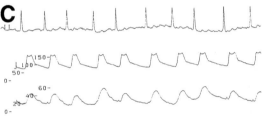

placed incorrectly at insertion time." Malpositioning, pinching, or kinking also occur with significant frequency. Pneumothorax and hemothorax are potential complications associated with catheter insertions (Fig. 13–32).

Radiographic confirmation of tube placement is essential at the time of insertion and thereafter as needed. Aberrant tip location is one of the most common complications associated with CV catheters. Additional medical imaging modalities may also prove useful when catheter placement is difficult or complications occur. For example, complications involving catheter fracture and subsequent migration can be resolved using angiography and fluoroscopy.

Recognition of catheter malposition requires thorough knowledge of CV structures and their branches. Typically, CV lines inserted from a right-sided approach will follow the course of the subclavian vein in lateromedial direction, then descend through the right brachiocephalic vein. From the right brachiocephalic vein, the catheter passes into the superior vena cava where it should terminate above the right

FIGURE 13–30. *A*, Pulmonary artery catheter passes through right atrium, right ventricle, and main pulmonary artery into the right pulmonary artery. *B*, Balloon of a pulmonary artery catheter inflated and wedged in a small pulmonary branch for wedge pressure measurement. *C*, Pulmonary artery pressure tracing. (From Moore DE: ET, CV, VAD, PA, Swan: What's It All About? Semin Radiol Technol 5(2):49, 1997. *A* and *B* originally from LifeART Collection Images, copyright 1989–1997 by TechPool Studios, Inc, Cleveland, OH.)

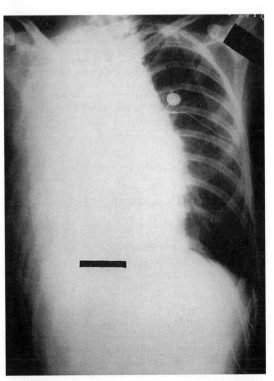

FIGURE 13–31. Right hydrothorax caused by displacement of a central venous line during dressing change; 1300 mL of IV fluids were evacuated via thoracentesis. (From Moore DE: ET, CV, VAD, PA, Swan: What's It All About? Semin Radiol Technol 5(2):49, 1997.)

help prevent occlusive problems. One of the most critical concerns of radiographers is catheter dislodgment, and this can be prevented only with increased awareness of the catheter's presence. Care must be exercised when handling patients with CV lines. Assessing the patient before performing radiographic procedures is essential to avert the possibility of line displacement (Fig. 13–31).

Regarding insertion problems, Eisenburg estimates, "up to one third of CV catheters are

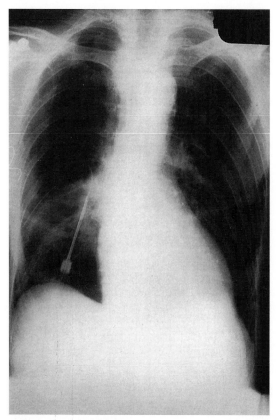

FIGURE 13–32. Pneumothorax on the right due to complications associated with central venous line insertion. Note a small angiographic catheter inserted to evacuate the pleural cavity and the oxygen tube across the lower field creating an artifactual distraction. (From Moore DE: ET, CV, VAD, PA, Swan: What's It All About? Semin Radiol Technol 5(2):49, 1997.)

atrium. Because of the right-sided position of the superior vena cava, as the catheter advances, its image should remain to the right of the vertebral column and should not cross midline (see Fig. 13–27B).

A left-sided approach involves a slightly longer catheter that is advanced lateromedially through the left subclavian vein to the left brachiocephalic vein. Because the left brachiocephalic vein courses in a relatively horizontal fashion as it crosses to the right of midline (see Fig. 13–27C), the catheter will traverse from left to right where it terminates in the superior vena cava with a short descending pattern. One problem associated with a left-sided approach is placement of the catheter tip in the thoracic duct. In this instance, the catheter does not cross midline. Checking for catheter position in orientation to the midline can be a simple way

to assess catheter position; right-sided approaches never cross midline, whereas a left-sided approach should always cross midline.

Although recognition of problems related to tubes and line usage is not specifically identified in the radiographer's scope of practice, an implied responsibility certainly exists. As techniques for patient care become more sophisticated, and as the team concept of health care management takes greater hold, practicing radiographers must direct attention to expanded learning opportunities to maintain clinical competency. In that regard, radiography remains a vital component of the health care team and improved patient care will result.

Summary

In summary, vital signs represent the primary mechanisms that function to maintain homeostasis. These mechanisms can adapt to changes within or outside of the body to maintain homeostasis. Therefore, the vital functions provide a relative constancy in the internal environment of the body to promote healthy survival. Assessment of vital signs is an objective noninvasive evaluation of the patient's immediate condition or response to therapy. Every health care professional should be competent in obtaining vital signs and understanding the significance of any abnormalities. Since the primary mechanisms that function to maintain homeostasis are represented by vital signs, accuracy in obtaining and recording the data is crucial.

The need for oxygen becomes critical to patients when the internal environment of the body is not consistent. Normally, 21% of oxygen maintains homeostasis; however, when the vital signs are abnormal, supplemental oxygen therapy is necessary. Supplemental oxygen therapy relieves the increased stress on the cardiopulmonary system.

Oxygen therapy may be administered by high-flow devices, such as air-entrainment masks, which deliver consistent concentrations of oxygen and supply entire inspiratory volumes as required by the patient. Oxygen therapy may also be delivered by low-flow devices, such as nasal cannulas, simple masks, aerosol masks, and nonrebreathing masks. Because of the variance of the patient's respiratory rate or change in breathing pattern, these devices provide neither consistent concentrations of oxygen nor the entire inspiratory volumes required by the patient.

Oxygen tents and oxyhoods are used to deliver oxygen to children requiring supplemental oxygen or humidity.

Ventilator patients require special care in handling, and ventilator alarms and settings must never be altered by the radiographic technologist.

It is important that radiographers understand the use and radiographic appearance of common chest tubes and lines, including endotracheal tubes, thoracostomy tubes, and central venous lines.

◀R REVIEW QUESTIONS

1 A patient presents to the emergency department with an oral temperature of 39.38°C. This finding is consistent with:
a) the normal temperature
b) hyperthermia
c) hypothermia
d) bradypnea

2 A patient is suspected to have suffered cardiac arrest. The pulse should be checked at the:
a) radial artery
b) brachial artery
c) carotid artery
d) femoral artery

3 The workload of the heart is significantly increased with:
a) hypertension
b) hypoxemia
c) tachypnea
d) all of the above

4 In the healthy adult the normal range for blood pressure is:
a) systolic 95 to 140 mm Hg, diastolic 60 to 90 mm Hg
b) systolic 60 to 90 mm Hg, diastolic 95 to 140 mm Hg
c) systolic 120 to 160 mm Hg, diastolic 80 to 100 mm Hg
d) systolic 60 to 80 mm Hg, diastolic 80 to 120 mm Hg

5 Monitoring vital signs helps evaluate which of the following?
a) homeostasis
b) response to therapy
c) life-threatening conditions
d) all of the above

6 Hypoxia is:
a) a drug that must be prescribed by a physician
b) necessary for cellular repair
c) a state describing oxygen-deficient tissue
d) necessary for cellular function

7 The body compensates for hypoxia by:
a) increasing the respiratory rate
b) increasing the depth of breathing
c) exhibiting cyanosis
d) both a and b

8 Which of the following devices can be classified as a high-flow oxygen delivery device?
a) air-entrainment mask
b) nasal cannula
c) simple mask
d) nonrebreathing mask

9 The device that delivers a specific inspiratory volume, respiratory rate, and concentration of oxygen is the:
a) air-entrainment mask
b) ventilator
c) nonrebreathing mask
d) nasal cannula

10 Oxygen therapy is administered for the purpose of:
a) relieving excessive work of the heart
b) relieving excessive work of breathing
c) relieving hypoxia
d) all of the above

BIBLIOGRAPHY

Bard Access Systems: Groshong Catheters. Salt Lake City, UT, Bard Access Systems, 1993.

Burton GC, Hodgkin J, Ward J: Respiratory Care. 4th ed. Philadelphia, JB Lippincott, 1997.

Carrasco C, Richli W, Charnsangave C, et al: Technical note: Repositioning misplaced central venous catheters. Cardiovasc Intervent Radiol 10:234, 1987.

Des Jardins: Cardiopulmonary Anatomy and Physiology. 3rd ed. Albany, New York, Delmar, 1997.

Eisenburg R: Fluid, electrolyte, and nutritional management of the surgical patient. *In* Diagnostic Imaging in Surgery. New York, McGraw Hill, 1987, p 1.

Erickson R: Mastering the ins and outs of chest drainage. Nursing 89:37, 1989.

Ferguson D: Cardiogenic shock. *In* Bennett C, Plum F (eds): Cecil Textbook of Medicine. Philadelphia, WB Saunders, 1996, p 477.

Freedman S, Bosserman G: Tunneled catheters: Technological advancements and nursing care issues. Nurs Clin North Am 28:851, 1993.

Heckman JD, et al: Emergency Care and Transportation of the Sick and Injured. 3rd ed. Chicago, American Academy of Orthopaedic Surgeons, 1981.

Infuse-a-Cath: Central Venous Catheter Nursing Manual. Beverly, MA, Strato Medical Corp, 1992.

Kacmarek RM, Mack C, Dimas S: The Essentials of Respiratory Care. 3rd ed. St. Louis, Mosby-Year Book, 1990.

Levitzky MG, Cairo J, Hall S: Introduction to Respiratory Care. Philadelphia, WB Saunders, 1990.

LifeART: CD-ROM Collections. Cleveland, OH, TechPool Studios Corp, 1994.

Potter PA, Perry AG: Basic Nursing Theory and Practice. 2nd ed. St. Louis, Mosby–Year Book, 1991.

Recht M, Burke D, Meranze S, et al: Simple technique for redirecting malpositioned central venous catheters. AJR Am J Roentgenol 154:183, 1990.

Scanlan CL, Spearman C, Sheldon R: Egan's Fundamentals of Respiratory Care. 6th ed. St. Louis, Mosby–Year Book, 1995.

Scott W: Complications associated with central venous catheters. Chest 94:1221, 1988.

Shapiro BA, et al: Clinical Application of Respiratory Care. 4th ed. St. Louis, Mosby–Year Book, 1991.

Sheldon R: Clinical application of the chest radiograph. *In* Wilkins R, Krider S, Sheldon R (eds): Clinical Assessment in Respiratory Care. St. Louis, Mosby, 1995, p 147.

Summerell N: Chest traumas: Causes of impaired gas exchange. *In* Nurse Review: A Clinical Update System. Vol 2. Springhouse, PA, Springhouse Group, 1989, p 137.

CHAPTER 14

INFECTION CONTROL

Jody L. Ellis, MPA, RT(R)

What man does not avoid contact with the sick, fearing lest he contract a disease so near?

OVID, 43 BC TO AD 17?

The Microbial World
Bacteria
Viruses
Fungi
Protozoan Parasites

The Establishment of Infectious Disease
Encounter
Entry
Spread
Multiplication
Damage
Outcome

The Chain of Infection
The Human Host
The Infectious Microorganism
The Mode of Transmission
The Reservoir

Nosocomial Infections
The Compromised Patient
Sources of Nosocomial Infection
Medical Personnel
Patient Flora
Contaminated Hospital Environment
Bloodborne Pathogens
Invasive Procedures

Microbial Control Within The Host
Constitutive Defenses of the Body
Normal Microbial Flora
Chemotherapy
Immunization

Environmental Control
Asepsis
Chemical Methods
Physical Methods
Handwashing
Standard Precautions
Handwashing
Gloving
Personal Protective Equipment
Needle Recapping
Biospills
Transmission-Based Precautions
Airborne Precautions
Droplet Precautions
Contact Precautions

Summary

OBJECTIVES

On completion of this chapter, the student will be able to:

1 Define the terminology related to infection control.
2 Identify the four basic infectious agents along with their unique characteristics.
3 Explain the steps involved in the establishment of an infectious disease.
4 Discuss the four factors involved in the spread of disease and the chain of infection.
5 Describe the various sources of nosocomial infection.

6 Explain the constituents of microbial control within the host.
7 Contrast medical and surgical asepsis.
8 List chemical and physical methods of asepsis.
9 Demonstrate the medically aseptic handwashing technique.
10 Describe the basic premises of standard precautions.
11 Relate types of transmission-based precautions with appropriate clinical situations.
12 Demonstrate contact precautions technique.

GLOSSARY

Asepsis: freedom from infection

Bacteria: in former systems of classification, a division of the kingdom Procaryotae, including all procaryotic organisms except the blue-green

Bloodborne Pathogens: disease-causing microorganisms that may be present in human blood

Chemotherapy: treatment of disease by chemical agents

Cyst: stage in the life cycle of certain parasites during which they are enclosed in a protective wall

Dimorphic: occurring in two distinct forms

Disease: any deviation from or interruption of the normal structure or function of any part, organ, or system (or combination thereof) of the body that is manifested by a characteristic set of symptoms and signs and whose etiology, pathology, and prognosis may be known or unknown

Disinfectant: chemicals used to free an environment from pathogenic organisms, or to render such organisms inert, especially as applied to the treatment of inanimate materials to reduce or eliminate infectious organisms

Eucaryotes: organisms whose cells have a true nucleus

Flora: microbial community found on or in a healthy individual

Fomite: object, such as a book, wooden object, or article of clothing, that is not in itself harmful but is able to harbor pathogenic microorganisms and thus may serve as an agent of transmission of an infection

Fungi: general term used to denote a group of eucaryotic protists—including mushrooms, yeasts, rusts, molds, and smuts—that are characterized by the absence of chlorophyll and by the presence of a rigid cell wall

Host: animal or plant that harbors or nourishes another organism

Iatrogenic: resulting from the activities of physicians

Immunity: security against a particular disease

Infection: invasion and multiplication of microorganisms in body tissues, which may be clinically inapparent or result in local cellular injury due to competitive metabolism, toxins, intracellular replication, or antigen-antibody response

Medical Asepsis: reduction in numbers of infectious agents, which in turn decreases the probability of infection but does not necessarily reduce it to zero

Microorganism: microscopic organism; those of medical interest include bacteria, viruses, fungi, and protozoa

Nosocomial: pertaining to or originating in the hospital; said of an infection not present or incubating prior to admittance to the hospital but generally occurring 72 hours after admittance

Pathogen: any disease-producing microorganism

Procaryotes: cellular organisms that lack a true nucleus

Protozoa: a subkingdom comprising the simplest organisms of the animal kingdom, consisting of unicellular organisms that range in size from submicroscopic to macroscopic; most are free living, but some lead commensalistic, mutualistic, or parasitic existences

Reservoir: alternate or passive host or carrier that harbors pathogenic organisms, without injury to itself, and serves as a source from which other individuals can be infected

Standard Precautions: precautions to prevent the transmission of disease by body fluids and substances

Sterilization: complete destruction or elimination of all living microorganisms, accomplished by physical methods (dry or moist heat), chemical agents (ethylene oxide, formaldehyde, alcohol), radiation (ultraviolet, cathode), or mechanical methods (filtration)

Surgical Asepsis: procedure used to prevent contamination of microbes and endospores before, during, or after surgery using sterile technique

Vaccine: suspension of attenuated or killed microorganisms (bacteria, viruses, or rickettsiae) administered for the prevention, improvement, or treatment of infectious disease

Vector: carrier, especially an animal (usually an arthropod) that transfers an infective agent from one host to another

Virion: complete viral particle, found extracellularly and capable of surviving in crystalline form and infecting a living cell; comprises the nucleoid (genetic material) and the capsid; also called viral particle

Virus: any of a group of minute infectious agents not resolved in the light microscope, with certain exceptions (eg, poxvirus), and characterized by a lack of independent metabolism and by the ability to replicate only within living host cells

The Microbial World

It has been well over 300 years since Anton van Leeuwenhoek first observed what he called "wee animalcules" under his crude microscope. At the time he reported his findings to the Royal Society of London, it was beyond anyone's imagination that these tiny creatures, known as microbes, could be anything more than a mere curiosity.

At the beginning of this century, the major causes of death in the United States were microbial infectious diseases. These diseases included pneumonia, tuberculosis, gastroenteritis, and diphtheria. Although today most microbial infections are under control, microbes still present a major threat to survival for the immunosuppressed individual. Furthermore, the threat of microbial disease in less developed countries still constitutes the major causes of death. Millions still die annually of illnesses such as malaria, cholera, and dysentery.

This last century has seen an explosion in knowledge of the sciences. The tiny amusing creatures of Leeuwenhoek's time have proved to be literally a matter of life or death. Microbes are essential to life through their ability to recycle organic and inorganic matter and devastating through their ability to produce disease. Most importantly, by studying these microbes at the molecular level, scientists have learned to identify them and determine their capabilities. Using this knowledge, many microbial functions can be controlled, making them beneficial or preventing potential harm.

It is important that the health care practitioner has an understanding of what infectious diseases are, how they are spread, and how they are controlled. Health care providers have been granted the responsibility not only to the patients entrusted to their care but also to the entire public sector.

Many **microorganisms** can grow in or on a host organism and cause disease. These diseases are known as infections. **Infection** refers to the establishment and growth of a microorganism on or in a host. It is only when the infection results in injury to the host that the host is said to have a disease. Infectious diseases are caused by pathogenic microorganisms. Most often, **pathogens** have the ability to do one of three functions extremely well. They can multiply in large numbers and cause an obstruction; they can cause tissue damage; and they can secrete organic substances called *exotoxins*. These exotoxins can produce certain side effects such as an extremely high body temperature, nausea, vomiting, or shock. Pathogens are divided into four basic infectious agents: bacteria, viruses, fungi, and protozoan parasites.

BACTERIA

Bacteria are microscopic, single-celled organisms with a simple internal organization (Fig. 14–1). Bacteria are procaryotic as opposed to eucaryotic organisms. **Procaryotes** lack nuclei and membrane-bound organelles, whereas **eucaryotes** have a true nucleus. Most of the cellular metabolic activities take place on the cytoplasmic membrane. Procaryotes do not have the capacity to ingest particulates or liquid droplets. Although bacteria are single celled, they may reside in the host in a group or cluster called a colony.

Bacteria are identified and classified according to their morphology, biochemistry, and genetic constitution. Morphology is considered a major criterion for classification. *Morphology* is the size or shape of the bacterium and is routinely determined by a simple staining technique called Gram staining. The medically important bacteria are classified into three general morphologies: cocci or spheres, bacilli or rods, and spirals.

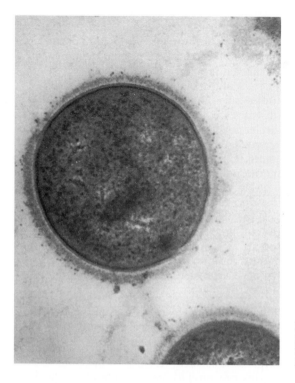

FIGURE 14–1. Transmission electron micrograph of a group B *Streptococcus* bacteria. (Reprinted with permission from Gorbach SL, Bartlett JG, Blacklow NR: Infectious Diseases. Philadelphia, WB Saunders, 1992, p 1421.)

Some bacteria have the ability to produce a highly resistant resting form known as an *endospore*. This structure is internal, as reflected in its name. Endospores are metabolically dormant structures that are highly resistant to the external environment. Spores possess extreme resistance to chemical and physical agents. They can remain viable for numerous years and then germinate in response to specific requirements. The endospore is a survival form of the bacterium that is produced, most often, in response to nutritional deprivation. Of all of the bacteria able to produce endospores, only two genera, *Bacillus* and *Clostridium*, are of medical importance. Some common bacterial infections encountered today are streptococcal pharyngitis (strep throat), *Klebsiella pneumoniae* infection (bacterial pneumonia), and *Clostridium botulinum* infection (food poisoning).

VIRUSES

Viruses are much simpler in form as compared with bacteria or animal cells (Fig. 14–2). Viruses are neither procaryotic nor eucaryotic. They are considered obligate intracellular parasites. Viruses cannot live outside a living cell. They lack the components necessary for their own survival because of their inability to synthe-size specific required proteins. Viruses depend on the host cell to provide these missing factors. A virus carries its own genetic information in the form of DNA or RNA, but never both. The DNA or RNA is surrounded by a protein coat called a *capsid*.

Viruses are characterized most generally by the chemical nature of their nucleic acid, their size, and their symmetry. Nucleic acids within a virus are, as stated earlier, either DNA or RNA, but these nucleic acids may be double or single, positive or negative stranded. Nucleic acids of differing viruses also possess varying weights. The size of a virus may vary from 20 to 250 nm. A nanometer is equal to 10^{-9} meters; therefore, direct observation of a virus is possible only through an electron microscope.

Viral infection is the result of a viral particle, also called a **virion,** attaching to a host cell and inserting its genome or genetic information into the host. The viral genome then redirects the host cell. The virus uses the organelles and metabolic functions of the host cell to produce new viruses. Once this process is completed, the new viral particles are released from the host cell. This sometimes results in the destruction of the cell. Some viruses have the ability to travel within the nervous system. They reappear sporadically and emerge at the nerve ending,

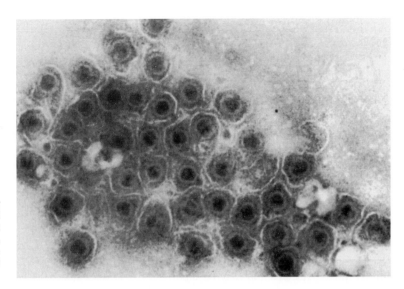

FIGURE 14–2. Varicella-zoster virus in vesicle fluid from a child with chickenpox. (Reprinted with permission from Gorbach SL, Bartlett JG, Blacklow NR: Infectious Diseases. Philadelphia, WB Saunders, 1992, p 1712.)

causing various symptoms. They then leave the site and travel up the nerve again. This pattern can be repeated several times and is known as a latent or dormant infection. A cold sore caused by herpes simplex is an example of a latent viral infection. Common viral diseases in humans include the common cold caused by the *Rhinovirus*, infectious mononucleosis caused by the Epstein-Barr virus, and warts caused by *Papillomavirus*.

FUNGI

Fungi (singular, *fungus*) can be macroscopic, as in the case of mushrooms and puffballs, or microscopic, such as yeasts and molds (Fig. 14–3). They are eucaryotic organisms with a nucleus and membrane-bound organelles. Fungi can be distinguished from bacteria by the fact that intracellular organelles can be visualized within the fungal cell. Fungal cells differ from animal cells in the type of sterol present in the cell membrane. The sterol present in animal cells is cholesterol. Fungi are also much larger than bacteria. Medically important pathogenic fungi are **dimorphic.** That is, they have the ability to grow in two distinct forms, either as a single-celled yeast or as a filamentous hyphae. A filamentous hyphae is better known as mold. Whether the organism is present in either form depends on the growth conditions. Fungi are classified according to the type and method of sexual reproduction.

A photomicrograph of a typical mold would reveal a structure similar to that of a plant or small tree. The molds produce tiny branches that extend into the air. It is here that spores are formed. These spores are called *conidia*. They are lightweight and resistant to drying,

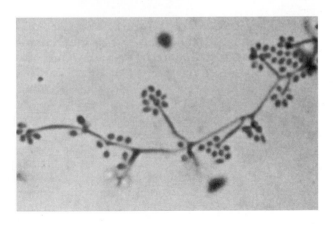

FIGURE 14–3. Daisy-like clusters of ovoid conidia, a fungus. (Reprinted with permission from Gorbach SL, Bartlett JG, Blacklow NR: Infectious Diseases. Philadelphia, WB Saunders, 1992, p 1924.)

and they are easily dispersed to new habitats. Diseases caused by fungi can be of four different classifications. The first is a superficial infection usually causing discoloration of the skin. Tinea nigra is a fungal infection that results in a painless black or brown discoloration of the palmar surface of the hand and the plantar surface of the foot. Second are the cutaneous infections, which involve the keratinized tissues of the hair, nails, and skin. The most common clinical infection in this group is tinea pedis, or athlete's foot. The growth pattern of this fungus forms a ring and is also known as ringworm. The third type is a subcutaneous fungal infection that enters the human host as a result of trauma to the skin. The fourth type is characterized by a systemic infection, which enters the circulatory and lymphatic systems and may be fatal.

PROTOZOAN PARASITES

Protozoa are unicellular organisms that are neither plants nor animals (Fig. 14–4). They are distinguished from bacteria by their greater size and the fact that they do not possess a cell wall.

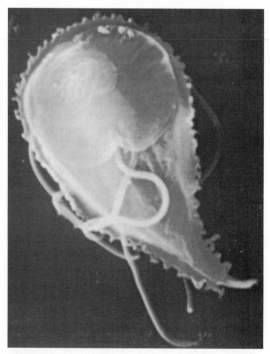

FIGURE 14–4. Scanning electron micrograph of *Giardia intestinalis*, a parasite. (Reprinted with permission from Gorbach SL, Bartlett JG, Blacklow NR: Infectious Diseases. Philadelphia, WB Saunders, 1992, p 1961.)

They are generally motile organisms and are eucaryotic. They are able to ingest food particles, and some species are equipped with rudimentary digestive systems.

Protozoa are classified according to their motility. The first group is classified by its slow, cellular flowing called *amoeboid locomotion*. Few amoebas are pathogenic. The motility of the second group is by a long *flagella*, a protein tail. The third group moves by the action of numerous short protein tails called *cilia*. Sporozoans constitute the fourth group. This group is unique in that they are nonmotile and, despite their name, do not form spores as bacteria and fungi do.

Some protozoa are able to form cysts, which permits them to survive while the parasite is out of a host. Cysts are resistant to chemical and physical changes.

Typical protozoan infections include *Trichomonas vaginalis* infection, a sexually transmitted disease that infects both males and females, and *Plasmodium vivax* infection (malaria).

The Establishment of Infectious Disease

From the time the infectious agent comes in contact with the host until the devastation of a disease is apparent, several complicated processes must be completed. These processes can be categorized into six steps. These six steps are the (1) encounter, (2) entry, (3) spread, (4) multiplication, (5) damage, and (6) outcome (Fig. 14–5). Remember that all six steps require the breaching of the host.

ENCOUNTER

The encounter involves the infectious organism coming into contact with the host. Each encounter varies according to the host and microorganism. Every individual and every microbe responds differently. Some organisms can infect the unborn child, although this is difficult, since the mother's womb is, microbically speaking, a sterile environment because of the selective passage allowed by the placenta. Still, some microorganisms are able to pass through the placenta to create what are called *congenital* infections. Examples of these infections are rubella and syphilis.

The initial encounter with infectious micro-

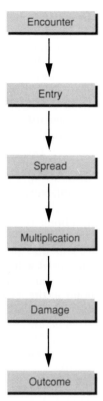

FIGURE 14-5. The establishment of an infectious disease is a six-step process.

organisms takes place during the normal birthing process. The child comes in contact with the microbial world that is present in the mother's vaginal canal. Fortunately, the newborn is born with antibodies obtained from the mother. These antibodies, plus those acquired through the mother's breast milk, provide the newborn with a sufficient immunologic base to cope with infection until its own immune system has matured. During the entire human life span, the body comes in contact with new organisms. Some are quickly eliminated, others are efficient colonizers. The colonizers either become part of the microbes normally found in the body or cause disease.

ENTRY

Much of the body is in contact with the external environment. The digestive, biliary, urinary, and respiratory systems are in direct connection with the exterior. In women, the peritoneal cavity is also exposed via the fallopian tubes. An infectious microbe can gain entrance into the human body by either ingression or penetration.

Ingression does not involve deep tissue penetration. Instead, these microorganisms adhere to the surface of the cell and excrete toxins that cause a distressed state within the system. Through the digestive system, infectious agents are ingested, most commonly through contaminated food or water. If the organism has the ability to survive the lower pH of the stomach and the small intestine, it may become anchored on the colon and cause a diseased state. The most common example of a symptom caused by an ingressive organism is diarrhea. Ingression can also take place in the respiratory system. Inhalation of contaminated aerosols or dust particles that are able to evade the powerful retrograde movement of the ciliary epithelium can lead to colonization within the lower respiratory tract. Pneumonia is contracted in this manner.

Penetration involves the microorganism invading past the epithelial barrier. This may take place in various forms. Some microbes are equipped with a special apparatus, like flagella. The bacteria that cause syphilis are able to penetrate using this mechanical device. Other microbes use vectors, such as mosquitoes or fleas, to penetrate into the tissue. Still others gain entry through tissue cuts and wounds. A phagocyte, which engulfs a foreign microbe, can transport it deeper into the tissue. In this instance, the human body itself is used to aid in penetration.

SPREAD

Spread is the propagation of the infectious organism. Spread can take place before or after multiplication. In either case, the most important barrier for the microbe to overcome in this step is the host's immune defenses. Dissemination is dictated by the logistics of both the host and the microbe. In other words, the site of microbial entry or the site where the microbe has taken up residence and the human anatomy at that site determine the spread of the microbe. For example, the viruses that cause the common cold are easily spread as aerosols through coughing and sneezing.

MULTIPLICATION

The number of microbes that gain entrance into the host is usually much too small to cause the symptoms of a disease. Most infectious agents must first multiply for their impact to be recognized. The time frame applied to this phenomenon is termed the *incubation period*, and its parameters are defined from the time the host's defenses have been overcome until the time a substantial population has been achieved.

DAMAGE

There are virtually uncountable ways in which an infectious agent can cause damage to a host. Damage can be either direct or indirect. Cell death caused by destruction of the host cells or by toxins or poisons secreted by the infectious agent are examples of direct damage. The growth phase of a microbe is characterized by exponential growth, and in a matter of hours there may be enough organisms present to cause a complete obstruction in a major organ system.

Infectious microbes can also damage a host indirectly by altering the metabolism of the host. These are represented by some of the most life-threatening diseases. Once a person has ingested the toxins secreted by the organism that causes botulism, it is only a matter of hours before death may result.

A microbe can also induce host responses. Indirectly, the host's inflammatory and immune responses can cause further cell destruction than that already achieved by the microbe. Usually, this destruction is minimal compared with the overall devastation that an infectious agent may induce. The sacrificing of a few cells is justified when the integrity of the entire human body is at stake.

OUTCOME

An encounter with an infectious agent can result in one of three outcomes: (1) the host gains control of the infectious agent and eliminates it; (2) the infectious agent overcomes the host's immunities to cause disease; or (3) the host and the infectious agent compromise and live in a somewhat anxious state of symbiosis.

The Chain of Infection

In 1876, Robert Koch, a physician, introduced the germ theory of disease. Before this

point, it was assumed that something was transmitted from an ill person to a well person. Up until the 16th century, evil spirits were a popular explanation for illness. In the 16th century, however, diseases were assumed to be spread by an unknown entity called a *contagion* and the disease was said to be *contagious*, a term still in use today. Through scientific experimentation, Koch was able to prove that specific organisms caused specific diseases. He was able to prove that a precise series of events must occur for microorganisms from an infected person to be transmitted to an uninfected person. His postulates forever changed the relationship between microorganisms and humans.

According to the postulates of Koch, four factors are involved in the spread of diseases. Each factor is considered a link in the chain, and each link is connected to the next to form a ring. If at any point in the infection the chain is broken, the cycle cannot continue and infection will cease. For infections to be transmitted, there must be (1) a host, (2) an infectious microorganism, (3) a mode of transportation, and (4) a reservoir (Fig. 14–6).

THE HUMAN HOST

Humans provide a favorable **host** environment for the growth of many microbes, because of the abundance of organic nutrients and metabolites found within the human body. Each region or organ of the body offers a different temperature, pH, or body fluid for microbial growth to occur. This diversity is optimal for the microbe with limited metabolic or aerobic requirements.

THE INFECTIOUS MICROORGANISM

Microorganisms include bacteria, viruses, fungi, and protozoa. These organisms have already been discussed.

THE MODE OF TRANSMISSION

Microorganisms can be transmitted either *exogenously*, from outside the body, or *endogenously*, from inside the body. Exogenously acquired diseases are those that result from an encounter with a microbe found in the environment. This transmission can be by either direct or indirect

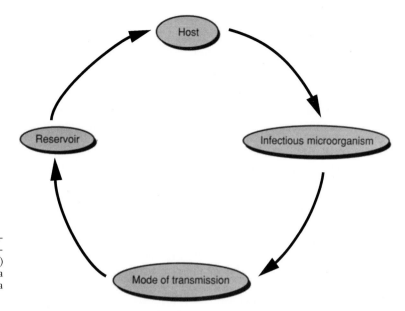

FIGURE 14–6. The chain of infection. For infections to be transmitted there must be (1) a host, (2) an infectious microorganism, (3) a mode of transmission, and (4) a reservoir.

host-to-host contact. There may also be indirect transmission through a vector or a fomite.

Direct host-to-host transmission occurs when an infected individual transmits an infection by any number of methods, such as hand holding, coughing, or sexual contact, to name just a few. Most importantly, direct contact involves touching of some sort. Sexually transmitted diseases use this route. Skin pathogens are also spread by the direct route. Staphylococcal infections can be spread by direct contact with the infected area, as demonstrated in impetigo infections.

Infective microbes are usually transported in a liquid medium. Secretions and excretions pick up organisms from infected areas and remove them during normal body functions. Body secretions like phlegm and aerosols from sneezes and coughs are common transportation media. Respiratory pathogens transmitted in the aerosols do not remain airborne and viable very long. Transmission is therefore considered to be of the direct route. Excretions, including urine and feces, are also pertinent carriers of microorganisms.

Some microorganisms require a **vector** to enter and exit the human host. A vector is usually an arthropod (mosquito, flea, tick, and so forth). When it consumes its blood meal from its human host, it can ingest an infectious microbe from the blood. When the vector goes on to obtain its next meal from a different individual, it can then transmit the infection to that individual. Lyme disease is transmitted by a vector, the deer tick.

A **fomite** is an inanimate object that has been in contact with an infectious organism. Food and water, radiographic equipment, and latex gloves can all serve as fomites.

Endogenous transmission is the result of encounters with organisms already present in or on the body, the normal flora. This usually happens when the normal flora of a specific area is transported to a different area. Staphylococci on the surface of the skin can invade deeper tissue through a laceration. In this case, the initial encounter with staphylococci may have been years earlier, but the infection was initiated as a result of the trauma. The primary encounter is termed the *colonization* and denotes the presence of a microbe. Do not assume because there is colonization, there is disease. Disease implies tissue damage and related symptoms.

THE RESERVOIR

A **reservoir** is the site where an infectious organism can remain alive and from which transmission can occur. People, animals, and inanimate objects can all serve as reservoirs.

A person who serves as a reservoir is called a *carrier.* A carrier is an infected individual who does not display the disease symptoms. Typhoid Mary is a classic example. Mary Mallon was a chronic carrier of *Salmonella typhi*, the organism that causes typhoid fever. She was employed in numerous households and institutions as a cook. She daily exposed other people to the pathogen, which led to an epidemic. After extensive investigations of numerous outbreaks, it was revealed that she was the source of each one. When tested, her bacteria count for this specific species was incredibly high. She continued to shed the organism for many years. It is assumed that her infected gallbladder supplied a continuous wave of organisms to her colon. Public health officials offered to remove her gallbladder, an operation she refused. Their only recourse was to imprison Mary to prevent further epidemics. After 3 years in prison, Mary was released on the promise that she cease to handle food and that she would continue to be monitored on a regular basis. Mary never appeared for her check-ups. She changed her name and continued to cook. For 5 more years, she caused another epidemic of typhoid fever. After another epidemiologic investigation, the source of infection was, once again, traced to her. She was imprisoned and remained there for 23 years until her death in 1938.

Animals can also serve as reservoirs. A common animal reservoir is the cow. Some diseases can be passed from the cow to a human host through the ingestion of milk. Pasteurization has helped to obliterate most of these pathogens.

Insects are another common reservoir. After an insect ingests a blood meal infected with pathogens, protozoa may complete their life cycles within the insect and are introduced into the host in a different stage of life. Such is the case for malaria, which is spread primarily by a mosquito vector. A dusty corner, contaminated linen, and food can serve as inanimate reservoirs.

Nosocomial Infections

It is a general conception that the hospital is a place where sick people can go to get better, and for the most part, this is true. However, approximately 5% of all hospital patients acquire an additional condition while in the hospital. These hospital-acquired conditions are known as **nosocomial** infections (*nosocomium* is the Latin word for hospital). These hospital pathogens follow the chain of infection, but the links are limited to those in contact with the microenvironment we know as the hospital. In the United States, billions of dollars are spent annually on nosocomial management, and such infections may contribute to nearly 100,000 deaths annually.

Within the health care field, there is yet another microenvironmet, that between the patient and physician. An infection that is the result of intervention with a physician is an **iatrogenic** infection. This type of infection is strictly limited to the physician, whether he or she is in the hospital or not.

The same organisms that cause nosocomial and iatrogenic infections may also be found elsewhere in the community, but the healthy population can usually combat these pathogens. Nosocomial pathogens are opportunistic. Given the right conditions—a patient with an impaired immune system, the ability to bypass anatomic barriers through burns, wounds, or surgery, and introduction through a catheter, syringe, or respirator—these pathogens thrive and exert their maximum biologic effects. Hospitals and their patients provide this optimal environment.

THE COMPROMISED PATIENT

Hospital patients have a greater sensitivity to infection. Many patients have weakened resistance to infectious organisms because of their admitting illness. These patients are said to be *compromised* or *immunosuppressed*. For example, organ transplant patients are given drugs to intentionally suppress their immune system. This is done to prevent the rejection of the transplanted organ, but it provides the opportunistic pathogen with a suitable host at the same time. The severity of the admitting condition corresponds to the risk of acquiring a nosocomial infection and vice versa. An outpatient having a mole removed has an extremely small chance of acquiring an infection as compared with the patient having emergency open heart surgery.

SOURCES OF NOSOCOMIAL INFECTION

Cross-infection within the hospital can come from a multitude of sources. The complexity of the hospital environment provides innumerable opportunities for the encounter of patients with infectious microbes.

Medical Personnel

Transmission between the hospital staff and the patient may be by direct skin-to-skin contact or indirect contact, by ingestion or inhalation. Unusual epidemics have been traced to hospital personnel. Food handlers can contaminate food eaten by the patient and a nurse can sneeze onto his or her hands and then touch a patient. Surgeons have been known to carry organisms in their facial hair. In one epidemic, the organisms were harbored in the carrier's vagina and were presumed to be aerosolized through normal body movement. The possibilities of transfer are endless. Medical personnel can continually serve as active colonizers or transient carriers, or they can become infected themselves.

Patient Flora

Microorganisms are almost always found in those regions of the body exposed to the external environment, such as the skin, gastrointestinal system, genitourinary system, and respiratory system. Potentially harmful bacteria such as staphylococci and streptococci are harbored in the nasopharynx of almost every healthy individual. When the individual is healthy, the relationship between the host and the microbe is either beneficial or neutral, but when the individual is compromised, the microbe seizes the opportunity to flourish and is harmful.

Contaminated Hospital Environment

Many microorganisms are endemic to the hospital environment. An example would be fungal infections acquired from the mildew that grows on moist walls. Also, infection can be acquired through improperly sterilized surgical equipment or contaminated intravenous solutions. Contamination through the hospital environment is often through fomites, such as instruments, fluids, food, air, and medications.

Bloodborne Pathogens

Bloodborne pathogens are disease-causing microorganisms that may be present in human blood. They may be transmitted with any exposure to blood or other potentially infectious material. For this reason, these pathogens will be considered nosocomial infections.

There are two bloodborne pathogens on the increase within the hospital setting, hepatitis B virus (HBV) and human immunodeficiency virus (HIV). A number of other bloodborne pathogens exist, such as those that cause hepatitis C, hepatitis D, and syphilis, but they are not as prevalent.

Hepatitus B virus causes illness primarily affecting the liver. Approximately 8700 health care workers contract hepatitis B each year. This infection results in swelling, soreness, and loss of normal function in the liver. HBV is a major cause of viral hepatitis.

The symptoms of hepatitis B include weakness, fatigue, anorexia, nausea, abdominal pain, fever, and headache. As the illness progresses, a yellow discoloration of the skin, called *jaundice*, may develop. In some cases, the disease may be asymptomatic and therefore may not be diagnosed.

A person's blood will test positive for the HBV surface antigen 2 to 6 weeks after symptoms of the illness develop. Approximately 85% of those infected will recover in 6 to 8 weeks, yet a blood test will always reveal that they have been exposed to the virus due to the presence of the HBV surface antigen.

A major source of HBV is the chronic active carrier of the virus. The carrier has the surface antigen present at all times. This may be the consequence of a problem with the immune system that prevents complete destruction of virus-infected liver cells. It is estimated that 1 to 1.25 million persons in the United States have chronic hepatitis B and are potentially infectious to others. The carrier can unknowingly transmit the disease to a susceptible host through a contaminated needle or other penetrating injury, and intimate contact. Each year, 200 health care workers will die of hepatitis B.

Human immunodeficiency virus is a virus that specifically infects the immune system T_4 blood cells in the human host. The presence of the virus renders the cells less effective in preventing disease. It is the virus that is responsible for acquired immunodeficiency syndrome.

Symptoms of HIV infection may include weight loss, fatigue, glandular pain and swelling, muscle and joint pain, and night sweats. People with HIV infection may feel fine and not be aware of their previous exposure to HIV for as long as 10 years. It may take as long as a year for the results of a blood test to become positive for HIV antibodies. Therefore, more than one test over a specified period of time may be required to determine infection after exposure to HIV.

Invasive Procedures

Invasive diagnostic or therapeutic interventions allow a microbe to gain entrance into an area of the body where it may not normally be able to overcome that person's defenses. These procedures give the microbe a free ride. The most common nosocomial infection, a urinary tract infection, is introduced by a Foley urinary catheter.

Other invasive procedures include any surgery and the insertion of such devices as needles, vascular catheters, endotracheal tubes, and endoscopes.

Microbial Control Within the Host

Microbes may be controlled within the host by different mechanisms. Some are part of the normal anatomy and physiology of the host. Others are introduced into the host, and still others are controlled by microbes themselves.

CONSTITUTIVE DEFENSES OF THE BODY

The human body has defense mechanisms with which a host can protect itself from microbial invasion. These defenses are categorized as mechanical, chemical, or cellular. The intact skin and the mucous membranes provide a mechanical and chemical barrier through which a microorganism must first pass. The sebaceous and sweat glands secrete moisture and fatty acids onto the skin that kill many bacteria and fungi. In addition, the mechanical process of the shedding of cells due to friction from rubbing the hands together during washing also provides a strong defensive system. Trauma such as a burn, abrasion, or another type of wound provide the obvious breaches to this barrier.

The mucous membranes of the respiratory, gastrointestinal, and genitourinary tracts and conjunctiva of the eye secrete a gel-like substance called mucus that traps foreign particles and prevents them from invading the adjacent tissue. Some epithelial cells are ciliated. The beating action of the cilia on the mucous membranes provides for the continuous movement of the fluid mucus to the exterior.

Tears continually bathe the eyes and urine cleanses the urinary tract. Both tears and urine are rich in lysosome, an enzyme that destroys the bacterial cell wall. The acidity of the stomach and the vagina also provides a competent barrier to invasion.

Despite these efficient chemical and mechanical barriers, microbes penetrate into the bloodstream and connective tissue daily. They gain entrance through everyday activity like eating, teeth brushing, scratching, and bowel movements. These daily attacks are survived through the cellular mechanism of defense, the phagocytic cell. The phagocyte is responsible for removing foreign particles, engulfing and destroying them through a process called phagocytosis. Phagocytosis is part of the inflammatory response.

NORMAL MICROBIAL FLORA

The human body contains thousands of species of microorganisms. Each of us is unique in that the types and amounts of each organism vary. Normal **flora** is defined as the microbial community found on or in a healthy individual. The normal flora for one person may be completely different from that of the next. Because of this microbial uniqueness, pathogenicity is not a black and white issue. What constitutes the normal flora of one person may be life-threatening to another. Although the normal flora may serve as the source of many opportunistic infections, in many areas of the body, the normal flora inhibits the attachment and colonization of many pathogens. The old saying, "Possession is nine tenths of the law" also applies to microbes. Those who have found their niche are reluctant to concede their occupancy to another organism, maintaining their physical advantage. Others secrete toxins that are inhibitory to other microbes.

CHEMOTHERAPY

Killing a microorganism outside the human body is a fairly simple task. To kill a microbe within the host requires the selective toxicity of a drug, also called selective **chemotherapy.** Most antimicrobial drugs have a single primary target, which most often are specific proteins, nucleic acids, and, in bacteria, the cell wall. Clinically useful antimicrobials must have the ability to inhibit reactions within the microbe but not interfere with the human cell with which the microbe is associated. Some chemo-therapeutic drugs are termed *static* because they inhibit growth but do not cause killing. Tetracyclines are examples of bacteriostatic drugs. Others are termed *cidal* because of their ability to kill susceptible microbes. Penicillins are examples of bacteriocidal drugs.

IMMUNIZATION

The awareness that individuals who survived an epidemic did not contract that disease again has been evident in history for many centuries. As early as the 10th century, the Turks were inoculating their infant daughters with extracts from the pustules of smallpox patients. If they survived, their value on the market as concubines for harems was increased because their bodies were not pocked or scarred from the disease. Modern immunology began with the experiments of Louis Pasteur. He developed vaccines for diseases including anthrax and rabies.

A **vaccine** is a mixture used to induce active **immunity** (the production of antibody). The importance of immunization is reflected in the marked drop in incidence of that specific disease after vaccination. The degree of immunity varies according to the patient and the quality and quantity of the vaccine. It is important to remember that rarely is immunization lifelong. In many cases, booster vaccines must be administered.

Environmental Control

Up to this point, the primary concern has been with the intimate relationship between the infectious microbe and the host. The constituents of the body, other microbes, medicines, and immunizations all contribute their defenses in the constant battle against infection. Each of these is important in ensuring the integrity of the host, but there is another important step not yet considered. In a world populated with millions and millions of people each with their own millions of microbes, it is important to focus attention on the bigger picture of environmental control. When one considers the number of microbes, the problem of environmental control seems overwhelming, yet it is one of the easiest methods of control.

Within the United States, recommendations and guidelines for environmental control of infectious diseases are issued by the United States Department of Health and Human Services (HHS) and by the Centers for Disease Control and Prevention (CDC). The established policies are enforced by the Department of Labor's Occupational Safety and Health Administration (OSHA). All rules and regulations are strictly enforced at both the state and federal levels. At the international level, the World Health Organization (WHO) serves to issue recommendations for infection control.

ASEPSIS

As radiologic technologists, we have the ability and the responsibility to prevent the spread of infectious organisms. Knowledge of the principles of sterilization and disinfection is fundamental. **Asepsis** means freedom from infection and can be divided into two categories: medical asepsis and surgical asepsis. **Surgical asepsis** is the procedure used to prevent contamination of microbes and endospores before, during, and after surgery using sterile technique. The absolute killing of all life forms is termed **sterilization.** If proper sterilization techniques are used, the probability of infection is theoretically zero. **Medical asepsis** involves a reduction in numbers of infectious agents, which in turn decreases the probability of infection but does not necessarily reduce it to zero. The microbes are not eliminated, however. Instead, their environment is altered so that it is nonconducive to growth and reproduction.

Each microbial species has an optimal temperature range for growth. Any variation above or below this range results in a blockage of growth. Most organisms that infect humans survive best at 37°C (98.6°F). An increase in metabolic activity, within the range, results in an increase in growth. Once above this range, the proteins or enzymes cannot perform their normal functions. A decrease within the range results in a slowing down of growth; once below the range, the protein loses its flexibility. This is one of the reasons the operating room is kept so cold.

Another important environmental effect on microbial growth is pH. Most human infectious microbes grow best at a neutral or slightly alkaline pH (7.0 to 7.4). Some prefer more acidic or alkaline conditions and seek those parts of the body that provide these conditions. Microbes are also sensitive to the presence or subsequent absence of oxygen. Consequently, environmental microbial control can be achieved through both physical and chemical means.

Chemical Methods

Chemicals that alter the environment available to the microbe are called **disinfectants.** This is an ambiguous term referring to either the inactivation or the inhibition of microbial growth. Disinfection may or may not entail the removal of bacterial endospores. If the disinfectant is applied topically, it is termed an *antiseptic.* Not only can disinfectants be classified according to whether they can be used on a living body, they can also be classified as to whether they kill or do not kill microbes. A *bacteriostatic* agent stops bacterial growth, and a *bacteriocidal* agent causes cell killing.

Chemical disinfectants common to the radiology department include the halogens chlorine and iodine, which are bacteriocidal. Chlorine is found in bleach. Because it is such a strong oxidizing agent, it is ordinarily used on inanimate objects. Iodine is used as the antiseptic in Betadine and Surgidine and is used in conjunction with alcohol swabbing. This antiseptic method is commonly used with invasive procedures. Alcohol cannot be used independently; although it is lethal to all vegetative cells, it cannot destroy endospores. Also common to the radiology department is hydrogen peroxide. This is used in a 3% solution as an antiseptic and is most effective in deep wounds. Ammonium-containing detergents are used as surface-active disinfectants throughout the hospital, and ethylene oxide is used for sterilization in the gas phase. Gas sterilization is used for electronic and plastic equipment that may be damaged by heat.

The effectiveness of chemical disinfectants is subject to concentration, temperature, time of exposure, types and numbers of microbes, and the nature of the object or person being treated. It is important to read all manufacturers labels carefully to ensure maximum effectiveness.

Physical Methods

Heat is the most frequently used method of sterilization. Moist heat is much more effective and rapid at killing than dry heat. Moist heat involves using steam under pressure. This is accomplished in a device known as an *autoclave.*

Effective killing of vegetative cells and endospores is accomplished at 121°C (250°F) at a pressure of 15 lb/in^2 for 15 minutes. Sterilization by dry heat is achieved in an oven. Dry heat requires a higher temperature for a longer time (160°C [320°F] for 120 minutes). Pasteurization involves moderate heating followed by rapid cooling. This process is used to kill heat-sensitive organisms in milk, beer, and wine. Pasteurization does not sterilize the liquid involved. Freezing can also kill certain organisms but is not a reliable form of sterilization. Ultraviolet (UV) light at 260 nm can produce maximal killing of microbes. UV light is used in germicidal lamps for control of airborne contaminates. UV light is restricted in its usage by its inability to penetrate glass, paper, body fluids, and thin layers of cells.

A host need not be a patient. The health care provider could also serve as a host. One of the simplest physical methods of microbial control, for the health care provider or the patient, is the use of barriers. Gloves, gowns, masks, protective eye wear or face shields all serve as barriers and defend against invasion by an infectious microbe.

HANDWASHING

The importance of handwashing in preventing the spread of infection is credited to Dr. Semmelweis of Vienna in 1846. He noted that when the medical students of the hospital went directly from class, in this case autopsies, to rounds in the hospital, the incidence of infection was high. What drew his attention to this practice was that when the students were on vacation the incidence of infection dropped significantly. He noted that the nurses attending the patients were not permitted in the autopsy room. He established a policy that no medical students would be allowed to examine patients until they had cleansed their hands with a solution of chloride of lime.

Handwashing is a routine practice in all patient care settings. It is the single most important means of preventing the spread of infection. Washing or scrubbing the hands involves the removal of contaminates (transients) as well as resident microorganisms. Handwashing is both a chemical and a physical process. Many soaps and detergents are bacteriocidal, but their application during handwashing is usually too brief to kill microbes. Depending on the condi-

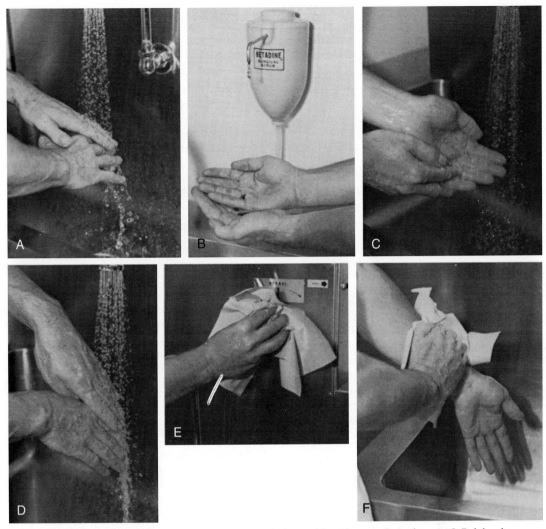

FIGURE 14–7. Proper handwashing. *A,* Wet hands thoroughly with water. *B,* Apply soap. *C,* Rub hands using a firm, vigorous rotary motion. *D,* Rinse, allowing the water to run down over hands. *E,* Turn off the water, using toweling on handles. *F,* Dry hands from elbow to fingertips.

tion of the skin and the numbers of microbes present, it may take as long as 7 to 8 minutes of washing to remove the transients. Resident microbes are much harder to remove because they are so firmly embedded. Soaps are effective at removing some fragile bacteria such as pneumococci and meningococci. An important and effective portion of handwashing appears to be the mechanical action of rubbing the hands together.

Because a radiologic technologist comes in contact with a myriad of patients on a daily basis, it is extremely important that handwashing be performed *before and after each patient.* This practice provides the simplest method of

environmental control. There is a specific protocol to be followed that is accepted as medically aseptic (Fig. 14–7):

1 Approach the sink. Consider it to be contaminated. Avoid contact with your clothing. Use foot or knee levers when available. If not, use toweling to handle all controls. Adjust water flow to avoid splashing. Adjust water temperature to comfort.

2 Wet hands thoroughly with water. During the entire procedure, keep hands lower than elbow. This advantageous use of gravity allows organisms to flow down the arm and off the fingertips.

3 Apply soap. Soap should be available in

liquid form and can be applied by use of foot or knee levers. Soap can also be dispensed from a pump.

4 Use a firm, vigorous, rotary motion. Begin at the wrist and work toward the fingertips. Rub palms, back of hands, between fingers, and under nails.

5 Rinse and allow water to run down over hands.

6 Repeat the entire process to cleanse from the elbow to the fingertips.

7 Turn off the water. Use toweling on handles if foot or knee levers are not available.

8 Dry from the elbow to the fingertips, never returning to an area.

STANDARD PRECAUTIONS

The Centers for Disease Control and Prevention (CDC) and the Hospital Infection Control Practices Advisory Committee (HICPAC) recently revised the isolation precautions for hospitals and other health care facilities. To clarify the confusion of such terms as universal precautions, body substance isolation precautions, and the old disease-specific isolation precautions, the CDC and HICPAC have reclassified infections, standardized terminology, and simplified precautions.

Standard precautions incorporates the features of both body fluid precautions and body substance isolation. Standard precautions should be used when performing procedures that may require contact with blood, body fluids, secretions, excretions, mucous membranes, and nonintact skin. Also included in this category are items soiled or contaminated with any of these substances. Because most patients in the radiology department have an unknown serostatus, all patients should be regarded as potentially infectious. Apply standard precautions to all patients regardless of diagnosis and infection status. Biosafety in the radiology department using standard precautions includes, but is not limited to, the following guidelines.

Handwashing

Hands must be washed before and after performing invasive procedures and after touching body fluids, blood, secretions, excretions, and contaminated items, regardless of whether gloves are worn. Gloves may have undetectable defects and may also be torn or damaged during use.

Gloving

Gloves must be worn during procedures that may involve contact with any patient's body fluids, blood, secretions, excretions, mucous membranes, nonintact skin, and contaminated items. Wear gloves during all vascular access procedures. Gloves must be promptly removed after use, before touching noncontaminated surfaces, and of course between patients.

Personal Protective Equipment

Personal protective equipment is provided by the hospital at no cost to the health care worker. This equipment provides a barrier between the patient and the health care provider to prevent exposure to the skin and mucous membranes. This equipment includes gloves, fluid repellent gowns, face masks, protective eyewear, and resuscitation masks and bags. Personal protective equipment must be utilized when contact with body fluids, blood, secretions, and excretions is possible.

Needle Recapping

An estimated 800,000 needle stick injuries and other injuries from sharp objects to health care workers occur annually in the United States. Avoid recapping used needles. If you must recap, apply the one-handed "scoop" technique or a needle-recapping device that holds the needle sheath. Place all used sharps into the designated puncture-resistant container, commonly called a *sharps container*.

Biospills

To clean biospills, wear gloves and the appropriate personal protective equipment. Blot the spill with paper towels and discard into a designated medical waste container. Clean the contaminated area with a bleach solution or a hospital-grade disinfectant.

TRANSMISSION-BASED PRECAUTIONS

Transmission-based precautions are applied whenever a patient is infected with a pathogenic organism or a communicable disease. Transmission-based precautions must also be applied when the patient is at risk of becoming infected, as are those who are immunosuppressed. Transmission-based precautions are used along with standard precautions, serving as a double protection, protecting both the patient and the health care practitioner. The transmission-based precautions have replaced the old category specific isolation precautions, such as contact and respiratory isolation. Isolation techniques have been revised and combined into three sets of guidelines. Keep in mind that under these guidelines, some infections and conditions fall into two categories.

Airborne Precautions

Pathogenic organisms that remain suspended in air for long periods of time on aerosol droplets or dust include tuberculosis, varicella (chickenpox), and rubeola (measles). Patients infected with pathogens that disseminate through the air are to be placed in a negative-pressure isolation room with the door closed. Health care practitioners should wear respiratory protection when entering the room. This type of respiratory protection should filter inspired air. An infected patient leaving his or her room should wear a surgical mask. Surgical masks filter expired air.

Droplet Precautions

When caring for patients who are infected with such pathogenic organisms as rubella, mumps, influenza, and adenovirus use droplet precautions. These pathogens disseminate through large particular droplets expelled from the patient while coughing, sneezing, or even talking. The pathogens infect another person through contact with the mouth, nasal mucosa, or conjunctiva.

Patients infected with these pathogens are placed in private rooms or with another patient infected with the same disease. The door may remain open because large droplets typically travel 3 feet before dropping to the ground. Health care practitioners should protect themselves by wearing a surgical mask when within 3 feet of the patient. Special ventilation precautions are not necessary. The patient should wear a surgical mask when leaving the room.

Contact Precautions

Use these precautions when caring for a patient infected with a virulent pathogen that spreads by direct contact with the patient or indirect contact with a contaminated object such as patient's dressings or bed rails. Conditions that require using contact precautions include methicillin-resistant *Staphylococcus aureus*, hepatitis A, impetigo, varicella, and varicella zoster.

This patient will be housed in a private room or with another patient infected with the same disease. The health care practitioner should properly don gloves before entering the room. The gloves will be removed and hands washed before leaving the room. A gown should be worn if the practitioner anticipates contact with the patient or his or her environment. Remove the gown before leaving the room. All radiographic equipment placed in the contaminated environment should be cleaned with an antiseptic solution.

When a patient requiring contact precautions is sent to the radiology department, the patient must wear appropriate barriers. In many cases the patient will wear a mask and an impervious gown. Staff in the department should be notified prior to receiving the patient. All radiographic equipment should be decontaminated with an antiseptic after the radiographic procedure is completed.

CONTACT PRECAUTIONS TECHNIQUE. There are many times when a radiologic technologist is required to perform examinations on patients who are on contact precautions. To maintain contact precautions usually requires teamwork. It is important to acquire the assistance of another health care provider. Contact precautions are maintained by the following steps (Fig. 14–8):

1 Determine the correct number of cassettes needed for the examination. Place each cassette into a protective bag. This may be either a plastic or cloth isolation bag. These bags should be available in the radiology department.
2 Move the portable machine to the isolated room.
3 Locate the isolation supplies for the room.
4 Remove all ornamentation (including watch, rings, earrings) and place them in your pocket.
5 Put on a lead apron.
6 Wash your hands as described previously.
7 Put on a clean gown, making sure it is sufficiently long to cover most of the uniform. Pick up the gown from the inside

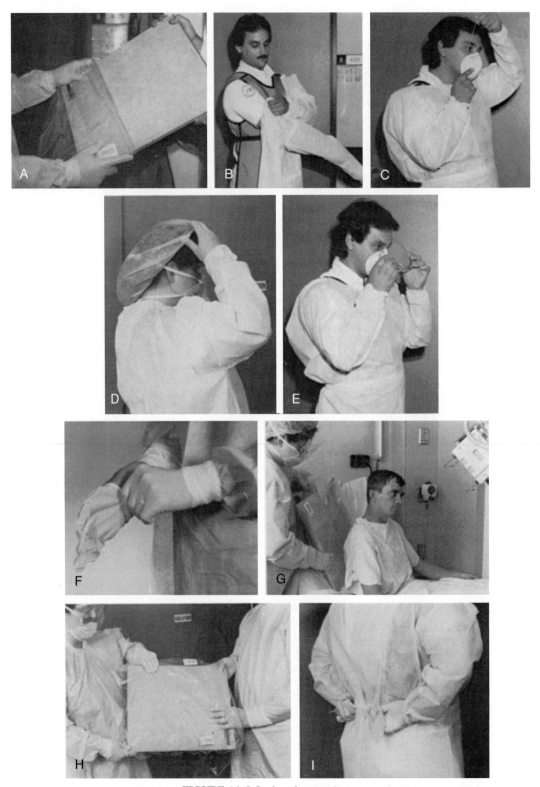

FIGURE 14–8 *See legend on opposite page*

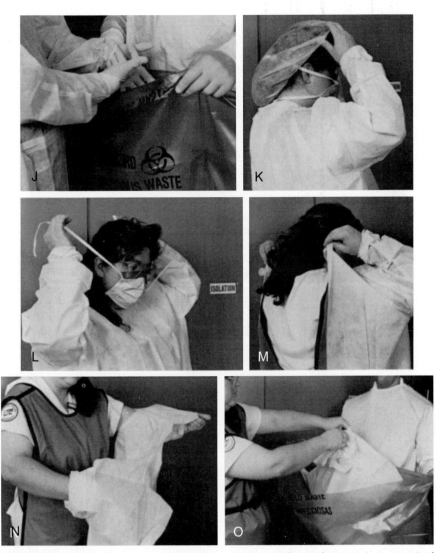

FIGURE 14–8. An appropriate contact precautions technique. *A*, Place each cassette in a protective bag. *B*, Put on a lead apron and then gown, never touching the outside of the gown with your hands. *C*, Put on a mask. *D*, Put on a cap. *E*, Put on protective glasses, if recommended. *F*, Put on nonsterile gloves. *G*, Position the bagged cassette beneath the patient. *H*, Fold the protective bag, never touching the inside while an assistant removes the cassette without touching the outside of the bag. *I*, Untie the gown at waist. *J*, Remove the gloves, turning them inside out. *K*, Remove the cap. *L*, Remove the mask by holding only the ties. *M*, Untie the neck of the gown. *N*, Turn the gown inside out without touching the outside of the gown. *O*, Place the gown in the appropriate receptacle.

near the armhole openings and gently shake it open. Put one arm in and then the other. First tie the neck strings, then tie the waist strings.

8 Put on a mask, tying it securely, and then a cap. Goggles may also be worn, if available.

9 Put on the gloves. These should be clean but need not be sterile. (See Chapter 15 if sterile gloving is required.)

10 Have the assistant put on a gown, gloves, and a cap.

11 Enter the isolated area and explain to the patient who you are and what you are doing. You will appear intimidating. A gentle word will go a long way at this point.

12 Position the patient and the cassette.

13 Have your assistant manipulate the machine and make the exposure.

14 Remove the cassette from behind the patient. Fold the edge of the protective bag back, never touching the inside. Have your assistant remove the cassette, never touching the outside. Place the covering into an appropriate container. Have your assistant remove the portable equipment from the room.

15 Untie the waist ties of the gown.

16 Remove your gloves. Remove the first glove with the other gloved hand, never touching the inside of the glove. Grasp the top of the glove and pull it inside out. Remove the other glove with the exposed hand, touching the inside only. Discard into an appropriate container.

17 Remove the cap and then untie the mask, touching the ties only, and remove the mask.

18 Untie the neck ties of the gown, and pull the gown forward and down from the shoulders. Pull the gown off so that the sleeves are inside out and the front of the gown is folded inward. Avoid touching the front of the gown. Discard into an appropriate container.

19 Wash your hands.

20 Have your assistant follow the same protocol. Clean the portable equipment with an antiseptic.

21 Wash your hands one last time.

Summary

Infection involves the establishment and dissemination of a microorganism on or in a host. Disease results when an infection causes physiologic damage to the host. Infectious diseases are caused by pathogenic microorganisms, which are divided into four basic infectious agents: bacteria, viruses, fungi, and protozoan parasites.

For an infectious agent to become established in a host, a breach of the host's defenses must occur. The establishment of infectious disease involves six steps: encounter, entry, spread, multiplication, damage, and outcome.

Four factors are involved in the spread of infectious diseases: the microorganism, the host, the mode of transmission, and the reservoir. Each factor is considered a link in the chain of infection. A break at any point in the chain results in the infectious disease's losing its ability to spread.

Nosocomial infections are those acquired in the hospital setting. Hospitals and compromised patients provide the optimal environment for nosocomial infections. Sources of this specific type of infection include the hospital proper and the medical personnel within, contaminated invasive diagnostic and therapeutic devices, and opportunistic microorganisms that are constituents of the normal flora.

The human body has mechanical, cellular, and chemical mechanisms that it uses to fight infection. The presence of the microorganisms included in the normal flora inhibits the attachment and colonization of new microbes. Chemotherapy and immunization have aided in the reduction and eradication of many infectious diseases.

Through asepsis, environmental control of infection is simple. Various chemical and physical methods may be used to achieve surgical or medical asepsis. The employment of the medically aseptic handwashing technique, standard precautions and transmission-based precautions has contributed significantly in reducing the probability of spreading infectious diseases.

Recommendations and guidelines are issued by the United States Department of Health and Human Services and by the Centers for Disease Control and Prevention. In turn, these guidelines are enforced by the Department of Labor's Occupational Safety and Health Administration. All rules and regulations are strictly enforced and reviewed to ensure the safety of every patient and health care provider within the clinical setting.

Students and practicing technologists are continuously challenged both physically and mentally by the microbial world. In this world of newfound, life-threatening diseases, education has become the key to survival. Health care providers must each make a personal commitment to infection control, so that, by collective effort, diseases can be conquered.

◀R REVIEW QUESTIONS

1 Microorganisms that cause infectious diseases can be classified as:
   a) lytic
   b) endogenous
   c) pathogenic
   d) nosocomial

2 The best method of preventing the spread of aerosol infections is by:

a) the patient's wearing a mask
b) the health care worker's wearing a gown
c) handwashing
d) all of the above

3 All of the following are types of indirect transmission except:
a) fomite
b) vector
c) aerosol
d) touching

4 The common cold is an example of an infection by a:
a) bacteria
b) virus
c) fungus
d) protozoa

5 The term that best describes the absolute removal of all life forms is:
a) antisepsis
b) medical asepsis
c) disinfection
d) sterilization

6 A person is bitten by a mosquito and develops an infection. This type of transmission is known as:
a) vector
b) fomite
c) nosocomial
d) iatrogenic

7 A health care worker is accidentally punctured with a contaminated needle. This type of transmission is known as:
a) vector
b) fomite
c) nosocomial
d) iatrogenic

8 An outpatient develops a staphylococcal infection after a surgical procedure. This type of transmission is known as:

a) vector
b) fomite
c) nosocomial
d) more than one of the above, but not all

9 An infectious microbe can gain entrance into the human body by:
a) ingression
b) penetration
c) both a and b
d) neither a nor b

10 Handwashing employs which of the following methods of infection control:
a) chemical
b) physical
c) sterile
d) a and b

BIBLIOGRAPHY

Balows A: Manual of Clinical Microbiology. 5th ed. Washington, DC, American Society for Microbiology, 1991.

Benson HJ: Microbiological Applications: A Laboratory Manual in General Microbiology. 5th ed. Dubuque, IA, William C. Brown, 1990.

Borton, D: Isolation precautions. Nursing January:49, 1997.

Brock TD, Madigan MT: Biology of Microorganisms. 5th ed. Englewood Cliffs, NJ, Prentice-Hall, 1988.

Gorbach SL, Bartlett JG, Blacklow NR: Infectious Diseases. Philadelphia, WB Saunders, 1992.

Lennette EH, Halonen P, Murphy FA: Laboratory Diagnosis of Infectious Diseases: Principles and Practice. Vol. 2. New York, Springer-Verlag, 1988.

Linne JJ, Ringsrud KM: Basic Techniques in Clinical Laboratory Science. 3rd ed. St. Louis, Mosby-Year Book, 1992.

National Safety Council: Bloodborne Pathogens Training Manual. Boston: Jones and Bartlett, 1992.

Prendergraph GE: Handbook of Phlebotomy. 3rd ed. Philadelphia, Lea & Febiger, 1992.

Schaechter M, Medoff G, Schlessinger D: Mechanisms of Microbial Disease. Baltimore, Williams & Wilkins, 1989.

Volk W, Benjamin D, Kadner R, Parsons JT: Essentials of Medical Microbiology. 4th ed. Philadelphia, JB Lippincott, 1991.

Walter JB: An Introduction to the Principles of Disease. 2nd ed. Philadelphia, WB Saunders, 1982.

CHAPTER 15

ASEPTIC TECHNIQUES

Steven B. Dowd, EdD, RT(R),(QM),(MR)(M)

Soap and water and common sense are the best disinfectants.

SIR WILLIAM OSLER (1849–1919)

OBJECTIVES

On completion of this chapter, the student will be able to:

1 Describe the use of a sterile drape to establish a sterile field.
2 List the steps in a surgical scrub.
3 Describe procedures for gowning and gloving.
4 List basic principles of sterile technique.
5 Describe the procedure for changing a dressing.
6 Provide care to a patient with a tracheostomy.
7 Provide care to a patient with chest tubes.
8 Describe the care of a patient with a urinary catheter.
9 Contrast intravenous and intra-arterial lines.
10 Assist the physician in pacemaker insertion.

GLOSSARY

Angiography: roentgenographic visualization of blood vessels following introduction of contrast material; used as a diagnostic aid in such conditions as cerebrovascular attacks (strokes) and myocardial infarctions

Arthrography: roentgenography of a joint after injection of opaque contrast material
Atelectasis: collapse of a lung
Auscultation: act of listening for sounds within the body, chiefly for ascertaining the condition of the lungs, heart, pleura, abdomen, and other organs, and for the detection of pregnancy

Foley Catheter: indwelling catheter retained in the bladder by a balloon inflated with air or fluid

Lithotomy Position: patient in dorsal decubitus position with hips and knees flexed and the thighs abducted and externally rotated; also called dorsosacral position

Microorganisms: microscopic organisms; those of medical interest include bacteria, viruses, fungi, and protozoa

Pneumothorax: accumulation of air or gas in the pleural space, which may occur spontaneously or as a result of trauma or a pathologic process, or which may be introduced deliberately

Purulent: consisting of or containing pus; associated with the formulation of or caused by pus

Sterile: aseptic; free from living microorganisms

Tracheostomy: surgical creation of an opening into the trachea through the neck; also used to refer to creation of an opening in the anterior trachea for insertion of a tube to relieve upper airway obstruction and to facilitate ventilation

Trendelenburg Position: position in which the patient is supine on the table or bed, the head of which is tilted downward 30 to 40 degrees, and the table or bed angled beneath the knees

Urinary Meatus: external urethral orifice; the opening of the urethra on the body surface through which urine is discharged

Voiding Cystourethrography: radiography of the bladder and urethra in which radiographs are performed before, during, and after voiding

Understanding aseptic (sterile) techniques is an important part of the professional practice of the radiologic technologist. Handwashing is recognized as the number-one priority for proper sterile technique. The concept of asepsis was discussed in Chapter 14. Along with knowledge of asepsis, it is important that the radiologic technologist never let his or her attitude toward asepsis become too casual. As in radiation protection, it is easy to become so familiar with equipment and procedures that some steps seem easier to leave out. Sloppy aseptic technique can never be tolerated. The purpose of aseptic technique is to reduce the number of harmful **microorganisms.** Surgical asepsis is protection against infection before, during, and after surgery by using sterile technique. Medical asepsis is the removal or destruction of infected material.

Among the numerous radiologic procedures requiring sterile technique are angiography, arthrography, hysterosalpingography, and radiography in the operating room. Other procedures described here require aseptic technique on the part of the technologist or an understanding of how aseptic technique was used for the specific procedure to better care for patients.

Sterile Draping

A **sterile** field is a microorganism-free area that can receive sterile supplies. Most often, it is established using a sterile drape. The first step in using a sterile drape is confirming that the package is sterile. If a package is not clean and dry, it is considered unsterile. If it appears to have been previously opened, or the expiration date has passed, it is also considered unsterile.

The procedure for opening a sterile package (eg, prepared in the hospital) containing a sterile drape on a surface such as a table is as follows (Fig. 15–1):

1 The package should be placed on the center of the surface with the top flap of the wrapper set to open away from the individual opening the package.

2 The first flap on the outside of the wrapper should be pinched between the thumb and index finger by reaching around (not over) the package. Some packages require that the uppermost flap at each corner be grasped. The flap should be pulled open and laid flat on the far surface.

3 Use the right hand to open the right flap and the left hand to open the left flap.

4 Grasping the turned-down corner, pull the fourth and final flap. If the inner surface of any of the package touches an unsterile object such as a sleeve, the entire pack and contents are considered unsterile and must be replaced.

A sterile package may also be opened as follows:

1 The package is held in one hand with the top flap opening away from the person opening the package.

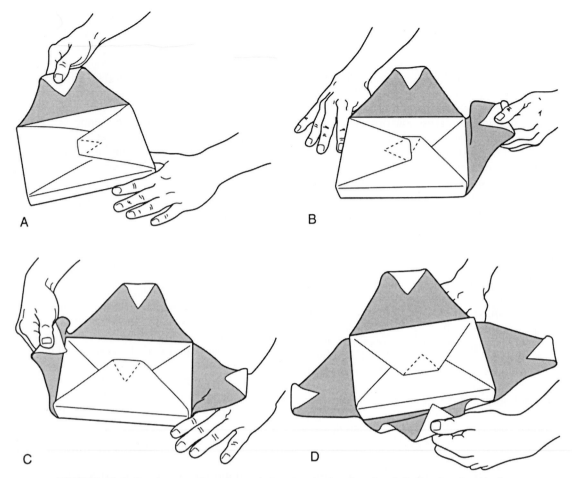

A

B

C

D

FIGURE 15–1. Opening a sterile package. *A*, Opening the first flap. *B* and *C*, Opening the side flaps. *D*, Pulling the last flap by grasping the corner.

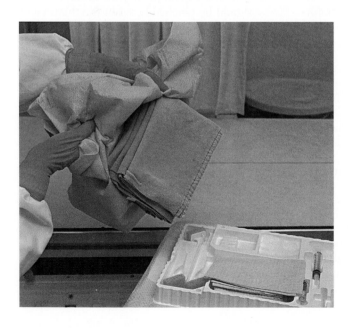

FIGURE 15–2. Dropping sterile towels onto a sterile field while keeping the nonsterile wrapping well away from the sterile field.

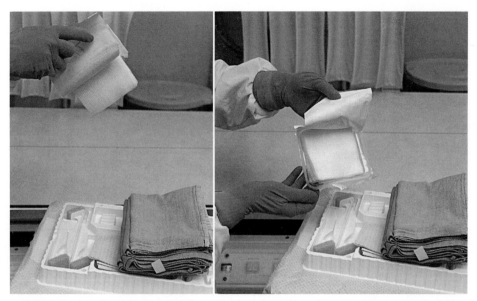

FIGURE 15–3. Opening commercially prepared sterile packs to drop sponges onto a sterile field.

2 The top flap is pulled well back and held away from both the contents of the package and the sterile field. Using the free hand to hold the flap against the wrist of the hand holding the package is an effective technique.

3 The contents are then dropped gently onto the sterile field from about 6 inches above the field and at a slight angle. These techniques help to make sure that the package wrapping does not touch the sterile field at any time (Fig. 15–2).

Commercial packages usually have specific directions for opening on the package. In general, there are packages with partially sealed corners, in which the container is held in one hand and the flap pulled back with the other, and those with partially sealed edges, in which both sides of the edge are grasped, one with each hand, and gently pulled apart (Fig. 15–3).

To establish a sterile field, the drape is plucked with one hand by the corner and opened. This corner is then used to fold back the top. Then the drape is lifted out of the cover and allowed to open freely without touching anything. Another corner of the drape is then picked up carefully and laid on a clean, dry surface with the bottom farthest from the person establishing the field (Fig. 15–4). Necessary sterile supplies can now be added to the field using the proper package-opening techniques.

Finally, sterile solutions are frequently poured into a metal or other container within the sterile field. Bottles containing sterile solutions are usually considered sterile on the inside but contaminated on the outside; thus, special care is needed in pouring these solutions. Always try to use the exact amount of solution. Once opened, the solution can be considered sterile only if used immediately. Once the container has been set down, it is no longer considered to be sterile, and a new container must be opened. Always confirm the name of the solution and its strength by checking three times. When possible, show the name to another person.

The procedure for pouring sterile solutions is as follows:

1 Remove the lid or cap from the bottle; place it on an unsterile surface with the top side down immediately to ensure the sterility of the inner surface.

2 The bottle should be held with the label uppermost so that poured solution cannot stain and obscure the label.

3 With as little of the bottle as possible over the field, hold it at a height of about 6 inches over the bowl (Fig. 15–5).

4 Pour the solution gently so that there is no splashing. Splashing of liquids can destroy a sterile field by allowing microorganisms to move from the unsterile table top through the wet drape that forms the bottom of the sterile field.

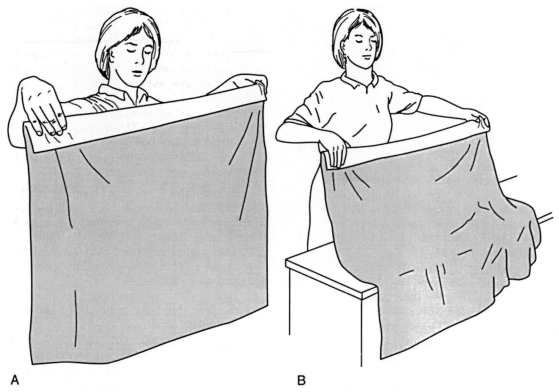

A   B

FIGURE 15–4. Establishing a sterile field. *A*, Holding the drape with one hand by the corner. *B*, Folding back the top to lift the cover and laying the drape on a clean, dry surface with the bottom farthest from the person establishing the field.

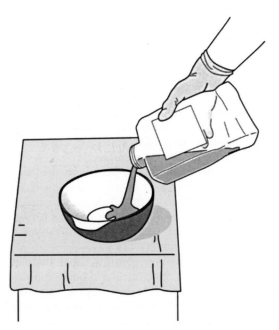

FIGURE 15–5. Pouring a sterile solution into a sterile bowl on a sterile field.

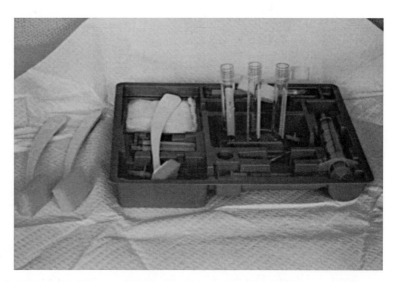

FIGURE 15–6. A typical myelography pack.

Sterile Packs

Commonly used sterile packs include myelography, minor procedure, and various special procedure packs used for procedures such as venograms, angiograms, and lymphangiograms. Items in the typical myelography pack are shown in Figure 15–6 and often include the following:

- injectable local anesthetic
- syringes and needles of various sizes
- sterile drape
- collection tubes (for spinal fluid)

A minor procedure pack, used for **arthrography** and biopsies, usually contains all of the above as well as a sterile gown. Although commercially prepared **angiography** packs are available, many hospitals prefer to make up their own trays. Typical supplies might include the following:

- needles to include three 18 gauge, one 20 gauge, one 22 gauge, and one 25 gauge (the larger gauge needles are used to inject local anesthetic)
- a plastic connector for test injections of contrast material
- one manifold (three stopcocks) for the contrast test, heparin drip, or saline flush
- a scalpel handle and a No. 10 scalpel blade used for arterial cutdown techniques
- a large number of gauze pads or topper sponges
- up to five 10-, 20-, or 30-mL Luer-Lok syringes for saline flush

- three 10-mL Luer-Lok syringes: two for contrast tests, one for local anesthetic
- forceps for sponges
- six sponges for preparation of the puncture site with anesthetic
- three stainless steel basins: one for saline solution, one for antiseptic, and one used as a waste basin; one emesis basin
- a straight clamp and a curved clamp for arterial cutdown techniques
- clamp to keep guide wire wrapped
- sterile screwdriver for tightening screws on manifolds

Surgical Scrubbing

Although individuals performing aseptic procedures wear gloves, the skin of their hands and forearms should be cleaned routinely to reduce the number of microorganisms in case a glove tears. A surgical scrub is required before participation in many interventional studies. The purpose of the surgical hand scrub is (1) to remove debris and transient microorganisms from the hands, nails, and forearms; (2) to reduce the resident microbial count to a minimum; and (3) to inhibit rapid rebound growth of microorganisms.

The sterile scrub consists of scrubbing with soap and water and a nail brush and often an immersion in a mild germicidal solution. There are two basic methods of surgical scrubbing: the numbered stroke method, in which a certain number of brush strokes are used for each finger, palm, back of the hand, and the arm; and the timed scrub. Although exact procedures and times for the scrub vary between settings and institutions, the following can serve as a guideline for the timed scrub:

1 Be sure that scrub brushes, antiseptic soap, and nail cleaners are available.
2 Remove all jewelry, including watch.
3 Wash hands and arms with antiseptic soap.
4 Clean subungual areas with nail file.
5 The sides of each finger, between the fingers, and the back and front of the hand should be scrubbed for 2 minutes.
6 The arm is now scrubbed with the hands higher than the elbows. Each side of the arm is washed to 3 inches above the elbow for 1 minute.
7 The process is now repeated for the other hand and arm. The hands remain above the elbows at all times.
8 The hands are dried as shown in Figure 15–7.

Sterile Gowning and Gloving

Gowns and gloves are put on after the surgical scrub. There are two methods of gowning: self-gowning and gowning another. Sterile gowning differs from gowning for isolation in that the focus is on surgical as opposed to medical asepsis. There are also two methods of gloving: self and another. A sterile surface is always required for sterile gloving.

SELF-GOWNING (Fig. 15–8)

1 Standing about 12 inches from the sterile area, pick up the gown by the folded edges and lift it directly up from the package.
2 Stepping back from the table, make sure no objects are near the gown. Grasping the gown at the neck band, hold it at arm's length, unfold it, and gently shake it.
3 Facing the inside of the gown and holding it by the shoulder seams, raise the arms up and slip them into the sleeves.
4 The gown may be adjusted by an unsterile worker standing behind and reaching inside the sleeves, grasping them, and pulling gently.
5 For the open method, the sleeves are pulled over the hands. For the closed method, the sleeves are pulled so that only the fingertips are visible.

6 An assistant fastens the back and waistband of the gown.

After the gown is on, only the sleeves and front of the gown down to the waist are considered sterile. To maintain sterile technique once in sterile gown and gloves, persons must pass each other back to back.

SELF-GLOVING

Self-gloving is performed after gowning. All jewelry should have been removed. The glove package should be opened facing the person who is going to wear the gloves with the right glove on the right side.

Closed Method (Fig. 15–9)

1 The hands are covered by the gown so that the fingers are covered by the sterile gown when grasping the gloves.
2 The glove of the dominant hand is picked up with the nondominant hand. (A right-handed person has a right dominant hand.)
3 The palm of the glove is placed on the palm of the dominant hand. The fingers of the glove face the elbow.
4 The bottom part of the cuff is grasped with the fingers of the dominant hand. The nondominant hand grasps the top part of the cuff and pulls it over the dominant hand.
5 The gloved hand picks up the other glove.
6 The ungloved hand holds the cuff through the sterile gown.
7 The gloved hand pulls the other hand into it.
8 The fingers are adjusted until comfortable.

Open Method (Fig. 15–10)

1 With the hands pushed through the sleeves, the cuff of the dominant hand glove is picked up with the nondominant hand. It is important not to touch the outside surface of the glove.
2 The dominant hand is slipped into the glove, and the glove is pulled on by the nondominant hand.
3 The gloved (and now sterile) dominant hand picks up the other glove by reaching under the cuff. It is important to touch only the outside surface of the glove with the sterile gloved hand.

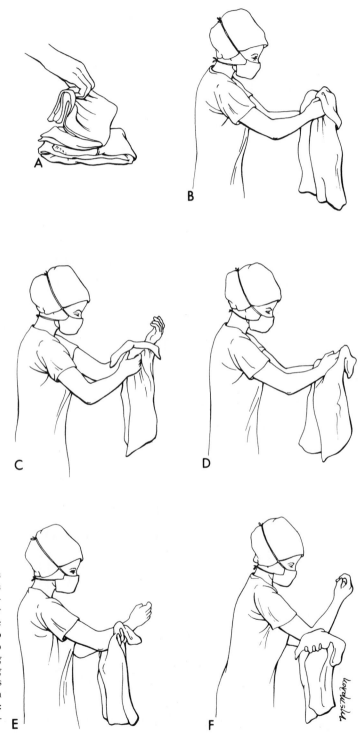

FIGURE 15–7. Drying hands and arms after a surgical scrub. *A*, A sterile towel is picked up. *B*, The towel is folded lengthwise. One end of the towel is used to dry one hand, using a blotting motion. *C*, The arm is rotated as it is dried from wrist to elbow. *D*, The dry hand is used to grasp the opposite end of towel to begin drying the other hand. *E*, The arm is dried using a blotting motion. *F*, Blotting proceeds to the elbow. (Reprinted with permission from Fuller JR: Surgical Technology: Principles and Practice, 3rd ed. Philadelphia, WB Saunders, 1994, p 71.)

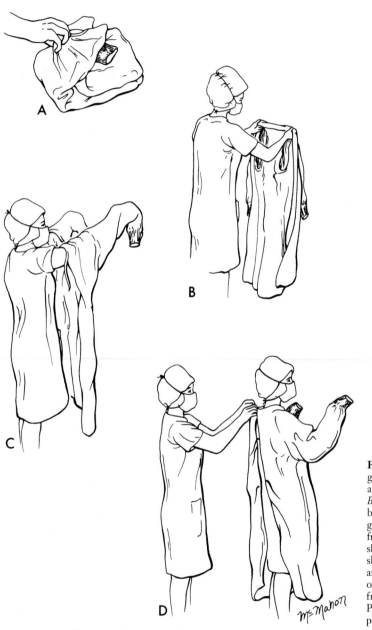

FIGURE 15–8. Self-gowning. *A,* The gown is picked up by the folded edges and lifted directly up from the package. *B,* The gown is grasped at the neck band, held at arm's length, unfolded, and gently shaken. *C,* The gown is put on from the inside by holding it by the shoulder seams, raising the arms up, and slipping them into the sleeves. *D,* An assistant fastens the back and waistband of the gown. (Reprinted with permission from Fuller JR: Surgical Technology: Principles and Practice, 3rd ed. Philadelphia, WB Saunders, 1994, p 72.)

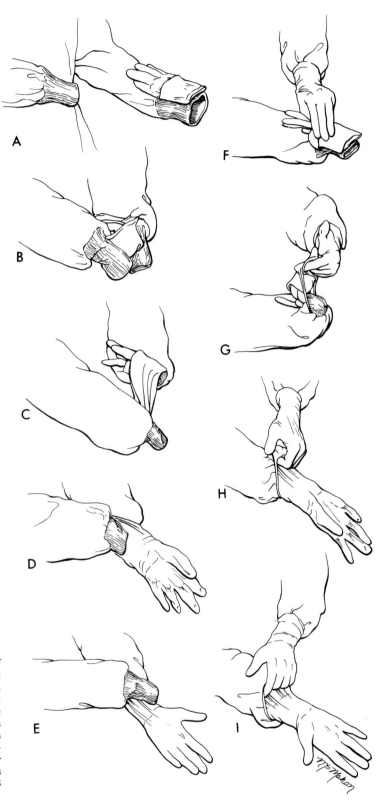

FIGURE 15–9. Self-gloving, closed method. *A,* The hands are covered by the gown so that the fingers are covered by the sterile gown when grasping the gloves. *B,* The glove of the dominant hand is picked up with the nondominant hand. *C,* The palm of the glove is placed on the palm of the dominant hand. *D,* The bottom part of the cuff is grasped with the fingers of the dominant hand. *E,* The nondominant hand grasps the top part of the cuff and pulls it over the dominant hand. *F,* The gloved hand then picks up the other glove. *G,* The ungloved hand holds the cuff through the sterile gown. *H,* The gloved hand then pulls the other hand into it. *I,* The fingers are adjusted until comfortable. (Reprinted with permission from Fuller JR: Surgical Technology: Principles and Practice, 3rd ed. Philadelphia, WB Saunders, 1994, p 73.)

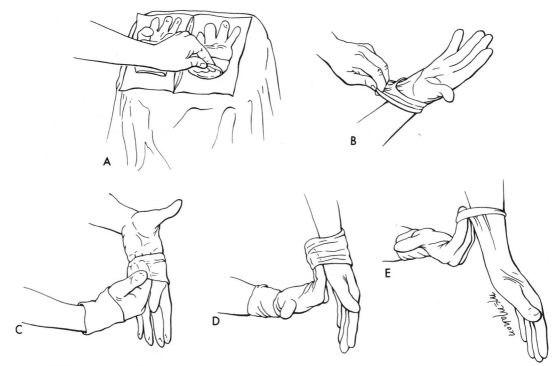

FIGURE 15–10. Self-gloving, open method. *A,* With the hands pushed through the sleeves, the cuff of the dominant hand glove is picked up with the nondominant hand without touching the outside surface of the glove. *B,* The dominant hand is slipped into the glove and the glove is pulled on by the nondominant hand. *C,* The gloved (and now sterile) dominant hand is used to pick up the other glove by reaching under the cuff, touching only the outside surface of the glove with the sterile gloved hand. *D* and *E,* The glove is then pulled onto the nondominant hand without touching the inside surface of the glove. (Reprinted with permission from Fuller JR: Surgical Technology: Principles and Practice, 3rd ed. Philadelphia, WB Saunders, 1994, p 74.)

4 The glove is then pulled onto the nondominant hand without touching the inside surface of the glove (which is actually the outside surface of the folded cuff).

GOWNING ANOTHER (Fig. 15–11)

1 The sterile person picks up the gown by the neck band, holds it at arm's length, and allows it to unfold.
2 The gown is held by the shoulder seams with the outside facing the sterile person.
3 The sterile gloves are protected by placing both hands under the back panel of the gown at the top shoulder seam.
4 The arms are slipped into the sleeves in a downward motion until the hands emerge from the sleeves.
5 Another person pulls the gown over the arms and shoulders and fastens the back and waistband of the gown.

GLOVING ANOTHER (Fig. 15–12)

1 The sterile person opens the package and picks up the gloves.
2 After informing the other person which hand to use, the sterile person grasps the cuff and pulls sideways to open the glove with the thumb facing the hand to be gloved. It is important to have an extremely good grasp on the cuff, since considerable force is exerted when the hand is pushed down into the tight glove.
3 The person putting the gloves on keeps the thumbs away from the glove to avoid possible contact and puts the hand in the glove using a downward motion.
4 The process is repeated for the other hand.

The procedure for removing gloves aseptically is also important to avoid contamination. The procedure to avoid touching the outside portion of the glove is shown in Figure 15–13.

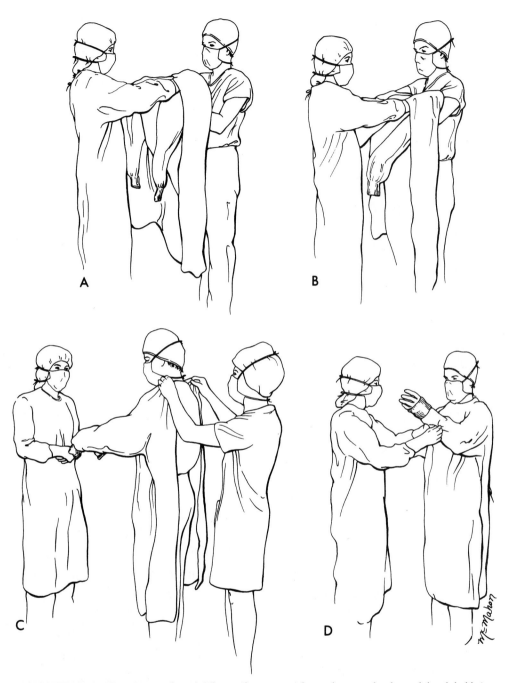

FIGURE 15–11. Gowning another. *A,* The sterile person picks up the gown by the neck band, holds it at arm's length, and allows it to unfold. *B,* The gown is held by the shoulder seams with the outside facing the sterile person while that person protects the sterile gloves by placing both hands under the back panel of the gown at the top shoulder seam. *C,* The arms are slipped into the sleeves in a downward motion until the hands emerge from the sleeves. *D,* Another person pulls the gown over the arms and shoulders and fastens the back and waistband of the gown. (Reprinted with permission from Fuller JR: Surgical Technology: Principles and Practice, 3rd ed. Philadelphia, WB Saunders, 1994, p 75.)

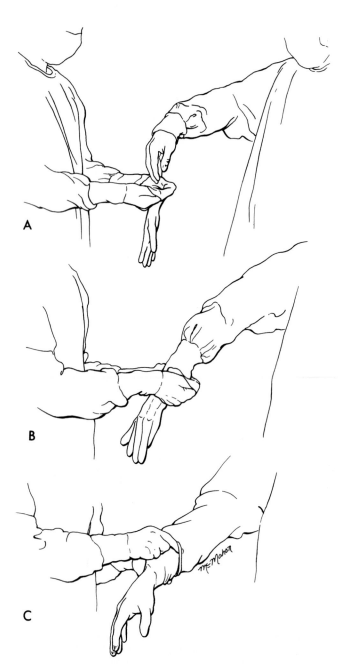

FIGURE 15–12. Gloving another. *A*, After informing the other person which hand to use, the sterile person grasps the cuff and pulls sideways to open the glove with the thumb facing the hand to be gloved. *B*, The person putting the gloves on keeps the thumbs away from the glove to avoid possible contact. *C*, The person putting the glove on pushes the hand in the glove, using a downward motion. (Reprinted with permission from Fuller JR: Surgical Technology: Principles and Practice, 3rd ed. Philadelphia, WB Saunders, 1994, p 76.)

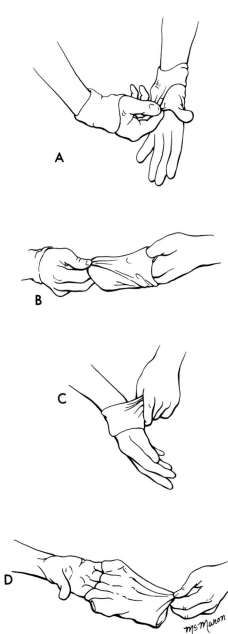

FIGURE 15–13. Removing gloves aseptically. *A*, Grasp the outside edge of the glove with the other gloved hand. *B*, Unroll the glove over the hand without letting the skin surface touch the outside of the glove. *C*, With the ungloved hand, grasp the opposite glove cuff, touching only the inside surface. *D*, Remove the glove by inverting it over the hand and discarding it. Throughout this procedure, the bare hand never touches the outside of the glove. (Reprinted with permission from Fuller JR: Surgical Technology: Principles and Practice, 3rd ed. Philadelphia, WB Saunders, 1994, p 76.)

BOX 15-1

Basic Principles of Sterile Technique

Only sterile items are used in sterile fields.

If in doubt about the sterility of an object, consider it unsterile. An unsterile object should be removed, covered, or replaced.

A sterile field must be continually watched to be considered sterile.

Create sterile fields as close to the time of use as possible.

Sterile persons should avoid unsterile areas.

Anything below the level of the table or the level of the waist, as well as the undersurface of the drape, is considered unsterile. Any item that falls below this area is considered to be contaminated.

Gowns are considered sterile on the sleeves and the front from the waist up. The back of the gown and below the waist is considered unsterile.

Persons in sterile gown and gloves must pass each other back to back.

A sterile person may touch only what is sterile.

Unsterile persons cannot reach above or over a sterile field.

Sterile materials must be kept dry. Moisture permits contamination. Packages that become wet must be resterilized or discarded.

If a solution soaks through a sterile field to a nonsterile field, the wet area may be redraped.

Sterile gloves must be kept in sight and above waist level.

Sterile Procedures

Box 15-1 lists the basic principles of sterile technique. The field includes the patient, table and other furniture covered with sterile drapes, and the personnel wearing sterile attire.

DRESSING CHANGES

Dressings are best changed in a team setting with another technologist or health care worker.

The physician is responsible for ordering dressing changes and reapplication. Be sure to secure privacy, explain the procedure to the patient, and secure consent before beginning the procedure. The equipment needed is as follows:

STERILE

- Disposable gloves
- Pack containing scissors, forceps, sterile towel, dressings, cotton-tipped swabs, and solution cup
- Antiseptic solution and sterile saline

UNSTERILE

- Plastic bag for discarded dressings
- Properly sized adhesive
- Pads to protect surrounding area from secretions
- Gowns are recommended by many texts if the wound is purulent; in a standard precautions environment, gowns are required at all times

All dressings are treated as if they were infected. Do not touch a dressing with bare hands. The procedure for changing a dressing is as follows:

1 The hands are washed, and patient privacy and consent are obtained. The adhesive tape surrounding the dressing must be removed. This is often a painful procedure, and a solvent such as baby oil might be needed to loosen the tape. Limit the amount of solvent to avoid contaminating the wound.

2 The dressing is removed with forceps or gloved hands, wrapped, and placed in the plastic bag. If the dressing does not come off easily, contact an appropriate individual (ie, department nurse, department supervisor, or physician) for additional instructions or to remove the dressing.

3 For reapplication, sterile technique is followed. The hands are washed, and the sterile towel is opened to use as a sterile field on which to place sterile dressings. The dressings are opened and placed on the sterile towel.

4 The tape is cut into the lengths that will be needed. Because the tape is not sterile, it is placed near but not on the sterile field.

5 Gloves are put on and the dressing is applied. The gloves are removed and the dressing is secured with the adhesive tape. The hands are washed again, the patient is

covered again, and the waste is disposed of according to the institutional policy.

TRACHEOSTOMIES

A **tracheostomy** is an operation performed under sterile technique that involves incising the skin over the trachea, then making a surgical wound in the trachea. This provides for an airway during upper airway obstruction. It is used in emergency situations and to replace the airway provided by an endotracheal tube that has been in place for several weeks. To prevent skin breakdown, tracheostomies are always covered with a dressing.

If at all possible, the first task in providing care to a patient with a tracheostomy is to establish communication. This usually consists of yes and no questions, hand signals, and simple sign language; less often, written communication methods are used. Because these patients are often extremely ill, they have difficulty in using written communication and little need for complicated messages.

The technologist caring for the tracheostomy patient must also be sensitive to unmet and inexpressible needs and the need to keep the patient's anxiety level low. Thus, these patients often have a great need to have procedures explained and repeated. A technologist may take a lot of time to explain a portable chest radiograph to a patient the first time and then slip into a routine of "We're going to take your chest x-ray now" each subsequent morning. The patient may have forgotten, in the midst of all the other procedures performed, exactly what that means. The patient may then consciously or unconsciously resist the procedure.

A tracheostomy should not be touched by the technologist except under conditions of sterile technique to minimize the possibility of infection. A tracheostomy must be suctioned often to remove secretions. This is usually a task of the nurse taking care of the patient, although in certain situations (eg, emergencies) this may be a task of the technologist. The patient must be well aerated with 5 to 10 breaths of oxygen before suctioning. This can be accomplished using an Ambu bag hooked to an oxygen source. Also prior to suctioning, the patency of the suction catheter must be tested by aspirating normal saline through the catheter. The procedure for suctioning is then as follows:

1 Insert the catheter in the stoma without suction until the patient coughs or resistance is met. Then, withdraw the catheter about 1 cm before beginning suctioning.

2 Suction should be applied intermittently and the catheter withdrawn in a rotating motion. Suctioning is activated by placing the thumb over the hole in the suction line to cause the suction to pull from the end of the tube where it is placed in the patient's body (Fig. 15–14).

3 The airway is assessed by **auscultation** of the lungs. A stethoscope is used to listen to the sounds of inspiration and expiration over the chest wall. Breath sounds are the result of free movement of air into and out of the bronchial tree. The duration, pitch, and intensity of sounds indicate whether breathing is normal or abnormal.

4 The procedure is repeated until the airway is clear. Never suction for longer than 15 seconds, and allow the patient to rest in between.

CHEST TUBES

Chest tubes are used to remove fluid, blood, and air from the pleural cavity. They assist in reinflating collapsed lungs (**atelectasis**) and al-

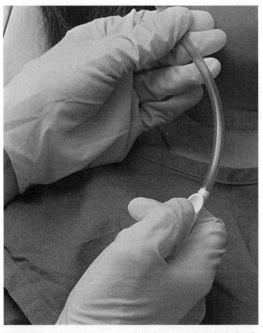

FIGURE 15–14. Suction tube showing thumb hole for activation of suctioning.

leviating pneumothorax, or air in the thoracic cavity. They are also used in cases of thoracotomy and open heart surgery. Normally, the pleural cavity contains no air or blood, containing instead a thin layer of lubricant that allows the pleurae to slide and move over one another without friction.

There are three compartments in chest drainage systems to which chest tubes are attached (Fig. 15–15). The first compartment is the collection chamber. It collects any fluid leaving the lung. The second compartment is the water seal chamber. It contains water and prevents air from the atmosphere from entering the cavity through the chest tube. The concept is similar to that of a drinking straw through which air can be blown (eg, into a glass of water) but none can return. The third compartment is the suction control chamber. It also contains water, the amount of which regulates the amount of suction. This suction removes unwanted air or fluid from the pleural cavity. Some units have an additional fourth chamber, a water seal vented to the atmosphere to prevent potential pressure build-up.

Radiographers often perform chest radiography, especially portable procedures, before and

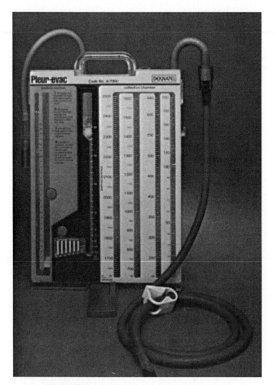

FIGURE 15–15. Chest drainage systems.

after the insertion of chest tubes to ensure proper placement. Figure 15–16 shows proper placement of chest tubes on a portable chest radiograph. Radiographers also make chest films to confirm that the tubes may be removed; these are sometimes taken in the radiology department. An initial radiograph confirms full lung expansion; a second is performed 2 hours after clamping to verify continued expansion. A third film is often obtained after removal of chest tubes to further confirm full lung expansion.

It is important to be careful when entering and leaving the patient's room after the tubes have been inserted; the tubes can be pulled from the body if caught by a mobile x-ray unit or tugged roughly during handling of the patient or cassette. Patients may also come to the radiology department by stretcher or wheelchair if they have had the chest tubes in place for a long time. *The exterior assembly of the chest tubes must always remain lower than the patient's chest.* Caution is necessary when moving and positioning the patient to prevent compromising the integrity of the tubes.

URINARY CATHETERS

Urinary catheterization is the insertion of a tube into the bladder using aseptic technique. The two main types of urinary catheters are the **Foley** (a retention balloon type) and the straight type (Fig. 15–17). On insertion of the Foley catheter, the balloon is filled with sterile water to hold the catheter in place. Any catheter that remains in place is also called an indwelling catheter. Urinary catheters can be used to:

- empty the bladder (ie, before surgery, radiologic or other examinations, or childbirth)
- relieve retention of urine or bypass obstruction
- irrigate the bladder or introduce drugs
- permit accurate measuring of urine output
- relieve incontinence

Sizes of catheters range from 8 to 18 in even numbers based on the French system. This system indicates the outer diameter of the catheter. Each unit on this scale is 0.33 mm; thus, catheters range in diameter from approximately 2.6 to 5.9 mm. It is better to choose a larger size when possible.

Because a urinary catheter can interrupt the body's defense mechanism against disease, a va-

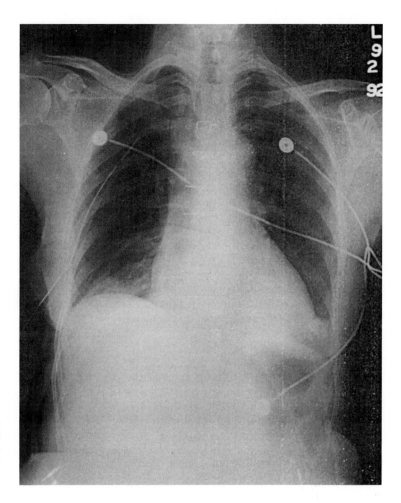

FIGURE 15–16. Radiograph verifying proper placement of chest tube in the right upper lobe of the lung. (Courtesy of University of Alabama at Birmingham Hospital, Birmingham, Alabama.)

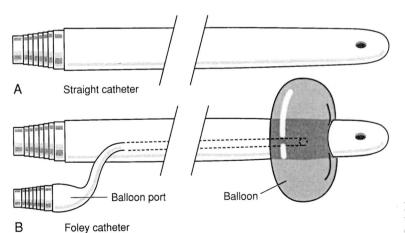

A   Straight catheter

B   Foley catheter

Balloon port

Balloon

FIGURE 15–17. The two main types of urinary catheters: straight (*A*), Foley (*B*).

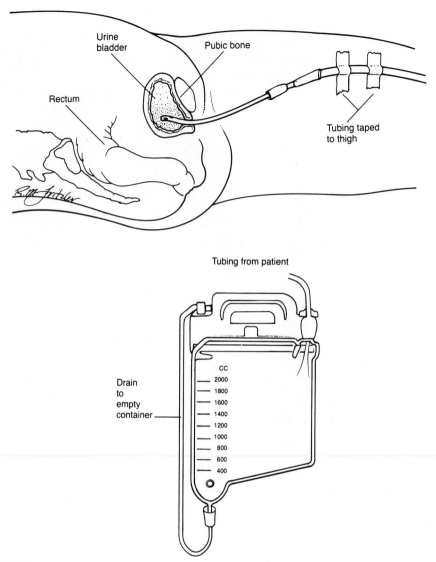

FIGURE 15–18. Proper placement of a urinary catheter in a female patient. (Adapted with permission from Craig M: Introduction to Ultrasonography and Patient Care. Philadelphia, WB Saunders, 1993.)

riety of catheters is available. Plastic catheters, for example, are suitable for short-term use only. Latex catheters can be used for 2 to 3 weeks and polyvinylchloride (PVC) catheters for 4 to 6 weeks, whereas the expensive pure silicone catheters are used only for long-term catheterization of 2 to 3 months.

The urine collection bag should be kept low (below the level of the bladder) to prevent reflux of urine back into the bladder. Failure to do this can lead to infection. This also facilitates drainage from the bladder by gravity. Bags should never drag on the floor. When transfer-

ring patients by wheelchair or stretcher, it is important to make sure that the drainage bag and tubing do not become entangled in wheels or caught on passing objects.

If the urine collection bag is emptied by the technologist, it is important to measure and record output unless otherwise noted. Do not forget to reclamp the stopcock after the bag has been emptied. In many cases, the patient's intake of fluids is also being recorded, so if the patient is given a drink of water or any other fluid, it should be recorded in the patient chart along with the recorded output. Always check with the nursing unit whenever there is a question of recording intake and output.

Technologists do not normally catheterize patients, although this varies depending on the setting. In some institutions, the radiographer might be responsible for catheterizing a patient undergoing a voiding cystogram as an outpatient. The equipment needed to perform urinary catheterization consists of a sterile catheter, a sterile collecting bag, a syringe with sterile water or saline, and a catheterization kit or the following supplies:

- sterile gloves
- antiseptic solution
- sterile cotton balls and sterile forceps
- lubricant (water-soluble jelly)
- container to receive urine
- sterile drape for sterile field

The procedure for performing urinary catheterization is as follows:

1 Wash hands, provide for patient privacy, explain the procedure, and secure consent.
2 Position female patients in the **lithotomy position;** position male patients supine and expose the genitalia.
3 Open the kit and put on the gloves, which will remain sterile during the entire procedure.
4 The sterile drape should be placed around the penis for a male patient or under the buttocks for a female patient.
5 If a Foley catheter is being used, test-inflate the balloon by injecting a small amount (about 1 mL) of sterile water into the balloon port of the catheter. If the balloon holds, deflate it. If it fails to hold, obtain a new Foley catheter.
6 Pour antiseptic over the cotton balls.
7 Coat the catheter tip with sterile lubricant.
8 Expose the **urinary meatus** using the nondominant hand. This hand is no longer considered sterile.
9 With female patients, separate the labia majora and minora. For male patients, hold the penis with the foreskin retracted.
10 Clean the urinary meatus with a cotton ball held by forceps. For males, circle the urinary meatus once and repeat. For females, wipe the labia minora from top to bottom and discard the cotton, then clean the urinary meatus from top to bottom. It is extremely important not to let the labia or foreskin contaminate the meatus before or after cleansing.
11 The catheter is now inserted slowly with the dominant hand until urine flows. For females, this is about 1½ inches (Fig. 15–18); for males, it is about 8 inches (Fig. 15–19). Always use a gentle pressure. Never force a catheter.

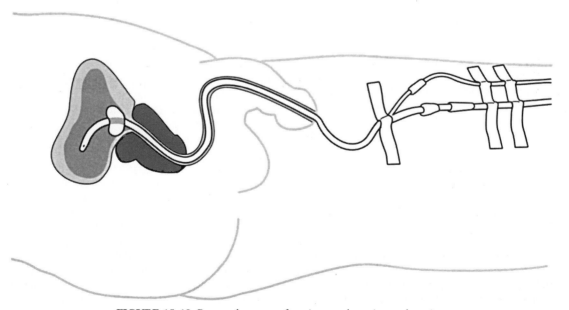

FIGURE 15–19. Proper placement of a urinary catheter in a male patient.

12 Reattach the syringe to the balloon port and fill the balloon. A light tug on the catheter ensures that the balloon is holding the catheter in place.

The radiologic technologist is often responsible for removing a urinary catheter after procedures such as **voiding cystourethrograms.** The materials needed to remove an indwelling catheter are a basin such as an emesis basin, scissors, and several paper towels. The procedure is as follows:

1 Wash hands, provide for privacy, explain the procedure to the patient, and secure consent.
2 Uncover the patient and place the basin under the catheter valve. Cut the tip of the balloon valve with the scissors, and allow the water from the balloon to drain into the basin.
3 Once the flow of water has ceased, place the towels under the catheter and pull gently. Stop and notify a physician or nurse if any resistance is noted.
4 When the catheter has been completely removed, wrap it in the towels, cover the patient, and discard the catheter.

Another type of urinary catheter is the suprapubic catheter. It is a closed drainage system inserted about 1 inch above the symphysis pubis into the distended bladder. The procedure is performed under general anesthesia. If the catheter is to be retained in place, it is sutured to the skin of the abdomen. Male patients may also have a condom catheter, a specially designed condom with a catheter at the end attached to a collecting bag. This allows an incontinent male patient the use of a catheter without the permanence or inconvenience of a Foley or straight catheter. This type of catheter is prone to infection at the tip of the penis and requires regular cleaning, care, and changing of the condom sleeve.

INTRAVENOUS AND INTRA-ARTERIAL LINES

Sterile technique is required for the insertion of lines (catheters) into veins and arteries. These are also called central venous and arterial lines. Intravenous lines are inserted for a variety of reasons, including the introduction of medications and intravenous fluids and the measurement of central venous pressure. The Swan-Ganz catheter, a specific type of intravenous catheter, is used to measure the pumping ability of the heart and other heart parameters. Other types of venous lines include the Intracath, Hickman, Briouvac, and Arrow-Howes triple lumen. Arterial lines include the radial arterial and femoral arterial. These lines are typically used for drawing blood and measuring blood pressure.

When performing special radiologic procedures, the radiologic technologist may encounter patients with arterial and venous lines in place. Also, fluoroscopy and portable chest radiography are often used to verify placement of the lines. The portable chest radiograph is also used to assess for pneumothorax. Gloves, masks, and gowns are typically worn. The patient is usually in the Trendelenburg position when the line is placed. Figure 15–20 demonstrates correct placement of a Swan-Ganz catheter.

PACEMAKERS

Permanent pacemakers are electromechanical devices inserted under the patient's skin to regulate the heart rate. Patients with symptomatic bradycardia (slow heart rate) are the most likely candidates for permanent pacemakers. A pacemaker can prevent bradycardia by sensing the heartbeats of a patient and pacing the heart when it does not initiate a heartbeat on its own.

Pacemaker units are about 1 inch in width, diameter, and thickness, weighing just a little over 1 ounce. The unit consists of a pulse generator and accompanying circuitry, and is connected to a lead. The tip of the lead contains a metal electrode that is put into contact with the heart. The electrode senses heartbeats and can also produce an electrical impulse to make the heart contract.

Using aseptic technique, the surgeon makes an incision at the level of the pectoral fascia, secures percutaneous access to a vein, and forms a pocket for the pulse generator. Before inserting the pacing lead, a needle and syringe are inserted into the subclavian vein for verification. Then, a guide wire is inserted through the needle to establish a pathway through the vein. The role of the radiographer is to assist the physician in placement through fluoroscopy. The position of the guide wire is verified under fluoroscopy. Then, an introducer sheath is used to place the pacing lead into the subclavian vein.

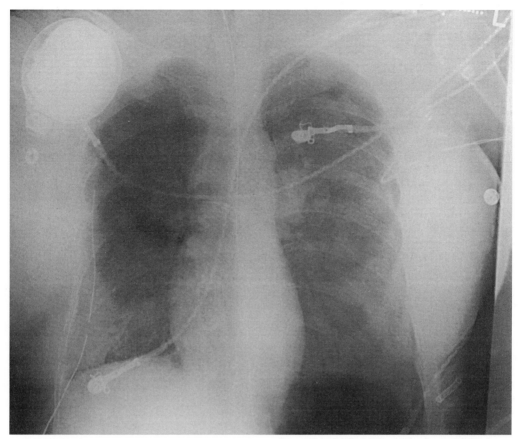

FIGURE 15–20. Radiograph verifying proper placement of a Swan-Ganz line. (Also note pacemaker and chest tube.) (Courtesy of University of Alabama at Birmingham Hospital, Birmingham, Alabama.)

Under fluoroscopy, the lead is advanced into the right atrium, the introducer sheath is withdrawn, and the lead is positioned in the apex of the right ventricle. At this point, the radiographer's role in the procedure is usually complete.

Temporary pacemakers are also usually connected to a transvenous pacing electrode, but the pacemaker is external to the patient's body. The fluoroscopic technique is similar to the permanent pacemaker insertion.

PORTABLE AND OPERATING ROOM RADIOGRAPHY

Radiography in the operating room requires strict attention to sterile technique. Specific guidelines are difficult to give because procedures vary greatly between surgeons and facilities. The one constant is the existence of a sterile corridor, the area between the patient drape and the instrument table. Radiographic cassettes are sometimes positioned under the table through a tunnel device; in other cases, they are enclosed in sterile covers and positioned by the physician.

In most cases, the radiography student observes procedures, especially at first, performed in the operating room. In some cases, the machinery is left outside the room until right before the procedure; in some, the surgeon or procedure demands that a set-up occur before the operation begins.

Neonatal Portable Radiography

For radiography of the neonate, there are two accepted methods of gonadal shielding: contact, which places lead directly on the baby's gonads, and shadow, which hangs a piece of lead in the beam (or places a piece of lead on the isolette), casting a shadow in the collimator light. Each has advantages and disadvantages. Shadow shielding, for example, requires low levels of ambient lighting for proper use. Contact shielding has the greatest potential for cross-infection.

Why is the potential for cross-infection so important? Sepsis and nosocomial infections are recognized as major threats that result in significant morbidity and mortality each year in the neonatal unit. Thus it is important, in neonatal radiography, to maintain asepsis as much as possible. The problem of cross-infection could be handled by keeping multiple pieces of lead in the wards and sterilizing after use; covering the lead with a pillow case or other protective covering, or assigning a piece of lead to each crib and cleaning after each patient. Each institution will probably decide, based on a number of factors, which method it finds to be the most usable.

Use of the C-Arm in Surgery

The use of the C-arm in surgery requires increased attention to maintaining a sterile field. There are basically three approaches to maintaining a sterile field, according to Bontrager (1997). Most common is draping the image intensifier and C-arm with what is known as a snap cover. A tension band is "snapped" in place when the image intensifier and C-arm are covered with a sterile cloth or bags. This approach allows the physician to manipulate the C-arm while maintaining a sterile field.

Hip pinnings or femur roddings may use an approach known as the shower curtain approach. On the patient's affected side, a sterile clear plastic sheet is suspended from a long horizontal metal bar attached to two vertical suspending rods. There is an opening in the middle of the sheet, which is attached using a special adhesive to the patient, allowing for access to the surgical site.

A third, but less common approach, is to drape the site with an additional sterile cloth. The C-arm is then brought over the anatomic area of interest. When the C-arm is no longer needed, it is removed, as is the cloth. This is a "stop-gap" measure in many cases, and is only useful when the physician does not need to manipulate the C-arm.

Summary

The purpose of aseptic technique is to reduce the number of harmful microorganisms. Surgi-

cal asepsis is protection against infection before, during, and after surgery by using sterile technique. Medical asepsis is the removal or destruction of infected material. A variety of radiologic procedures require sterile technique.

A sterile field is a microorganism-free area that can receive sterile supplies. The patient is the center of the sterile field. The field includes the patient, table and other furniture covered with sterile drapes, and the personnel wearing sterile attire.

Commonly used sterile packs include myelography, minor procedure, and special procedure packs. Minor procedure packs are used for arthrography and biopsy.

The purpose of the surgical hand scrub is to remove debris and transient microorganisms from the hands, nails, and forearms; to reduce the resident microbial count to a minimum; and to inhibit rapid rebound growth of microorganisms.

Gowns and gloves are put on after the surgical scrub. There are two methods of gowning: self-gowning and gowning another. Sterile gowning differs from gowning for isolation in that the focus is on surgical as opposed to medical asepsis. There are also two methods of gloving: self and another.

All dressings are treated as if they were infected and are not touched with bare hands. Dressings are best changed with an assistant.

A tracheostomy involves incising the skin over the trachea, then making a surgical wound in the trachea. This provides for an airway during tracheal obstruction. If at all possible, the first task in providing care to a patient with a tracheostomy is to establish communication.

Chest tubes are used to remove fluid, blood, and air from the pleural cavity. Special caution is needed when dealing with a patient with chest tubes to keep the drainage system below the chest and to maintain the integrity of the tube.

Urinary catheterization is the insertion of a tube into the bladder using aseptic technique. The two main types of catheters are the Foley (a retention balloon type) and the straight type.

Intravenous and intra-arterial lines are inserted for a variety of reasons, including introduction of medications and pressure measurements. The radiographer may assist the physician in determining the placement of the line with fluoroscopy or a portable chest radiograph.

Pacemakers are electromechanical devices inserted under the patient's skin to regulate the heart rate. Pacemakers are further subdivided into permanent, which are inserted in a pocket of skin, and temporary, which sit outside the patient's body. Both types use a transvenous pacing electrode that is monitored on fluoroscopy for proper placement.

Operating room radiography procedures vary greatly between surgeons and institutions. The one consistency is existence of a sterile corridor, the area between the patient drape and the instrument table.

◀R REVIEW QUESTIONS

1 A pacemaker prevents bradycardia by:
 1. Sensing the patient's heartbeats
 2. Pacing the heart when it does not contract
 3. Producing electrical impulses
 a) 1 and 2 only
 b) 1 and 3 only
 c) 2 and 3 only
 d) 1, 2, and 3

2 What type of catheter is the Foley?
 a) retention balloon
 b) straight
 c) coiled
 d) self-cleansing

3 When handling sterile gloves with a nonsterile hand, which of the following is not considered sterile?
 a) the outside of the cuff
 b) the inside of the cuff
 c) the fingertips of the glove
 d) the thumb of the glove

4 Outside air is prevented from entering the pleural cavity through the chest tube by the:
 a) collection chamber
 b) water seal chamber
 c) suction control chamber
 d) first compartment

5 The number-one priority for good sterile technique is:
 a) sterile drapes
 b) gowns
 c) handwashing
 d) saline solution

6 The first rule of caring for a tracheostomy patient is:
 a) watch for secretions
 b) establish communication

c) contact the nurse in charge of the patient.
 d) attempt to finish the procedure as quickly as possible

7 The purpose of the surgical hand scrub is to:
 1. remove debris and transient microorganisms from the hands, nails, and forearms
 2. destroy infected material
 3. inhibit rapid rebound growth of microorganisms
 a) 1 and 2 only
 b) 1 and 3 only
 c) 2 and 3 only
 d) 1, 2, and 3

8 Urine should flow in a female patient when the catheter has been inserted approximately:
 a) 1½ inches
 b) 2½ inches
 c) 4½ inches
 d) 8½ inches

9 What parts of a gown are considered sterile?
 1. sleeves
 2. front from the waist up
 3. back below the waist
 a) 1 and 2 only
 b) 1 and 3 only
 c) 2 and 3 only
 d) 1, 2, and 3

10 Which of the following are types of intravenous lines?
 1. Swan-Ganz
 2. Femoral
 3. Hickman
 a) 1 and 2 only
 b) 1 and 3 only
 c) 2 and 3 only
 d) 1, 2, and 3

BIBLIOGRAPHY

Askin DF: Bacterial and fungal infections in the neonate. J Obstet Gynecol Neonat Nurs 24:635–643, 1995.
Ballinger P: Merrill's Atlas of Radiographic Positions and Radiologic Procedures. 7th ed, vol 1. St. Louis, CV Mosby, 1991.
Bontrager KL: Textbook of Radiographic Positioning and Related Anatomy. 4th ed. St. Louis, Mosby-Year Book, 1997:556.
Craig M: Introduction to Ultrasonography and Patient Care. Philadelphia, WB Saunders, 1993.

Donowitz LG: Nosocomial infection in neonatal intensive care units. Am J Infect Control 17:250–257, 1989.

Dugan L: What you need to know about permanent pacemakers. Nursing 21(6):46–52, 1991.

Ehrlich RA, McCloskey ED: Patient Care in Radiography. 3rd ed. St. Louis, CV Mosby, 1989.

Fuller JR: Surgical Technology: Principles and Practice. Philadelphia, WB Saunders, 1981.

Goodman LR, Putnam CE (eds): Intensive Care Radiology: Imaging of the Critically Ill. St. Louis, CV Mosby, 1978.

Kozier B, Erb G, Olivieri R: Fundamentals of Nursing: Concepts, Process, and Practice. 4th ed. Menlo Park, CA, Addison-Wesley, 1991.

Levitsky MG, Cairo JM, Hall SM: Introduction to Respiratory Care. Philadelphia, WB Saunders, 1990.

Marlowe JE. Surgical Radiography. Baltimore, University Park Press, 1983.

Rees-Williams C, Meyrick M, Jones M: Making sense of urinary catheters. Nurs Times 84:46–47, 1988.

Snopek AM: Fundamentals of Special Radiographic Procedures. 3rd ed. Philadelphia, WB Saunders, 1993.

Strodtbeck F: Viral infections of the newborn. J Obstet Gynecol Neonat Nurs 24:659–667, 1995.

Torres LS: Basic Medical Techniques and Patient Care for Radiologic Technologists. 5th ed. Philadelphia, JB Lippincott, 1997.

Tortorici MR. Fundamentals of Angiography. St. Louis, CV Mosby, 1982.

CHAPTER 16

NONASEPTIC TECHNIQUES

Steven B. Dowd, EdD, RT(R),(QM),(MR)(M)

As it takes two to make a quarrel, so it takes two to make a disease, the microbe and its host.

CHARLES CHAPIN
THE PRINCIPLES OF EPIDEMIOLOGY

OBJECTIVES

On completion of this chapter, the student will be able to:

1 Describe the insertion, care, and removal of nasogastric tubes.
2 Assist a patient with the use of the male urinal.
3 Assist a patient with a bedpan.
4 Describe the common types of enemas.
5 Describe the procedure for a cleansing enema.
6 State the need for patient teaching regarding the barium enema—preparation, procedural, and postprocedural.
7 Differentiate between the single-contrast and double-contrast barium enemas.
8 Describe the procedure for a colostomy barium enema.
9 State the needs of a colostomy patient undergoing a barium enema.

GLOSSARY

Barium: bulky, fine white powder, without odor or taste and free from grittiness, $BaSO_4$, used as a contrast medium in roentgenography of the digestive tract

Bedpan: vessel for receiving the urinary and fecal discharges of a patient unable to leave his or her bed

Colostomy: surgical creation of an opening between the colon and the surface of the body; also used to refer to the opening, or stoma, so created

Defecation: evacuation of fecal material from the intestines

Emesis Basin: kidney-shaped vessel for the collection of vomitus

Enema: a liquid injected or to be injected into the rectum

Enterostomal Therapist: health professional (usually a nurse) with special training and certification in the care of ostomies and related concerns

Flatus: gas or air evacuated through the anus

Fowler's Position: position in which the patient's head is raised 18 or 20 inches above the flat position; the knees are also raised

Low-Residue Diet: diet that gives the least possible fecal residue, such as gelatin, sucrose, dextrose, broth, and rice

Lumen: cavity or channel within a tube or tubular organ (pl. lumina)

Nasogastric (NG) Tube: tube of soft rubber or plastic inserted through a nostril and into the stomach; for instilling liquid foods or other substances or for withdrawing gastric contents

Ostomate: one who has undergone enterostomy or ureterostomy

Perineum: region between the thighs, bounded in the male by the scrotum and anus and in the female by the vulva and anus

Purgation: catharsis; relief of fecal matter effected by a cathartic

Sims' Position: position in which the patient lies on the left side with the right knee and thigh flexed and the left arm parallel along the back

Stoma: opening established in the abdominal wall by colostomy, ileostomy, and so forth

Urinal: vessel or other receptacle for urine

Viscosity: physical property of liquids that determines the internal resistance to shear forces

Understanding nonaseptic techniques (the use of nasogastric tubes, male urinals, bedpans, enemas, and colostomies) is important to the professional practice of the radiologic technologist. Most of these techniques are performed with patients who are very sick or in great discomfort. The radiologic technologist functions in this area in a variety of roles—patient teacher, patient advocate, nurse, and physician extender, to name but a few. In a health care environment that often seems impersonal and more concerned with procedures than with the patients receiving them, technologists need to develop abilities of compassion, caring, and competency to be that excellent practitioner that we all strive to be. Adlai Stevenson once said that understanding human needs was half the job of meeting them. Students need to develop the competencies for patient care in nonaseptic techniques as well as sensitivity to patient needs.

Nasogastric Tubes

Nasogastric (NG) tubes are plastic or rubber tubes inserted through the nasopharynx into the stomach. The primary use of an NG tube is for decompression or removal of **flatus** and fluids from the stomach.

The two most common NG tubes used for gastric decompression are the Levin and the Salem-sump tubes (Fig. 16–1). The Levin tube is a single-**lumen** tube with several holes near its tip. The Salem-sump tube is a radiopaque double-lumen tube. One of the lumina provides an air vent; the other is for the removal of gastric contents. Other types of NG tubes include the Cantor, Keofeed, Miller-Abbott, and Sengstaken-Blakemore.

A patient with an NG tube in place usually suffers from discomfort. It has been stated that the discomfort of an NG tube often exceeds that of the surgical procedure that accompanies it. Keeping the patient reassured and informed is of the utmost importance in ensuring that the procedure is therapeutic and securing patient cooperation. Care must be taken to prevent accidental withdrawal of the tube after it has been inserted.

INSERTION OF A NASOGASTRIC TUBE

Most often, a physician or nurse is responsible for the insertion of an NG tube. The materials needed for passage of an NG tube are

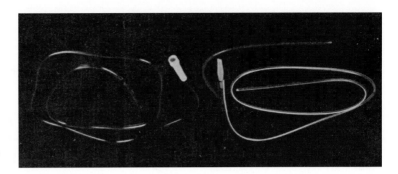

FIGURE 16–1. Levin *(left)* and Salem-sump *(right)* nasogastric tubes.

- rubber or plastic tube, usually a 14- to 16-French (4.7- to 5.3-mm) lumen for an adult patient
- a basin of ice to make the rubber tube more rigid, facilitating passage
- emesis basin
- clean, disposable gloves
- towel
- glass of water with a drinking straw
- 20- to 50-mL aspirating or bulb syringe
- water-soluble lubricating jelly
- tape to hold the tube in place at the nose (butterfly tape or 1-inch hypoallergenic tape)
- stethoscope
- clamp, drainage bag, or a suction machine if suction is to be used
- facial tissues

The procedure for inserting an NG tube is as follows:

1 Identify the patient and explain the procedure. Make sure consent for the procedure has been obtained.
2 Place the patient in a high Fowler's position with pillows supporting the head and shoulders. The tissues and the **emesis basin** should be close for patient use. The procedure is begun by externally measuring the distance from the nose to the stomach. Levin tubes have black markings on them that indicate how far the tube has been inserted.
3 The tube is lubricated at the distal end with the water-soluble lubricating jelly just before insertion. The patient is instructed to swallow water through a straw as the procedure begins. If the patient is unable to take fluids, air may be swallowed through the straw. The tube should go down easily with little force. The patient should be encouraged to swallow. The proper position is shown in Figure 16–2.

Tube placement can be verified by a variety of means, including fluoroscopy. Most often, a syringe is attached to the end of the tube and the diaphragm of the stethoscope is placed over the upper left quadrant of the abdomen just below the costal margin. Ten to 20 mL of air is injected while the abdomen is auscultated. A whoosing sound indicates the tube is in the stomach. As a further check, the syringe can be gently aspirated back to obtain gastric contents.

The tube is usually secured using the butterfly method (Fig. 16–3):

1 Cut two pieces of tape approximately 2

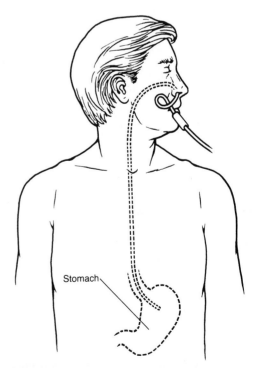

Stomach

FIGURE 16–2. Proper nasogastric tube position. (Reprinted with permission from Craig M: Introduction to Ultrasonography and Patient Care. Philadelphia, WB Saunders, 1993, p 69.)

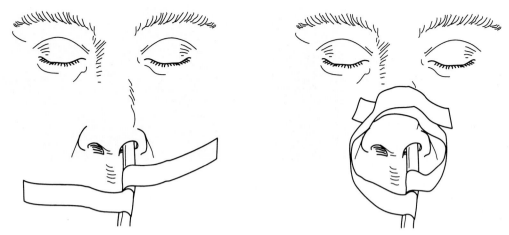

FIGURE 16–3. Taping nasogastric tube properly with 1 inch of hypoallergenic tape.

inches long and tear one lengthwise. Leave the other piece intact.
2 Wrap the intact piece of tape around the tubing.
3 Crisscross the two pieces of tape at the front of the tubing, and place them over the bridge of the nose. A second piece of tape may be placed over the first two to hold them in place.

Levin tubes must be secured so that they are not accidentally withdrawn. There should be no pulling pressure on the tube. Eating or drinking after the insertion of a gastric tube is not allowed unless specifically ordered by the physician. Sometimes patients are allowed to chew gum or suck on small ice chips to increase irrigation and to relieve dryness of the throat.

REMOVING A NASOGASTRIC TUBE

The items needed to remove an NG tube are

- emesis basin
- tissues and several thicknesses of paper toweling
- impermeable bag for disposal
- clean, disposable gloves

The procedure for removing an NG tube is as follows:

1 Identify the patient and explain the procedure. Make sure that consent has been secured.
2 Wash hands, then turn off and disconnect the suction apparatus if one is in place.

3 Gently remove the tape from the patient's nose, and make certain that the tubing is free from the patient's facial skin.
4 Put on clean gloves and ask the patient to take in a deep breath as the tube is gently withdrawn. Wrap the tube in the paper toweling, and place it in the disposal bag. If there is any resistance, stop the procedure and ask for assistance in the tube withdrawal from an appropriate individual, usually a supervisor or the department nurse.

TRANSFERRING A PATIENT WITH A NASOGASTRIC TUBE

When NG tubes are used for gastric decompression, they are usually connected to an intermittent gastric suctioning device. If a patient is to be transferred, it must first be confirmed that the physician has given an order allowing the transfer and the interruption of the suction. The length of time that suction can be interrupted safely also must be known. If it is for only a short time, suction must be re-established in the radiology department. This can be accomplished either by taking the patient's portable suction machine to the radiology department or by using suction available in the department (Fig. 16–4). Before transferring the patient, the amount of suction pressure required must be determined. The amount of pressure ordered varies, and the correct level can be determined by reading the physician's orders or by asking the nurse in charge of the patient.

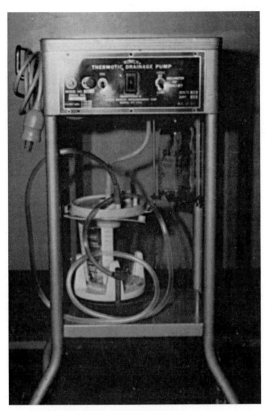

FIGURE 16–4. Portable suction unit.

In discontinuing suction on a single-lumen tube, the following materials are needed:

- pair of clean, disposable gloves
- clamping device
- package of sterile gauze sponges
- two rubber bands

The procedure for discontinuing suction is as follows:

1. Explain the procedure to the patient, making sure that consent has been given.
2. Wash hands.
3. Open the package of sponges and put on the gloves.
4. Turn off the suction.
5. Clamp or plug the gastric tube with the clamp or stopper, place one gauze pad over the end of the tube, and secure it with a rubber band.
6. Cover the connecting end of the suction tubing or the adapter with the other sponge, and secure it with a rubber band. This gauze covering will keep both ends of the tubing clean while not in use.

7. Secure the suction tubing on the machine so that it will not fall onto the floor, and make certain the NG tube will not be dislodged during the transfer.

If the suction is to be restarted in the radiology department on arrival, set the suction pressure gauge, turn on the suction, and reattach it to the tubing. This procedure is repeated when transferring the patient to the nursing unit.

A double-lumen tube must never be clamped closed with a hemostat or regular clamping device, because this may cause the lumina to adhere to each other and destroy the double-lumen effect. To prevent leakage from this type of tube, the barrel of a piston-like syringe may be inserted into the suction-drainage lumen, and it is then pinned to the patient's gown with the barrel upward.

Urinals

The male **urinal** (Fig. 16–5) is made of plastic or metal and is shaped so that it can be used by a patient who is supine, lying on his right or left side, or in **Fowler's position**. The urinal may be offered to the male patient who is not ambulatory—that is, confined to a stretcher or wheelchair or unable to walk.

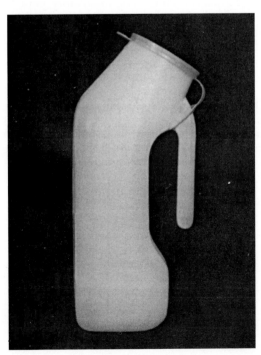

FIGURE 16–5. Male urinal.

If the patient is able to help himself, the radiographer simply hands him an aseptic urinal and allows him to use it, providing privacy whenever possible. When he has finished, the radiographer should put on clean, disposable gloves, remove the urinal, empty it, and rinse it with cold water. It is then placed with the soiled supplies to be resterilized. The patient should be offered a wash-cloth with which to wash his hands. The radiographer should then remove the gloves and wash hands.

Some patients require assistance in using a urinal. The radiographer would then proceed as follows:

1 Put on clean, disposable gloves, and raise the cover sheet sufficiently to permit adequate visibility while being careful not to expose the patient excessively.
2 Spread the patient's legs and place the urinal between them. Place the penis into the urinal far enough so that it does not slip out, and hold the urinal in place by the handle until the patient finishes voiding. Remove the urinal, empty it, remove the gloves, and wash your hands.

Bedpans

The patient who is not ambulatory must be offered a **bedpan** for **defecation;** a non-ambulatory female patient requires a bedpan for both defecation and urination. In the radiology department, clean bedpans are stored in a specific area. Bedpans must be sterilized between uses.

There are two types of bedpans (Fig. 16–6). The standard bedpan is made of metal or plastic and is about 2 inches high. If a patient has a fracture or another disability that makes it impossible to use a pan of this height, a fracture

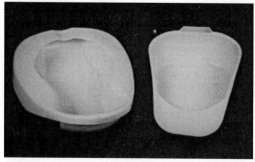

FIGURE 16–6. Standard, or regular *(left)* and fracture *(right)* bedpans.

pan is used. It has a shallow upper end about ½ inch deep.

Handwashing is important and should be performed both before and after assisting the patient with a bedpan. If the pan is cold, run warm water over it, then dry it. Patient privacy must be secured and respected. Always place a sheet over the patient. The procedure for assisting a patient with a bedpan is as follows:

1 Remove the bedpan cover and place it at the end of the table. Sometimes it is best to have a chair nearby on which to place the pan.
2 If the patient is able to move, place one hand under the lower back, asking the patient to raise his or her hips. Place the pan under the hips. Be sure the patient is covered with a sheet.
3 If the patient is able to sit up, this is ideal. If possible, the patient's head should be elevated 60 degrees.
4 Balance is poor while on a bedpan, so do not leave the patient alone for a long period. In most cases, it is necessary to leave the patient alone, but be sure to indicate how help may be summoned.
5 When the patient has finished using the bedpan, put on clean, disposable gloves. Have the patient lie back, place one hand under the lumbar area, and instruct the patient to raise up at the hips.
6 Then, remove the pan, cover it, and empty it in the designated area. Rinse it clean with cold water, and return it to the area where used equipment is placed. Offer the patient a wet paper towel or washcloth to wash hands and a paper towel to dry them. Remove the gloves and wash your hands.

When a patient requires more assistance with a bedpan than can be provided by one person, it becomes necessary to have an assistant. The procedure is as shown in Figure 16–7:

1 Both persons put on nonsterile gloves.
2 The assistant should stand at the opposite side of the table.
3 Turn the patient to a lateral position.
4 Place the pan against the patient's hips, then turn the patient back to a supine position while holding the pan in place. Be certain that the hips are in good alignment on the pan. Place pillows under the patient's shoulders and head and remain nearby in case assistance is needed.

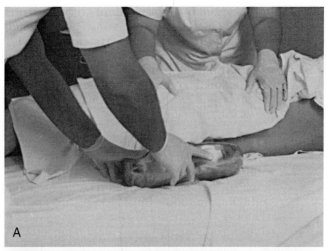

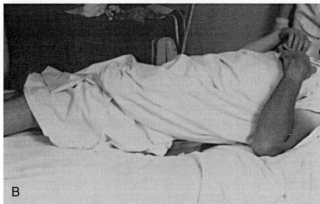

FIGURE 16–7. Two-person method of bedpan placement with helpers wearing gloves. *A,* Turn patient onto side and position bedpan. *B,* Turn patient onto back.

5 When the patient has finished, put on clean gloves and reverse the procedure to remove the pan.

The patient may require assistance in cleaning the **perineum.** Clean, disposable nonsterile gloves must be worn. Several thicknesses of tissue should be folded into a pad. Wipe the patient's perineum clean and dry. For female patients, be sure to wipe from the mons pubis toward the rectal area to avoid contaminating the genital area. Cover the pan, empty it, and place it in the soiled equipment area for resterilization. Remove the gloves and wash your hands.

Enemas

CLEANSING ENEMA

A cleansing **enema** is used to promote defecation. For an examination such as a barium enema to best demonstrate pathology or to verify normal structures and function, the bowel should be clear and free of fecal material. The fluid instilled in a cleansing enema breaks up the fecal mass, stretches the rectal wall, and initiates a defecation reflex. The types of enemas are as follows:

Tap water (hypotonic): Plain tap water may be used to cleanse the colon but should not be repeated because of the potential development of water toxicity or circulatory overload.

Hypertonic solution: This is often used when the patient cannot tolerate large amounts of fluid. It pulls fluid from the interstitial spaces around the colon. A small amount (120 to 180 mL; 4 to 6 oz) is usually effective. Available commercially under the name Fleet Enema.

Saline: Physiologic (normal) saline is the safest, especially for infants, children, and the elderly, as the fluid is of the same osmolarity as the interstitial spaces of the colon. One teaspoon of salt can be combined with 500 mL (1 pint) of water to prepare this solution.

Soapsuds solution: Pure castile soap may be added to either tap water or normal saline, depending on both patient condition and frequency of administration. Soap should be added to the enema bag after water is in place. Soapsuds enemas promote peristalsis and defecation but produce mild irritation of the bowel.

Oil retention: This uses an oil-based solution. It permits administration of a small volume (120 to 140 mL) to be absorbed by the stool. It should be retained, if possible, for 1 hour. The absorption of oil softens stool for easier evacuation.

In some departments, radiographers administer cleansing enemas to patients the morning of the examination to ensure a good preparation. In fact, some feel that only radiographers and radiologists have a full understanding of the need for a clean colon, and the way in which fecal matter will interfere with the examination. Gelfand and colleagues (1991) note that, in relation to the cleansing enema, "nursing personnel or busy hospital orderlies usually cannot be depended on to perform this task with the necessary diligence." The radiographer may also be responsible for instructing the patient in proper preparation for examinations that require bowel preparation. In any case, an understanding of the cleansing enema procedure facilitates an understanding of the barium enema procedure, which is standard practice of the radiographer. The materials needed for administering a cleansing enema to an adult patient are as follows:

- plastic container that holds 1000 to 1500 mL of fluid. This may be a bucket or a plastic bag with attached tubing (Fig. 16–8 illustrates popular types of empty enema sets).
- plastic tubing with a 22 or 26 French (7.3 to 8.7 mm) lumen about 4 feet long with a smooth, perforated tip and a clamping device
- liquid castile soap (5 to 30 mL)
- water-soluble lubricant
- paper or cloth pad to place under the patient's hips, paper towels to receive the enema tip, and a towel to protect the table
- bedpan

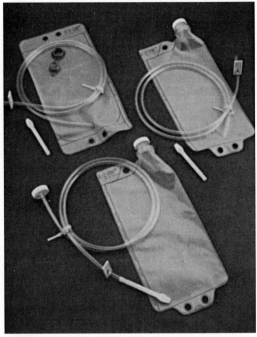

FIGURE 16–8. Empty barium enema sets. (Courtesy of E-Z-EM. Inc., Westbury, New York.)

- clean, disposable gloves
- drape sheet to cover the patient

The procedure for administering a cleansing enema to an adult patient is as follows:

1 Make sure that the examination has been ordered and that consent has been secured.

2 Inform the patient that a cleansing enema has been ordered and why it has been ordered, and explain the procedure.

3 Attach the tubing to the container if this has not been done, and close the clamp.

4 Prepare the enema solution at a sink capable of providing hot and cold water. The water used should be warmed to approximately 105°F (41°C). Fill the container with 1000 mL of water. If a soapsuds enema has been ordered, place the soap in the container and mix it.

5 Open the clamp, allowing some of the fluid to run through the tubing into the sink. This displaces the air so that it will not run into the colon and ensures proper functioning of the set.

6 Drape the patient with the drape sheet and position the patient in a left **Sims' position** (left anterior oblique). Arrange

the drape sheet so that only the area of the buttocks that must be exposed for insertion of the enema tip is visible. Place a towel under the patient's hip to protect the table.

7 Put on gloves. Lubricate the tip of the tube if it is not prelubricated.

8 Tell the patient when the tube is about to be inserted.

9 Lift the patient's right buttock with the heel of the hand to expose the anus. (Fig. 16–9*A*)

10 Ask the patient to slowly exhale and gently insert the enema tip into the rectum toward the umbilicus (anteriorly and superiorly) no more than 3 to 4 inches (Fig. 16–9*B*). Make certain that the anus is visualized as the tip is inserted to prevent injury to the patient. Forceful application of the tube may damage the mucous membranes. If problems are encountered in inserting the tip, a qualified professional such as another radiographer, a supervisor, or the department nurse should be asked to attempt the insertion. The patient may also assist.

11 Explain to the patient that the enema is about to begin. Let the patient know that there may be some cramping as the fluid runs in. Cramping often occurs when the sigmoid colon has been filled (usually after administration of 200 to 400 mL of fluid). Let the patient also know that the enema will be stopped until the cramping stops. The patient should be instructed to breathe through the mouth rapidly. Also inform the patient that the fluid should be retained as long as possible. A stepping stool should also be positioned to assist the patient off the table, and the patient should be told of its presence.

12 When the tip is inserted, hold it in place with the nondominant hand and release the tube clamp with the other hand. Then, raise the container of fluid 18 inches above the table.

13 Allow the fluid to run in slowly. It should take about 10 minutes for all the fluid to be used. The patient is asked to lie supine and then turn onto the right side to cleanse the transverse and ascending colon. The quantity of fluid that a patient can retain will vary, but if possible, at least 500 mL of fluid should be used. If less than 400 mL of fluid has been used

in an adult patient, it is fairly certain that any feelings of fullness reported by the patient are due to cramping.

14 Do not allow air to enter the rectum. Clamp off the tube before this can occur.

15 Gently remove the enema tip, wrap it in a paper towel, and place it in the enema container. Dispose of the set in the appropriate receptacle, and remove the gloves.

16 The patient should rest quietly on the table for at least 10 minutes before going to the toilet to expel the enema. Stay close by to assist the patient. If the patient cannot make it to the toilet, a bedpan may be used; be sure to follow proper procedure in using a bedpan (outlined earlier).

In some departments, the patient is told not to flush the toilet until the expelled material has been assessed. Others allow the patient to report the color, quantity, and consistency of the fecal material. Preparation for some studies requires that a second or even a third enema be administered so that the bowel is thoroughly cleansed. This process is called giving enemas "until clear" and means that the enema fluid returns with no fecal matter present. This procedure is not usually repeated more than three times because the patient's fluid balance may be jeopardized.

SELF-ADMINISTERED CLEANSING ENEMA

The radiographer may be required to instruct the patient in personal preparation for large bowel cleansing. In most cases, the physician ordering the examination will have provided the patient with instructions relative to preparation. If this is not the case, the radiology department will have specific routine instructions, based on the radiologists' order, to be provided to the patient. Patients vary in their understanding of and willingness to accept procedures and preparations; in some cases, it may be necessary to refer the patient to a supervisor or back to the personal physician.

OTHER ASPECTS OF PREPARATION

Bowel preparation is the least standardized aspect of barium enema examinations, but it is

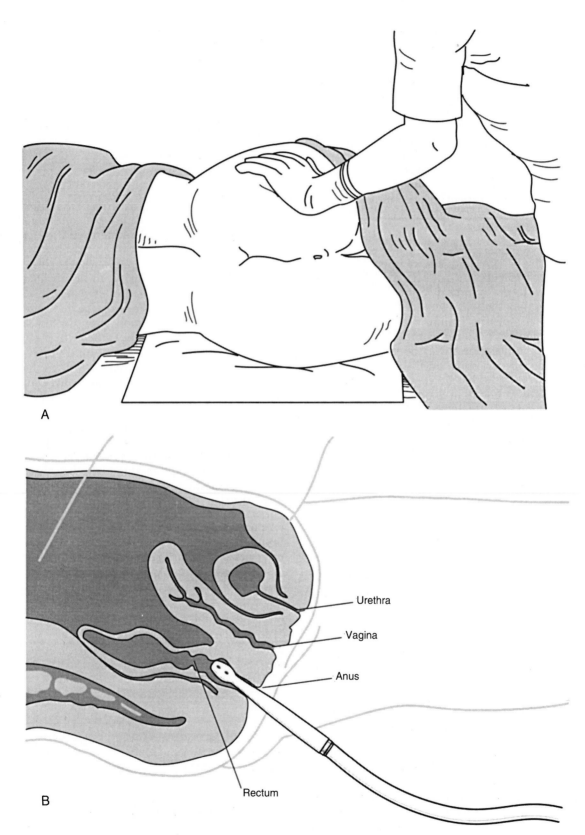

FIGURE 16–9. Insertion of an enema tip. *A*, Lift the patient's right buttock with the heel of the hand to expose the anus. *B*, Insert the enema tip into the rectum toward the umbilicus (anteriorly and superiorly) no more than 3 or 4 inches.

also one of the most important. See Boxes 16–1 and 16–2 for some representative preparations. Most often, preparation consists of:

Dietary restrictions, usually in the form of a minimal- or **low-residue diet.** This severely restricts the patient's intake of milk, overcooked meat, and eggs, and it avoids fruit and vegetables.

Purgation using a variety of laxatives, including castor oil, bisacodyl, or magnesium citrate

Overhydration. A clear liquid diet is often prescribed for the 24-hour period before a barium examination. This includes carbonated beverages, clear gelatin, clear broth, and coffee and tea with sugar. Whole-grain cereals, bread, vegetables, fried foods, and milk would be excluded.

Cleansing water enema as previously described

Diabetic patients require special preparation. Diabetic low-calorie drinks may be added to the standard regimen, and insulin-dependent diabetic patients often forgo their normal morning insulin dose until after the examination has been completed.

It has also been noted that elderly patients as a group (particularly the frail elderly) probably require increased education and counseling for

BOX 16–1

Sample Inpatient Bowel Preparation

1. Clear liquid diet for the 24 hours before the examination; no milk or milk products
2. Push fluids, with the patient drinking one full glass of water every hour, if possible. Chart fluid consumption.
3. One hour after lunch, and 3 hours before bisacodyl is given, give 3 oz of milk of magnesia with water.
4. 25 mg of bisacodyl 3 hours after milk of magnesia
5. Nothing by mouth after midnight
6. Fleet enema at 6:00 AM the day of examination
7. Postprocedural: Push fluids and give 2 oz of milk of magnesia to facilitate passage of barium

BOX 16–2

Sample Outpatient Bowel Preparation

BROWN METHOD

On the day before barium enema:
1. Clear fluids only from noon
2. One full glass of water every hour until 10 PM
3. 300 mL of cold magnesium citrate at 4 PM
4. 5 mg of bisacodyl at 6 PM
5. Nothing by mouth after midnight

PICOLAX METHOD

On the day before barium enema:
1. Before breakfast: One packet of Picolax. Be sure to drink plenty of fluids throughout the day.
2. Breakfast: One boiled egg, slice of white bread with honey, one cup of tea or coffee (milk allowed)
3. Lunch: Grilled or poached fish or chicken, small portion of cooked rice, plain yogurt, one cup of tea or coffee (may be sweetened; no milk); no potatoes, vegetables other than the rice, and no fruit
4. Take the second packet of Picolax at 4 PM.
5. Take a late supper (7–9 PM) of clear broth.
6. Clear fluids only after supper

STANDARD BOWMAN GRAY PREPARATION

(Originators of this method report a 97% success rate in patient preparation)
1. Clear liquid diet 24 hours before examination.
2. 8 ounces of water each hour day before examination.
3. 300 mL of magnesium citrate solution, 4 PM day before examination.
4. 60 mL of castor oil 8 PM day before examination.
5. Day of examination: 1500 mL cleansing enema in radiology department. Waiting times after cleansing: 30 minutes for single-contrast examination; 60 minutes for double-contrast.

preparation for barium enemas (Gurwitz et al, 1992; Grad et al, 1991). This is not typically due to the fact that they are, as is stereotypically presented, "senile." However, their familiarity with, and ability to perform, certain portions of the preparation may be compromised. If assessment indicates that the patient will not or may not be able to perform certain aspects of the preparation, it may be necessary to contact the radiologist or the patient's referring physician.

It is also important to note that there are bowel preparations and there are people preparations. That is, viewing the patient as a bowel rather than a person may lead to a substandard examination because of the lack of patient understanding and cooperation. If, in patient instruction, the radiographer focuses on reciting facts rather than ensuring that the patient understands the preparation, the examination may be less than adequate as a result of poor preparation.

One good technique to ensure understanding is to have the patient repeat back the instructions. Do not fall into the trap of thinking that a simple "yes" really means the patient understands. Be sure that he or she knows and understands the words as well as the meaning of the procedures. It is not uncommon, for example, for patients to arrive for a barium enema and to exclaim, "What! Another enema! I had three last night!" not knowing that these initial enemas were preparations for the morning examination.

BARIUM ENEMA

The **barium** enema is given in an examination used to diagnose pathologic conditions of the colon or lower gastrointestinal tract. A much larger catheter is required than is used for cleansing enemas to allow the barium, which is of greater **viscosity,** to be instilled into the lower bowel. The catheter may have a plain tip or an inflatable cuff attached (Fig. 16–10). The cuff is inflated after the tip is inserted to hold the catheter in place and to prevent involuntary expulsion of barium.

Facilities and physicians vary widely in their use of inflatable cuffs (balloon catheters). Some do so routinely, always inflating the cuff, whereas others always use the cuff but inflate only out of necessity. Still others believe they should be used only when absolutely necessary. Damage to the rectal wall from improper use of balloon catheters is the most common complication of a barium enema. Balloons should never be overinflated (the amount recommended varies from 30 to 90 mL of air) and are contraindicated in cases of rectal narrowing. Other complications include breaks in the gastrointestinal mucosa due to trauma or disease,

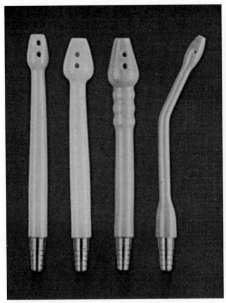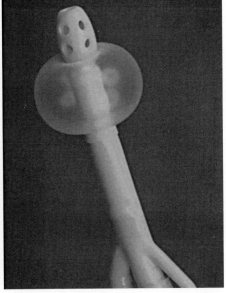

FIGURE 16–10. *Left,* Plain barium enema tip. (Courtesy of E-Z-EM, Inc., Westbury, New York.) *Right,* Barium enema tip with an inflatable cuff.

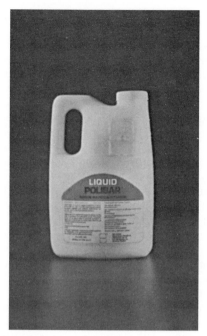

FIGURE 16–11. Commercial barium suspension. (Courtesy of E-Z-EM, Inc., Westbury, New York.)

which permits barium to enter the peritoneal cavity or bloodstream. Disease conditions such as ulcers, cancer, and diverticulitis can create minute asymptomatic perforations that can blow out under pressure. Then, peritonitis or venous emboli may cause serious complications, including death, as well as fibrosis or barium granuloma. In addition, allergic reactions to Latex tips and cuffs have also been reported.

Barium solution is usually available in a prepared, prepackaged powder (which must be mixed with water) or suspension (Fig. 16–11). Barium suspensions and solutions should have the following characteristics:

- allow for rapid flow
- allow for good adhesion to the mucosa
- provide adequate radiographic density in a thin layer
- have even, plastic coating
- lack foam or artifacts

The quantity of barium solution prepared is large. Most bags hold 3000 mL and the actual amount prepared varies. The barium solution may be prepared using warm or cold water. Advocates of the use of cold water hold that this method will reduce irritation to the colon and helps the patient to "hold" the enema. Some also advocate the use of salt (2 teaspoons per 1000 mL of water) to prevent fluid overload. Because of radiologist preferences in terms of viscosity and density, there is no one correct way to mix barium. Let the patient know that the entire 3000 mL in the bag may not be administered.

Since greater pressure is required to secure an adequate flow rate, the bag is usually suspended at a greater distance (up to 30 inches) above the table. Excessive height may cause severe abdominal cramping and rupture of diverticula in the colon as a result of excessive fluid pressure. The initial portion of the procedure is much the same as for the cleansing enema.

Follow the same instructions for inserting the tip as were given in the section on the cleansing enema. The patient may lie in a supine position while waiting for the radiologist.

Patient instruction and reassurance are of utmost importance. Patients must know that they will receive a variety of instructions and also that the radiologist will give a variety of instructions to the radiographer that the patient may ignore. Also, patients may not understand the difference between the cleansing enemas they have received and the barium enema.

It is important that the patient understand the need (1) to keep the tip firmly in the rectum, (2) to relax the abdominal muscles to reduce intra-abdominal pressure, and (3) to use deep oral breathing to prevent spasms and cramps. As with the cleansing enema, the patient must know that the procedure will be suspended if cramping occurs.

Student radiographers should carefully observe the interactions between radiographers, radiologists, and patients to develop their own style of patient instruction during the procedure. Although the basic information is consistent from patient to patient, the way it is communicated may vary according to special needs.

DOUBLE-CONTRAST BARIUM ENEMA

In many facilities, the double-contrast barium enema (the addition of air or carbon dioxide to provide for two contrasts—barium and the air) has become routine. It is especially indicated in diarrhea and high-risk cases—for example, the patient with polyps, a family history of colorectal cancer, or personal history of cancer or rectal bleeding. The patient often receives an injection of a smooth-muscle relaxant such as glucagon immediately before the examination to relieve bowel spasm.

A typical routine for a double-contrast barium enema begins with the patient in a prone position and the table tilted slightly head-down. Barium (about 300 mL) is instilled into the splenic flexure, and air is then insufflated (added). This pushes the barium to fill the transverse colon. The bag is lowered and the head of the table is raised to drain the rectum. This also traps barium in the transverse colon. The patient may be turned to the right side and more air added to bring barium around the hepatic flexure. The patient is then turned prone to bring the barium to the cecum. Once the colon is filled with barium and distended with air, a variety of radiographic views are taken.

Other means of performing double-contrast examinations described in the literature include Miller's seven-pump method; Pochazevsky and Sherman's single-stage, closed system; and Welin's double-stage or Malmo technique, in which the barium is added, the patient evacuates the barium, and air is added. Various radiologists also have their own routines.

SINGLE-CONTRAST BARIUM ENEMA

Single-contrast barium enemas are indicated in certain situations:

- Colon configuration is of prime importance.
- Only gross pathology must be shown.
- Fistulas are suspected.
- Acute appendicitis or diverticulitis is suspected.
- An intussusception is to be reduced.
- A volvulus or acute obstruction is to be evaluated.
- The patient is not movable or cooperative, or is extremely debilitated.

In a typical single-contrast barium enema, the suspension is run in slowly with compression applied to the abdomen. About 1500 mL of barium is required for the average adult barium enema. Spot views of the cecum, flexures, and the sigmoid colon are taken. A variety of views of the abdomen (typically anteroposterior, posteroanterior, and decubitus), a 30-degree caudal angulation of the sigmoid colon, and a lateral rectal view are taken. The excess barium is drained back into the bag, the tip is removed, and the patient is sent to the toilet to evacuate as much of the barium as possible. A postevacuation film is then taken, usually with the patient in the prone position.

When removing a rectal catheter that has an inflatable cuff attached, the cuff must be deflated before the catheter is removed. The barium is sometimes removed by gravity flow before the catheter tip is removed, and air is then permitted to escape from the cuff. After this, the catheter is gently removed. If there is any resistance, it may be necessary to summon another individual (another radiographer, a supervisor, the department nurse, or in extreme cases, the radiologist) to remove it.

When perforation of the bowel is suspected, water-soluble iodine compounds are the only acceptable contrast media (rather than barium). These compounds, such as Gastrografin, are also used in a variety of other cases in which administration of barium sulfate can prove hazardous. These would include delineation of an anastomosis in the immediate preoperative period, outlining of the distal colon and rectum in cases of megacolon and Hirschsprung's disease, and when there is a high risk of barium impaction. Water-soluble contrast agents are hypertonic, which means they draw fluid into the bowel. This can cause diarrhea and a sudden reduction in blood volume, particularly dangerous in neonates and in patients with Hirschsprung's disease.

The patient is assisted to the toilet after barium enemas. Patients are often dehydrated as a result of the preparation for a barium enema. This can lead to a postural drop in blood pressure, which could cause the patient to become dizzy and fall. It may also be necessary to allow the patient to evacuate some of the barium into a bedpan before moving.

POSTPROCEDURAL INSTRUCTIONS

Postprocedural instruction to the patient is necessary after a barium enema because barium retention can cause fecal impaction or intestinal obstruction. Barium has hydroscopic qualities, which means that it will absorb fluid from the bowel. Extreme dehydration as a result of preparation for the examination is another possible postprocedural complication. In geriatric patients, fluid imbalance may lead to altered mental status.

Stools are often white or very light colored

until all of the barium is expelled. Some physicians regularly prescribe a laxative medication or an enema after barium studies. In any case, the lack of a bowel movement within 24 hours indicates that the personal physician should be contacted. The importance of eliminating the barium cannot be overly stressed to the patient.

The patient should increase fluid intake and dietary fiber for several days unless medically contraindicated. The patient should be instructed to rest after the examination. Weakness or fainting; abdominal pain, constipation, or rectal bleeding; not passing flatus; and polyuria, nocturia, or abdominal distention all indicate that the personal physician should be contacted immediately.

Colostomies

Because of trauma or pathology such as cancer, diverticulitis, and ulcerative colitis, formation of a **stoma** (mouth) from the bowel to the outside of the body may be necessary. Permanent **colostomies** are performed when a portion of bowel is removed. A temporary colostomy is performed to heal or rest a diseased portion of bowel.

There are several types of colostomies. A descending or sigmoid colostomy is a permanent colostomy in which the diseased portion of the colon or rectum is removed. A transverse colostomy has a portion of the transverse colon removed. In a double-barrel colostomy, two stomas are formed: the proximal delivers stool, the distal produces mucus. The longer a colostomy has been in place, the greater the consistency of stool.

The radiographer must recognize that an ostomy produces a major change in a patient's body image and that many persons with new colostomies go through the grieving process. The loss of a bowel can be viewed in the same light as any other loss, including death. That is, patients typically pass through various stages, including denial, anger, bargaining, depression, and, finally, acceptance.

Caring for a patient with a new ostomy requires sensitivity and a matter-of-fact attitude, two seemingly separate entities. These must be reconciled for effective care of the ostomy patient. Barbara Mullen, author of *The Ostomy Book* and an **ostomate,** has said that she appreciated plain speaking over half-hearted platitudes after her own ostomy. Even a hint of

revulsion or hesitancy can be interpreted negatively by the patient. The radiography student who has never seen an ostomy should observe routines until technical competency, a matter-of-fact attitude (plain speaking), and sensitivity can be combined.

A patient with a colostomy needs special instructions for adequate preparation. Usually, the stoma is irrigated the night before and the morning of the examination. Irrigation is a type of "enema" for the colostomy that should prevent expulsion of feces for 24 hours. Dietary and laxative preparations also vary depending on the ostomy. The ostomate must be instructed, for example, not to take bismuth subgallate tablets—as he or she may normally do to control odor—because these are radiopaque. If available, an **enterostomal therapist** instructs the patient in preparation. Ostomy patients should be instructed to bring an extra pouch with them if they are coming from outside the hospital.

ADMINISTERING A BARIUM ENEMA TO A PATIENT WITH A COLOSTOMY

Most colostomies are performed because of cancer. About 10% of patients who have their bowels removed because of cancer have recurrences, which necessitate follow-up studies.

The colostomy patient will have a dressing or drainage pouch in place over the area of the stoma. The dressing must be removed by a radiographer wearing clean gloves, then placed in a plastic bag and disposed of in a receptacle intended for contaminated waste. The gloves are then removed, and hands are washed. A drainage pouch should be removed and put aside in a safe place to be reused. Gloves are put on again. The patient may want to do this or provide direction for the procedure. The pouch must be kept clean and dry.

The procedure for administering a barium enema to a patient with a colostomy is somewhat different from that for the regular examination, because of the lack of a sphincter. The main problem with barium administration through a colostomy is trying to prevent leakage without damaging the colostomy. A cone-shaped tip with a long drainage bag that attaches to it is frequently the tip of choice. Nipple colostomy tips and double-barrel (dual tubing that allows for simultaneous study of the proximal and distal colonic loops) colostomy tips are

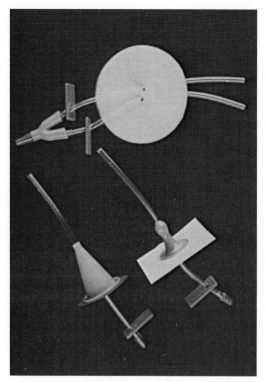

FIGURE 16–12. A variety of colostomy tips. (Courtesy of E-Z-EM, Inc., Westbury, New York.)

also available (Fig. 16–12). Sometimes, a small catheter with an inflatable cuff is used. If the patient has had the ostomy for some time, self-insertion of the tip may be preferred.

The radiographer typically lubricates the tip of the cone and hands it to the patient for insertion. If the patient is unable to do so, the task is performed by the radiologist, who also tapes the device in place. Clean, disposable gloves should be put on. A much smaller amount of barium solution is often needed, especially when the study is done for the distal portion of the remaining colon.

Once the cone or catheter has been inserted, the diagnostic procedure is similar to that for other patients. An intravenous smooth-muscle relaxant is usually necessary to prevent peristalsis, which continually empties the colon. About 250 mL of barium is usually used. Care must be taken, if air insufflation is used, not to overdistend the colon. So as not to traumatize the stoma site, prone views are not performed.

When the procedure is completed, the drainage bag can be attached to the cone and the barium drained. When the drainage is com-

plete, the ambulatory patient may be escorted to the toilet with the drainage bag still in place to be cleaned; the ostomy pouch is then replaced.

Ostomates are often independent if they have had the ostomy for a long time. It is important that the patient be allowed a certain degree of self-control in addition to the direction given to the patient by the radiographer and the physician.

Summary

Nasogastric tubes, male urinals, bedpans, enemas, and colostomies are a part of the daily practice of a radiographer. The detailed routines are described here as they are commonly performed in hospitals and other health care facilities; the actual routine at any given institution may vary slightly.

The radiographer is most likely to encounter the Levin and Salem-sump nasogastric tubes. Patients with nasogastric tubes in place usually suffer from discomfort and require a good deal of assurance. The radiographer may assist in inserting nasogastric tubes and is sometimes responsible for their removal. Before moving a patient with a nasogastric tube, the radiographer must be sure of the length of time that suction may be discontinued.

Urinals are used by male patients unable to walk or stand for urination. They must be rinsed between uses by the same patient, and sterilized after each patient. Bedpans are used by female patients for urination and defecation and by male patients for defecation only. There are two basic types, the standard bedpan and the fracture bedpan. It is important to maintain a patient's sense of dignity and privacy when using a bedpan.

In some departments, radiographers or other workers in the department are responsible for administering cleansing enemas as a means of bowel preparation. There are five basic types of cleansing enemas: tap water (hypotonic), hypertonic solution, physiologic (normal saline), soapsuds, and oil retention. Radiographers function as patient educators in informing patients of the standardized bowel preparation used at their institution. These preparations usually include dietary restrictions, purgation, overhydration, and cleansing enemas. The professional radiographer focuses on patient understanding of the procedure rather than simply reciting facts to the patient.

The barium enema is given in an examination to diagnose potential pathology of the colon. The barium used is more viscous than water and is administered differently than the water enema. Patient instructions before, during, and after the procedure are necessary to ensure a diagnostic outcome without postprocedural complications. The two main types of barium enemas are the single-contrast examination, where only barium is used, and the double-contrast examination, where both barium and air are used to outline the colon.

Colostomies are formed by bringing a portion of the colon to the outside in the form of a stoma, or mouth. Patients with ostomies require special care that often comes only through observation and experience. Allowing as much patient control as possible while maintaining control over the examination, as well as not showing signs of revulsion or hesitancy, is important. Administration of a barium enema in a patient with a colostomy is different than in a regular patient because of the lack of a sphincter and the sensitivity of the stoma site.

◀R REVIEW QUESTIONS

1 The two most common types of nasogastric tubes are:
1. Levin
2. Salem–sump
3. Miller–Abbott
4. Cantor
a) 1 and 2
b) 2 and 3
c) 2 and 4
d) 1 and 4

2 How can leakage from a double-lumen tube be prevented?
a) Clamp with a hemostat
b) Clamp with a regular clamping device
c) Use a piston-like syringe
d) Leakage is not a problem with a double-lumen tube

3 Bedpans should be:
a) rinsed between uses
b) sterilized between uses
c) disposed of after use
d) none of the above

4 Hypertonic solution is used when:

a) fluid must be of the same osmolarity as that of the interstitial spaces of the colon
b) stool must be softened
c) the patient cannot tolerate large amounts of fluid
d) infant safety is a primary concern

5 The normal adult patient should be able to tolerate _____ of fluid from a cleansing enema.
a) 200 mL
b) 500 mL
c) 1000 mL
d) 1500 mL

6 If cramping occurs during a barium enema:
a) the patient should be told to use deep oral breathing
b) the enema should be stopped
c) the bag should be raised
d) a and b

7 Desirable characteristics of a barium suspension include:
1. rapid flow
2. good mucosal adhesion
3. thick layering
a) 1 only
b) 1 and 2 only
c) 1 and 3 only
d) 1, 2, and 3

8 A postural drop in blood pressure can occur after a barium enema as a result of:
a) a reaction from the barium
b) dehydration
c) trapping of barium in the transverse colon
d) none of the above

9 With a double-barrel colostomy, the proximal stoma delivers _____ and the distal stoma delivers _____.
a) stool/mucus
b) mucus/stool
c) mucus/flatus
d) solids/fluids

10 About _____ of colostomy patients have recurrences of cancer.
a) 10%
b) 20%
c) 30%
d) 40%

BIBLIOGRAPHY

Ballinger P: Merrill's Atlas of Radiographic Positions and Radiologic Procedures. 7th ed, vol 2. St Louis, CV Mosby, 1991.

Bartram CI: The large bowel. In Whitehouse GH, Worthington BS (eds): Techniques in Diagnostic Imaging. 2nd ed. Boston, Blackwell Scientific Publications, 1990.

Craig M: Introduction to Ultrasonography and Patient Care. Philadelphia, WB Saunders, 1993.

Ehrlich RA, McCloskey ED: Patient Care in Radiography. 3rd ed. St Louis, CV Mosby, 1989.

Gelfand DW, Chen DYM, Ott DJ: Preparing the colon for the barium enema examination. Radiology 178:609–613, 1991.

Grad RM, Clarfield AM, Rosenboom M, et al. Adequacy of preparation for barium enema among elderly outpatients. Can Med Assoc J 144:1257–1261, 1991.

Gurwitz JH, Noonan JP, Sanchez M, et al. Barium enemas in the frail elderly. Am J Med 92:41–44, 1992.

Miller RE: Barium pneumocolon: Technologist-performed "7-pump" method. AJR 139:1230–1232, 1982.

Mullen BD, McGinn KA: The Ostomy Book. Palo Alto, Bull, 1980.

The perils of a barium blowout when contrast medium escapes from the GI tract. Emerg Med 16:57–60, 1984.

Pochazevsky R, Sherman S: A new technique for roentgenologic examination of the colon. AJR 89:787–796, 1963.

Robinson SB, Demuth PL: Diagnostic studies for the aged: What are the dangers? J Gerontol Nurs 11:6–12, 1985.

Torres LS: Basic Medical Techniques and Patient Care for Radiologic Technologists. 5th ed. Philadelphia, JB Lippincott, 1997.

Troupin RH: Diagnostic Radiology in Clinical Medicine. 2nd ed. Chicago, Year Book, 1978.

CHAPTER 17

MEDICAL EMERGENCIES

Joanne S. Greathouse, EdS, RT(R), FASRT

Important to proper evaluation of the critically ill patient is a spirit of cooperation and ongoing communication.

LAWRENCE GOODMAN AND CHARLES PUTMAN INTENSIVE CARE RADIOLOGY, 1978

OBJECTIVES

On completion of this chapter, the student will be able to:

1 Define terms related to medical emergencies.
2 List the objectives of first aid.
3 List general priorities in working with patients in acute situations.
4 Explain the purpose of an emergency cart and its contents.
5 Explain the four levels of consciousness.
6 Describe the signs and symptoms of various medical emergencies.
7 Discuss methods of avoiding the factors that contribute to shock.

8 Discuss factors that contribute to the development of hypoglycemia.
9 Describe the appropriate procedure for handling patients with various medical emergencies.
10 Describe the correct procedure for administration of cardiopulmonary resuscitation.
11 Demonstrate appropriate principles of cardiopulmonary resuscitation.

GLOSSARY

Aura: subjective sensation or motor phenomenon that precedes and marks the onset of a paroxysmal attack, such as an epileptic attack

Cardiopulmonary Resuscitation (CPR): artificial substitution of heart and lung action as indicated for cardiac arrest or apparent sudden death resulting from electric shock, drowning, respiratory arrest, and other causes

Cerebrovascular Accident (Stroke): condition with sudden onset caused by acute vascular lesions of the brain; it is often followed by permanent neurologic damage

Emergency: unexpected or sudden occasion; an urgent or pressing need

Epistaxis: nosebleed; hemorrhage from the nose

Hemorrhage: escape of blood from the vessels; bleeding

Hyperglycemia: abnormally increased concentration of glucose in the blood

Hypoglycemia: abnormally diminished concentration of glucose in the blood

Lethargy: abnormal drowsiness or stupor; a condition of indifference

Nausea: unpleasant sensation, vaguely referred to the epigastrium and abdomen, and often culminating in vomiting

Pallor: paleness; absence of skin coloration

Shock: condition of profound hemodynamic and metabolic disturbance characterized by failure of the circulatory system to maintain adequate perfusion of vital organs

Syncope: temporary suspension of consciousness due to generalized cerebral ischemia; faint or swoon

Urticaria: vascular reaction, usually transient, involving the upper dermis, representing localized edema caused by dilatation and increased permeability of the capillaries, and marked by the development of wheals; also called hives

Vertigo: illusion of movement; sensation as if the external world were revolving around the patient or as if the patient were revolving in space

Vomiting: forcible expulsion of the contents of the stomach through the mouth

Wound: bodily injury caused by physical means, with disruption of the normal continuity of structures

Wound Dehiscence: separation of the layers of a surgical wound; it may be partial, or superficial only, or complete, with disruption of all layers

The Medical Emergency

DEFINITION AND OBJECTIVES OF FIRST AID

An **emergency** is a situation in which the condition of a patient or a sudden change in medical status requires immediate action. Emergency actions on the part of the radiologic technologist as a whole have the objectives of preserving life, avoiding further harm to the patient, and obtaining appropriate medical assistance as quickly as possible. Although instances in which a radiologic technologist is called on to initiate emergency measures are infrequent, it is incumbent on the technologist to be able to recognize emergency situations, to maintain a calm and confident presence, and to take appropriate action. The recognition of need for assistance is a critical first step; it is important that the technologist be able to recognize when such assistance might be warranted.

GENERAL PRIORITIES

Although most patients are sent to the radiology department only after they have been stabilized, some patients are not stable, and the status of others may change while they are in the department. Radiologic technologists should never underestimate their ability to contribute to a patient's survival and well-being by quick thinking and appropriate action. The technologist should keep in mind the following priorities when working with patients in emergency situations:

1 Ensure an open airway.
2 Control bleeding.
3 Take measures to prevent or treat shock.
4 Attend to wounds or fractures.
5 Provide emotional support.
6 Continually re-evaluate and follow up appropriately.

EMERGENCY CART

Familiarity with the location of emergency equipment in the radiology department is an important part of being able to respond appropriately. Most radiology departments have at least one emergency cart (often referred to as a crash cart). This cart is a wheeled container of equipment and drugs typically required in emergency situations (Fig. 17–1).

The cart itself and its contents—drugs and equipment needed to handle typical life-threatening emergencies—are similar from institution to institution (Box 17–1). The ready availability

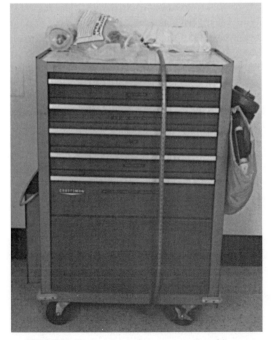

FIGURE 17–1. A typical emergency "crash" cart.

BOX 17–1

Equipment and Drugs Typically Found on an Emergency Cart

STANDARD EQUIPMENT

Backboard	Suction bottle
Stethoscope	Hemostat
Blood pressure cuff	Scissors
Ambu bag	Surgeon's gloves, various sizes
Laryngoscope	
Flashlight	Syringes, variety of sizes
Batteries	
Extension cord	Needles, variety of sizes
Oxygen flow meter	
Tourniquet	Stopcocks and connectors, variety
Airways	
Endotracheal tubes	Tongue blades
Nasopharyngeal tubes	Sterile gauze
	Adhesive and paper tape
Suction catheters	
Levine tubing	Alcohol swabs
Jelco cannulas	Surgical lubricant
Trach tubes	Blood collection tubes
Cut-down tray	

DRUGS AND SOLUTIONS

Epinephrine—bronchodilator
Atropine—anticholinergic
Bretylium tosylate (Bretylol)—antiarrhythmic
Digoxin (Lanoxin)—antiarrhythmic
Diphenhydramine (Benadryl)—antihistamine
Dobutamine (Dobutrex)—stimulant
Dopamine (Intropin)—stimulant
Furosemide (Lasix)—diuretic
Isoproterenol (Isuprel)—bronchodilator
Lidocaine (Xylocaine)—antiarrhythmic
Nitroglycerin—vasodilator
Norepinephrine bitartrate (Levophed)—vasoconstrictor
Phenytoin (Dilantin)—anticonvulsant
Procainamide (Pronestyl)—antiarrhythmic
Propranolol (Inderal)—antiarrhythmic
Sodium bicarbonate—fluid replacement
Sodium nitroprusside (Nitropress)—vasodilator
Verapamil (Isoptin)—vasodilator

of emergency equipment and drugs reduces the time required to respond to medical crises. A radiologic technologist's orientation to a department should include learning the location of emergency carts and a familiarity with the contents and organization of the carts at that particular institution.

Head Injuries

Victims of head trauma are often seen in the radiology department. Although it is not the radiologic technologist's responsibility to diagnose head injuries, it is useful to have a knowledge of categorization so a basic assessment can be made and changes in a patient's status noted. Although there are several ways of categorizing head injuries, the simplest form of classification is by level of consciousness.

LEVELS OF CONSCIOUSNESS

The patient with the least severe injury is classified as alert and conscious. This patient can typically respond fully to questions and other stimuli. A more seriously injured patient is drowsy but can be roused to response with loud speaking or gentle physical contact. Even more serious injury produces a patient who is unconscious and reacts only to painful stimuli. These patients typically do not respond to verbal stimuli but react to stimuli such as pinches and pinpricks. The most serious condition is that of a patient who is comatose and unresponsive to virtually all stimuli.

INDICATIONS OF DETERIORATING SITUATIONS

The technologist should quickly assess a patient when the procedure is begun so that it is readily noticeable if the patient deteriorates from one level of consciousness to another. Findings in an alert or drowsy patient that can signify a deteriorating head injury include irritability, **lethargy,** slowing pulse rate, and slowing respiratory rate.

When working with an intoxicated patient with a head injury, the technologist is cautioned against assuming the patient has passed out merely from inebriation. If there is any doubt about the cause of the patient's loss of consciousness, it is far better to assume a more serious head injury and to obtain medical assistance than for a patient to suffer further deterioration needlessly.

RESPONSE TO DETERIORATING SITUATIONS

If the radiologic technologist recognizes a deteriorating head injury, the first priority is main-

taining an open airway while moving the patient as little as possible. The procedure should be stopped and medical assistance obtained quickly. It is also helpful to obtain vital signs while waiting for help to arrive.

Shock

DEFINITION AND TYPES

Another situation typically encountered with emergency patients is shock. **Shock** is a general term that indicates a failure of the circulatory system to support vital body functions. There are several types of shock:

- *hypovolemic*—due to loss of blood or tissue fluid
- *cardiogenic*—due to a variety of cardiac disorders, including myocardial infarction
- *neurogenic*—due to spinal anesthesia or damage to the upper spinal cord
- *vasogenic*—due to sepsis, deep anesthesia, or anaphylaxis

The technologist is most likely to encounter hypovolemic shock or anaphylactic shock, a special type of vasogenic shock, as a result of reaction to contrast media administered in the course of a procedure.

PREVENTION

Several factors can contribute to the likelihood that a patient will experience shock or to the degree of shock experienced. Any sudden change in body temperature is one such factor. That is why it is important to keep patients covered to maintain normal body temperature; it is equally important not to overheat the patient.

Pain, stress, and anxiety also contribute to the development of shock. Handling patients gently during a procedure not only is an important aspect of good psychological care but also can be a factor in the patient's physical condition. The technologist should also work calmly and confidently, even in a situation of maximum stress; this helps reassure emergency patients and can contribute to their overall physiologic well-being.

SIGNS AND SYMPTOMS

Signs and symptoms that a patient might be going into shock include restlessness, apprehension or general anxiety, tachycardia, decreasing blood pressure, cold and clammy skin, and **pallor.** If the radiologic technologist believes that such a situation is developing, he or she should stop the procedure, ensure maintenance of the patient's body temperature, call for medical assistance, and measure the patient's vital signs while awaiting assistance.

CONTRAST MEDIA REACTIONS (ANAPHYLACTIC SHOCK)

Anaphylactic shock is a type of vasogenic shock and is most commonly encountered in the radiology department in connection with the administration of iodinated contrast media. Although there is a great deal of debate about the nature of contrast media reactions, there is at least some agreement that these reactions have an element of allergic reaction. While such reactions are not common, neither are they so rare as to warrant complacency on the part of the technologist. Reaction to contrast media can range from mild to severe. Because the most severe reaction can result in death due to cardiac arrest, contrast media should not be administered without first taking an adequate history.

In general, the longer it takes for a reaction to develop, the less severe it is. Accordingly, the most severe reactions typically arise very quickly. It is possible, however, for a severe delayed reaction to occur. Thus, it is important to constantly monitor patients who have had contrast media injections.

Mild reactions are similar to other allergic reactions. Patients develop localized itching and **urticaria** (hives) and may experience nausea and vomiting. Generalized itching and hives are indicative of a systemic reaction, which is generally more serious. While none of these are serious in and of themselves, they may signal the onset of a more serious reaction. The physician should be notified immediately in the event of any reaction. Most often, a mild antihistamine is administered to counter the allergic reaction.

The most serious reactions might include laryngeal edema, shock, and cardiac arrest. All of these are life-threatening and should be handled accordingly. The physician must be notified at once and vital signs taken. Patients who suffer cardiac arrest should be treated with cardiopulmonary resuscitation.

Diabetic Crises

Many patients who undergo radiologic procedures are required to have had gastrointestinal preparation, which might include a special diet or fasting. Most patients can tolerate this preparation fairly easily (if not necessarily comfortably), but such alterations in dietary patterns can be particularly troublesome for diabetic patients.

In the normal patient, the body adjusts its insulin production and excretion to meet the demands made on it by the body's intake of carbohydrate. In some diabetic patients (type I, typically juvenile in onset), however, the insulin is given exogenously and the patient must adjust dietary intake to balance the insulin taken. The gastrointestinal preparation can create havoc with that balance.

HYPOGLYCEMIA

Hypoglycemia is a condition in which excessive insulin is present. This can be the result of a patient's taking the usual dose of insulin before a gastrointestinal study and then not having a normal breakfast. The brain requires glucose for normal metabolism. If no food is eaten, the administered insulin depletes the body's energy store, leading fairly quickly to insulin shock (sometimes called an insulin reaction). Patients who are experiencing this condition are intensely hungry, weak, and shaky and may sweat excessively. They may also become confused and irritable, sometimes to the point of aggression and mild hostility. Most patients, especially those who have lived with the condition for a time, recognize the condition before it becomes serious. The patient needs a quick form of carbohydrate. Some patients carry glucose tablets with them. If these are not available, any form of carbohydrate should be administered as long as the patient is conscious. Orange juice sweetened with sugar, a sugared soft drink, a candy bar, or any form of carbohydrate can be used. Because physical activity continues to deplete the patient's energy stores, the patient should be encouraged to sit quietly until the food has had a chance to take effect, usually 10 to 15 minutes. No food or fluid should be given to an unconscious patient. If a hypoglycemic patient becomes unconscious, immediate medical attention is required.

HYPERGLYCEMIA

Hyperglycemia is a condition of excessive sugar in the blood and is the characteristic typically associated with diabetes. This condition develops gradually, generally over a period of hours or days, so it is not likely to be seen by a technologist. These patients exhibit excessive thirst and urination, dry mucosa, rapid and deep breathing, and drowsiness and confusion. If untreated, the condition leads to diabetic coma. The patient needs insulin, so if this condition is suspected, the technologist should get medical help.

Respiratory Distress and Respiratory Arrest

ASTHMA

Another medical crisis that occasionally occurs in the radiology department is respiratory distress. Patients with asthma seem to particularly react in stressful situations, such as they might experience in a radiology department. A patient in respiratory distress generally exhibits wheezing, a result of dilatation of bronchi on inspiration and collapse on exhalation. Because this is a chronic condition, many patients carry an aerosol inhaler or other form of bronchodilator. The radiologic technologist should stop the procedure, assist the patient to a sitting position (to support easier respiration), and attempt to reassure the patient. If the patient has medications available, the technologist should allow the patient to use them. If not, medical assistance should be obtained.

A calm, confident manner is important when faced with a patient suffering from an asthmatic attack. When the patient begins to suffer respiratory distress, the anxiety is likely to increase, which further interferes with respiratory function. Thus, the technologist's calm handling of the situation not only can comfort the patient but may be a factor in limiting the severity of the problem.

CHOKING

Radiologic technologists should also be familiar with the Heimlich maneuver. This maneuver is used in situations in which a person appears to be choking. The technologist should first

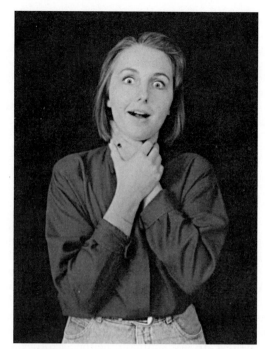

FIGURE 17–2. The universal distress signal for choking.

ascertain that the patient is choking by asking the question "Can you speak?" Patients with partial obstruction can verbalize their problem, but complete obstruction prevents the patient from speaking. An individual who is choking and cannot verbalize a response generally clutches the throat with both hands and becomes red in the face. This signal is the universal distress signal for choking (Fig. 17–2). In cases of either partial or complete obstruction, the patient should be encouraged to cough. If coughing is unsuccessful in dislodging the obstruction, the Heimlich maneuver should be used.

HEIMLICH MANEUVER

The purpose of the Heimlich maneuver is to increase intrathoracic pressure sufficiently to propel the lodged object out of the throat. To apply, the rescuer stands behind the victim and wraps both arms around him or her, clutching one fist with the other hand. The thumb side of the fist is placed in the midline of the victim's abdomen, above the navel and well below the sternum. With the rescuer's elbows held out from the victim, pressure is exerted inward and upward (Fig. 17–3). Although each thrust

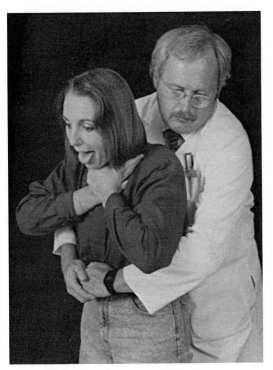

FIGURE 17–3. The Heimlich maneuver.

should be administered separately, the procedure may be repeated quickly 6 to 10 times, or until the obstructing object is expelled.

An unconscious patient should be placed in the supine position. The rescuer kneels astride the victim and places the heel of one hand as described above. The second hand is placed directly on top of the first, and pressure is applied in a quick upward thrust (Fig. 17–4). These maneuvers should not be used with

women in advanced stages of pregnancy or with infants or small children. Variations of the Heimlich maneuver have been developed for these situations.

Modification for Pregnant Patients

Abdominal thrusts could be dangerous for women in late stages of pregnancy, so chest thrusts are used instead. The rescuer again stands behind the patient but places his or her arms under the victim's armpits and around the victim's chest. The thumb side of the fist is placed in the center of the sternum, the second hand is placed over the fist, and backward thrusts are given (Fig. 17–5).

Modification for Infants

In infants younger than 1 year of age, a combination of back blows and chest thrusts is recommended. The infant is held by the rescuer along his or her arm with the head lower than the trunk and supported by holding the victim's jaw. With the arm holding the infant resting on the rescuer's thigh, the rescuer uses the heel of the hand to deliver four back blows between the infant's scapulae. While continuing to support the head and neck, the infant is turned over and four chest thrusts are given with two or three fingers (Fig. 17–6). To determine the location of the hand for chest thrusts, the index finger is placed on the sternum just below the intermammary line. Two or three fingers are used to perform the chest thrusts.

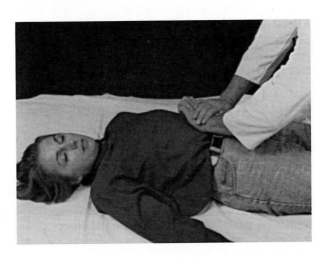

FIGURE 17–4. The Heimlich maneuver on an unconscious victim.

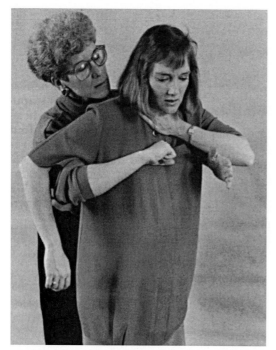

FIGURE 17–5. The Heimlich maneuver adapted for a woman in an advanced stage of pregnancy. (Courtesy of George Greathouse.)

Cardiac Arrest

SIGNS AND SYMPTOMS

Death from cardiac arrest has been reduced significantly in the past 30 years because of the advent of **cardiopulmonary resuscitation (CPR).** Patients who are experiencing cardiac arrest generally complain of crushing chest pain, often described as feeling like an elephant is standing on one's chest. The pain may also radiate down the left arm.

CARDIOPULMONARY RESUSCITATION

The radiologic technologist should be familiar with an institution's protocol for cardiac emergencies. On realization that a patient has suffered cardiac arrest, the appropriate alert should be initiated before the beginning of CPR.

Cerebral function is generally impaired if the brain is deprived of oxygen for more than 4 to 6 minutes, so CPR must be initiated immediately on verifying that cardiopulmonary distress

exists, but it is vitally important that these procedures be performed only after it has been determined that true cardiopulmonary distress exists. CPR provides external support for circulation and respiration and consists of three primary aspects—the ABC's: *a*irway, *b*reathing, and *c*irculation. The following abbreviated protocol is based on the standards and guidelines of the American Medical Association.

One-Person Rescue

1 *Establish unresponsiveness* by gently shaking and shouting at the victim (Fig. 17–7*A*). If these actions fail to rouse the person, call for help and proceed with CPR.
2 *Position the patient* on his or her back on a hard surface to facilitate CPR. A radiographic table is suitable. If the patient is lying on a stretcher, the backboard from the emergency cart should be used.
3 *Open the airway* by tilting the head back. This helps prevent the tongue from falling back and obstructing the airway. Place one

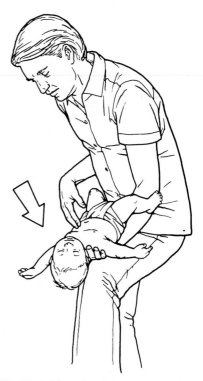

FIGURE 17–6. The Heimlich maneuver on an infant. Position the infant face up over the forearm. Use two or three fingers to perform the *abdominal* thrust. (Reprinted with permission from Craig M: Introduction to Ultrasonography and Patient Care. Philadelphia, WB Saunders, 1993.)

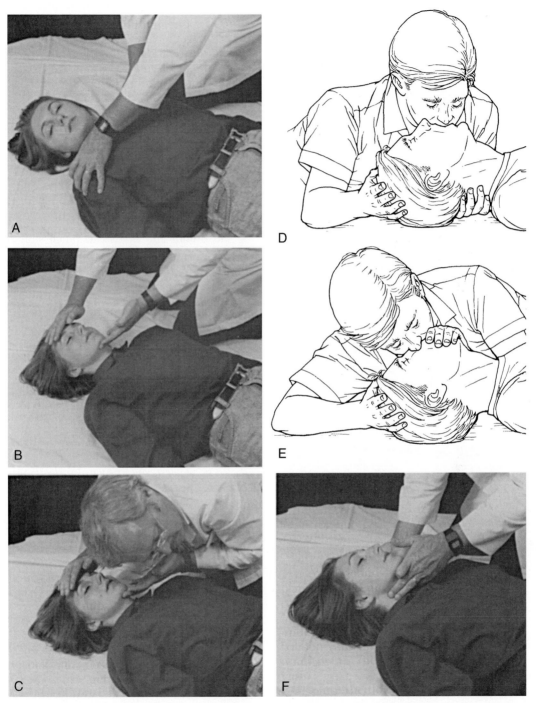

FIGURE 17–7. Cardiopulmonary resuscitation—one-person rescue. *A,* Establishing unresponsiveness of victim. *B,* Head tilt/chin lift. *C,* Proper position for establishing breathlessness. *D,* Mouth-to-mouth rescue breathing. *E,* Mouth-to-nose rescue breathing. *F,* Establishing circulatory inadequacy by palpating the carotid artery.

Illustration continued on following page

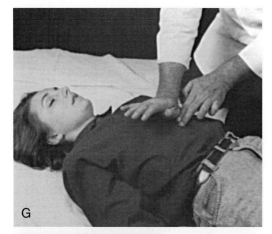

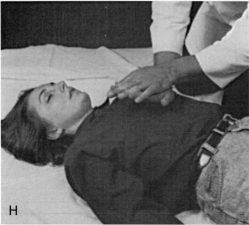

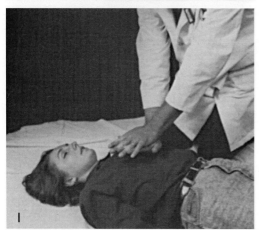

FIGURE 17–7 *Continued. G,* Correct placement of hand along sternum. *H,* Correct placement of hands for external chest compressions. *I,* Locked elbows with the arms extended directly over the patient's sternum to apply compression straight down from the shoulders. (*D* and *E* reprinted with permission from Craig M: Introduction to Ultrasonography and Patient Care. Philadelphia, WB Saunders, 1993.)

hand on the victim's forehead and apply firm backward pressure while placing the fingers of the other hand beneath the bony part of the chin and lifting upward (Fig. 17–7*B*). The lips should be close together, but the mouth should not be completely closed.

4 *Establish breathlessness* by placing an ear over the patient's nose and mouth and looking toward the patient's chest (Fig. 17–7*C*). In this position, listen for breath sounds, look for any rise and fall in the chest, and feel for flow of air from the victim's nose. If there is no breath, proceed with rescue breathing.

5 *Perform rescue breathing.* Put the palm of the hand on the victim's forehead and use the thumb and fingers to pinch shut the victim's nostrils. Take a deep breath and seal your lips around those of the victim, or place a face mask tightly over the nose and mouth (Fig. 17–7*D*). Initially, blow two deep breaths, each of 1 to 1½ seconds, into the patient's mouth or into the mask, taking another breath between the ventilations. If the mouth is damaged or clogged, it is possible to seal the victim's mouth closed and to seal your lips around the nose of the victim (Fig. 17-7*E*).

6 *Establish circulatory inadequacy* by palpating the carotid artery (Fig. 17–7*F*). If, after 5 to 10 seconds, the pulse is absent, proceed with closed chest compressions.

7 *Perform chest compressions* by positioning yourself to one side of the patient and placing the hands properly. This is done by using the hand to find the lower edge of the rib cage and running the middle and index fingers along the lower edge to the point where the ribs meet the sternum. Place the middle finger at this notch and then place the heel of the other hand on the sternum next to the index finger (Fig. 17–7*G*). The heel of the hand should rest along the length of the sternum. The other hand is placed on top of the first, and the fingers of both are interlaced and extended to prevent their tips from applying inadvertent pressure on the ribs (Fig. 17–7*H*). The elbows are locked with the arms extended directly over the patient's sternum, and compression is applied straight down from the shoulders (Fig. 17–7*I*). The force

applied should be sufficient to depress the sternum 1½ to 2 inches in an adult. Pressure should be released after each compression to allow the sternum to return to its original position, but the hands should not be lifted from the sternum.

Fifteen compressions should be alternated with two ventilations; the compressions are given at a rate of 80 to 100 per minute. After four complete cycles of compressions and ventilations (15:2 ratio), take no more than 7 seconds to re-evaluate the patient. If breathing and pulse are still absent, continue CPR, checking every few minutes for the return of pulse and breathing.

Two-Person Rescue

The protocol for CPR with two rescuers is similar, but each rescuer independently performs compressions or ventilations with periodic switches of position. One rescuer is at the victim's side and performs chest compressions. The second rescuer is at the victim's head and maintains the open airway and provides breathing, usually mouth to mask (Fig. 17–8).

Compressions are delivered at the rate of 80 to 100 per minute, with a 2- to 3-second pause for two ventilations after every five chest compressions. When rescuers become fatigued, an organized switch of positions should take place.

Infant Rescue

The CPR procedure for infants and children is basically the same as that for adults, with

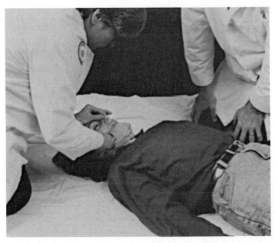

FIGURE 17–8. Position of two rescuers for two-person cardiopulmonary resuscitation.

adjustments made in the volume of air delivered during artificial breathing and the placement of the hands and the depth of depression of the sternum during external chest compressions. When breathing for a pediatric victim, the volume of air should be just enough to cause the rise and fall of the chest.

When performing chest compressions on infants, the index finger should be placed on the sternum just under the point where it intersects with the intermammary line. Using the second, third, and fourth (or only the third and fourth) fingers, compress the sternum to a depth of ½ to 1 inch at a rate of 100 per minute. In a child up to 8 years of age, the hand placement is the same as for an adult. The chest, however, is compressed with only one hand to a depth of only 1 to 1½ inches.

CONSIDERATIONS

CPR is not indicated in all situations of cardiac arrest. If there is any doubt as to its appropriateness, it should be initiated. It is clearly *not* indicated in instances in which the patient, the patient's family, or the patient's physician has specifically requested that resuscitation should not be done. In these cases *DNR* (do not resuscitate) should be clearly indicated on the patient's chart.

Once begun, basic life support should (and for legal reasons, must) be continued until the victim resumes spontaneous respiration and circulation, a physician or other responsible health care professional calls a halt, or the rescuer is too exhausted to continue.

Improperly performed CPR can be not only ineffective but also hazardous. Possible complications from CPR include rib fractures, fractured sternum, pneumothorax, lacerated liver and spleen, and fat emboli. The incidence of complications can be reduced (but not eliminated) by adherence to guidelines.

The American Medical Association recommends that health professionals be taught all CPR skills, including single-rescuer, two-rescuer, and infant. The professional technologist is encouraged to become familiar with all required skills and to achieve certification in all CPR procedures.

Cerebrovascular Accident

A cerebrovascular accident (stroke) may occur in patients in the radiology department. Strokes are more likely in the elderly (over 75 years of age) but can occur in any adult. The onset of a stroke may be sudden or may develop gradually over a period of several hours. Warning signs include paralysis on one or both sides, slurred speech or complete loss of speech, extreme dizziness, loss of vision (particularly if only in one eye), and complete loss of consciousness. The symptoms are sometimes only temporary.

If the radiologic technologist observes any of these signs or symptoms, even if only temporarily, they should be reported to a nurse or physician. Because the potential for paralysis or loss of consciousness is present, the patient should not stand or be moved before further medical assessment can be made. If the patient loses consciousness, CPR may be required and should proceed as described.

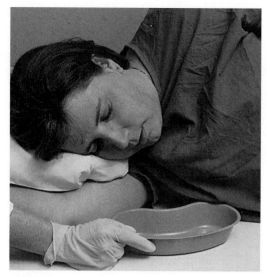

FIGURE 17–9. Lateral decubitus position to prevent aspiration of vomitus.

Minor Medical Emergencies

NAUSEA AND VOMITING

Other minor incidents may happen in the radiology department that, although not threatening serious injury, should nevertheless be handled expeditiously. **Nausea** and **vomiting** are frequent occurrences. Nausea tends to be both a psychological and a physiologic reaction. Patients who feel nauseous often report that feeling to the health care worker. Patients who follow instructions to breathe slowly and deeply through their mouths often become calmer, and nausea and vomiting are avoided.

If the technique does not work and vomiting does occur, it is important that the patient be in a position in which aspiration of vomitus into the lungs is not likely. Recumbent patients should be helped into a lateral decubitus position if possible (Fig. 17–9). If such movement of the patient is contraindicated (eg, a fracture of an arm or leg), the patient should be assisted in turning his or her head to the side. All patients should be provided with an emesis basin and moist cloths.

EPISTAXIS

Epistaxis, or nosebleed, is another common occurrence. Again, this is seldom life-threatening. Patients should lean forward and pinch the affected nostril against the midline nasal cartilage with digital pressure (with the fingers). Pa-

tients should not be put in a recumbent position or instructed to tilt the head backward because this allows the blood to flow down the throat, resulting in the patient's swallowing it. If gentle pressure fails to stop the blood flow, a moist compress may also be applied. This will stop most nosebleeds. If it is not effective within 15 minutes, medical assistance should be obtained.

VERTIGO AND SYNCOPE

Many otherwise healthy patients who have been bedridden or who have had limited mobility for a period often experience **vertigo** (dizziness) or **syncope** (fainting). Vertigo is also often a precursor to syncope. A patient who experiences vertigo should be assisted to a seated or recumbent position. This prevents injury from falling due to problems with equilibrium. Patients who arise from a radiographic table often experience vertigo as a result of orthostatic hypotension, so care should be exercised not to rush these patients, letting them sit on the side of the table for a few minutes before they are escorted from the radiography room.

Syncope is a self-correcting, temporary state of shock and the result of lack of blood flow to the brain. Treatment is aimed at increasing blood flow to the head. The patient should be assisted to a recumbent position, with the feet elevated. Any tight clothing should be loosened. These actions assist in increasing overall blood flow. A moist cloth may also be applied to the forehead. Patients should remain recumbent until such time as they feel strong enough to undergo the remainder of the procedure or return to their rooms.

SEIZURES

Seizures are one of the most frightening events a radiologic technologist might experience. Seizures are caused by a variety of factors, few of which are clearly understood, and may range from mild to severe. A patient who undergoes a mild seizure may experience a brief loss of consciousness or may only stare into space for a brief time. This patient may be only slightly confused and weak after such an episode, but the procedure should nevertheless be postponed until another time.

More severe seizures are characterized by involuntary contraction of muscles, on either one or both sides of the body. This may last for only a minute or up to several minutes. The patient may drool from his or her mouth because of loss of control. The goal is to prevent the patient from injuring himself or herself to the extent possible. No attempt should be made to restrain the patient, since the involuntary movements make this not only ineffective but dangerous. Likewise, no health care worker should ever place his or her hand in a patient's mouth to prevent a backward tongue drop.

Seizure patients often experience an **aura,** a physical or mental warning of an impending seizure. The aura is unique for each individual but can be an important help to both the patient and the health care professional. If sufficient warning is given, the patient should be moved to the floor away from objects against which he or she could hit his or her head. A pillow should be placed under the head so it is not banged against the floor. The same precautions should be taken with all seizure patients, although the absence of a warning aura requires the technologist to be more creative in minimizing the potential for patient harm.

After a seizure, the technologist should be sure that the patient has an open airway, clearing mucus from the mouth as necessary. The patient typically is weak and perhaps disoriented and generally has no memory of the seizure.

While these experiences are often startling, it is helpful to the patient's caregiver to note a few things about the seizure itself. First, make note of where the seizure began, whether it was one-sided or two-sided, and its length. These pieces of information are often important clues in determining the nature of the seizure and may prove helpful in later management and treatment.

FALLS

Despite appropriate assistance and care, a patient may occasionally fall while in the radiology department. In such a situation, the technologist should attempt to minimize the physical impact of the fall to the extent possible and then proceed with appropriate emergency action as indicated by the patient's condition.

Wounds

HEMORRHAGE

Some patients may come to the radiology department with **wounds** sustained previously or during surgery. Such wounds may **hemorrhage** (ie, bleed outside a vessel). The technologist should always make note of the condition of dressings. If they are clean at the outset of a procedure but become saturated, attention is needed. The saturated dressing should not be removed. Pressure should be applied directly over the saturated dressing, preferably with an additional sterile bandage pressed against it. Clotting may take up to 10 minutes, so the pressure may need to be maintained for some time. Once the bleeding appears to be under control, the bandage should be tied or taped into place.

When a bleeding wound is on an extremity, the affected extremity may be placed above the level of the heart unless there are other problems that would contraindicate such a procedure. This slows the blood flow to the extremity and results in less blood loss.

BURNS

The radiologic technologist may be called on to perform radiologic procedures on patients with burns. A burn injury disrupts the normal protective function of the skin, so it is imperative to maintain sterile precautions. Burns are typically extremely painful injuries, so extra gentle care in handling is also indicated.

DEHISCENCE

Wound dehiscence is uncommon but may happen. This refers to a situation in which a patient's sutures separate and allow abdominal contents to spill out of the peritoneal cavity. No attempt should be made to replace tissues inside the wound, but a sterile covering should be used to cover the area. The patient should be placed in a seated position, somewhat bent forward to relieve any additional pressure on the wound. Medical attention should be obtained quickly.

Summary

The thought of some of these medical emergencies may seem somewhat frightening, but most of them are uncommon. They do occur with enough regularity, however, that it is important for the technologist to be aware of typical signs and symptoms associated with the various conditions. The radiologic technologist should be prepared to deal with major medical emergencies, including head injuries, shock, diabetic crises, respiratory distress or arrest, and cardiac arrest. Minor emergencies that may be encountered include nausea and vomiting, epistaxis, syncope and vertigo, seizures, falls, and problems with wounds. An alert technologist who obtains medical assistance quickly may significantly reduce a patient's morbidity and may also play a role in saving a life.

In addition to the technical knowledge necessary, it is also important for the radiologic technologist to respond to all of these situations in a calm, confident manner. It is difficult to think and act appropriately in such periods of stress, but being able to do so is important to the overall outcome. Moving too quickly and risking a mistake is not worth the potential harm that could be caused.

◀R REVIEW QUESTIONS

1 In working with a patient, which of the following would be the first priority for attention?
a) providing an open airway
b) splinting a fractured extremity
c) controlling bleeding
d) treating shock

2 Which of the following signs or symptoms is typically associated with a deteriorating head injury?
a) increasing pulse rate
b) increasing respiratory rate
c) lethargy
d) thirst

3 Which of the following actions would help prevent a patient from going into shock?
a) minimizing pain
b) providing emotional support
c) maintaining a normal body temperature
d) all of the above

4 A patient suffering from hypoglycemia needs which of the following?
a) rest
b) insulin
c) carbohydrates
d) a and c

5 Where should the heel of the hand be placed when doing chest compressions during CPR on an adult?
a) near the sternal angle
b) at the xiphoid process
c) two fingers above the xiphoid process
d) anywhere along the length of the sternum

6 *Syncope* is a medical term for which of the following?
a) dizziness
b) fainting
c) hemorrhage
d) nosebleed

7 Which of the following is typically associated with shock?
a) decreasing pulse rate
b) decreasing blood pressure
c) fever
d) flushed face

8 The Heimlich maneuver is used in response to which of the following situations?
a) asthmatic crisis
b) cardiac arrest
c) choking
d) wound dehiscence

9 How long can the brain be deprived of oxygen before cerebral function impairment is likely?

a) 30 seconds
b) 60 seconds
c) 2 minutes
d) 4 to 6 minutes

10 Which of the following actions is the most appropriate in handling a patient who begins a violent seizure?
a) Restrain the patient in any way possible.
b) Ensure an open airway, putting your hands into the victim's mouth if necessary.
c) Attempt to prevent the patient from injuring himself or herself.

d) All of the above.

BIBLIOGRAPHY

American Medical Association: Standards and guidelines for cardiopulmonary resuscitation (CPR) and emergency cardiac care (ECE). JAMA 255:2905–2931, 1986.
Copass MK, Soper RG, Eisenberg MS: EMT Manual. 2nd ed. Philadelphia, WB Saunders, 1991.
Grant HD, et al: Emergency Gare. Englewood Cliffs, NJ, Prentice-Hall, 1989.
Judd RL, Ponsell DD: Mosby's First Responder. 7th ed., St. Louis, CV Mosby, 1995.
Thompson JM, et al: Mosby's Manual of Clinical Nursing. 3rd ed. St. Louis, CV Mosby, 1993.

CHAPTER 18

PHARMACOLOGY

Nadia A. Bugg, PhD, RT(R)

A desire to take medicine is, perhaps, the great feature which distinguishes man from other animals.

SIR WILLIAM OSLER (1849–1919)

OBJECTIVES

On completion of this chapter, the student will be able to:

1 Recognize common definitions and nomenclature associated with pharmacology.
2 Recognize the various classifications of drugs.

3 Describe the actions, indications, and precautions related to various drugs.
4 List the "five rights" of drug administration.
5 List the methods of drug administration.
6 Prepare intravenous drugs for injection.
7 Perform venipuncture using appropriate universal precautions.
8 Describe documentation procedures related to drug administration.
9 Define abbreviations commonly used in drug administration.

GLOSSARY

Ampule: small sealed glass container that holds a single dose of parenteral solution in a sterile condition

Analgesic: drug that relieves pain without causing a loss of consciousness

Anaphylaxis: condition of shock caused by hypersensitivity to a drug or other substance that results in life-threatening respiratory distress and vascular collapse

Anesthetic: drug that produces a loss of feeling or sensation

Anticholinergic: drug that blocks the passage of impulses through the parasympathetic nerves

Arrhythmia: any variation from the normal rhythm of the heart beat

Atherosclerosis: condition in which there is thickening of the wall of a blood vessel caused by the deposit of plaque (atheroma)

Bolus: a concentrated mass of pharmaceutical preparation

Bronchodilator: drug that causes expansion of the lumina of the air passages of the lungs

Coagulation: process of clot formation

Contraindication: any condition that renders the administration of some drug or some particular line of treatment improper or undesirable

Diuretic: drug that promotes the excretion of urine

Drug: any chemical compound administered to humans as an aid in the diagnosis, treatment, or prevention of disease

Edema: presence of abnormally large amounts of fluid in the tissues of the body

Emetic: drug that causes vomiting

Extravasation: discharge or escape of fluid from a vessel into the surrounding tissue

Generic Name: drug name that is usually descriptive of its chemical structure but is not protected by a trademark

Grand Mal Seizure: condition in which a sudden loss of consciousness is immediately followed by generalized convulsions

Hematoma: localized collection of blood in the tissue due to a break in the wall of the blood vessel

Hypertension: persistently high arterial blood pressure, usually exceeding 140 mm Hg systolic and 90 mm Hg diastolic

Idiosyncratic Reaction: unusual response to a drug that is peculiar to the individual

Infiltration: diffusion of fluid into a tissue; often used interchangeably with *extravasation*

Intramuscular: within the muscle tissue

Intravenous: within a vein

Laxative: agent that acts to promote evacuation of the bowel

Microorganism: microscopic organism such as a bacterium or a virus that is too small to be seen without a microscope

Neoplastic: pertaining to new or abnormal growths that are uncontrolled and progressive (either benign or malignant)

Parenteral: not through the gastrointestinal tract but by injection through some other route

Peristalsis: waves of contraction that propel contents through the gastrointestinal tract

Petit Mal Seizure: mild convulsion that may or may not be associated with a loss of consciousness

Pharmacist: one who is licensed to prepare and dispense drugs

Pharmacology: science that deals with the origin, nature, effects, and uses of drugs

Physiologic Dependency: compulsion to take a drug continuously to prevent withdrawal symptoms

Schizophrenia: chronic mental disorder characterized by periods of withdrawn or bizarre behavior

Side Effect: consequence other than the one for which a drug is used

Subcutaneous: beneath the skin

Sublingual: beneath the tongue

Therapeutic: pertaining to the art of healing

Thromboembolic Disorders: conditions involving the partial or complete obstruction of a blood vessel

Topical: applied to a certain area of the skin and affecting only the area to which it is applied

Transdermal: entering through the skin

Vasoconstrictor: drug that causes constriction of the blood vessels

Vasodilator: drug that causes the dilation of the blood vessels

Venipuncture: puncture of a vein

Vial: small glass bottle containing multiple doses of a drug

Introduction to Pharmacology

The preparation of drugs is often a responsibility of radiologic technologists. Under the direction of a licensed practitioner, usually a radiologist, the technologist is frequently required to administer drugs in the radiology department. Increasingly, the radiologic technologist is expected to have a broad knowledge of drugs, including their classification, actions, interactions and reactions, and principles and methods of administration, as well as the skills necessary to assist with drug administration in a number of different clinical situations. This knowledge is essential to good patient care and competent professional practice. As the role and responsibilities of the radiologic technologist continue to expand in the area of drug administration, the information presented in this chapter will provide a fundamental theoretical framework within which the level of knowledge may increase.

A **drug** is any chemical substance that produces a biologic response in a living system. More specifically, a drug is a substance used as medicine to aid in the diagnosis, treatment, or prevention of disease. The science concerned with the origin, nature, effects, and uses of drugs is called **pharmacology.**

DRUG NOMENCLATURE

A *nomenclature* is a classified system of names. In pharmacology, drugs are classified in a number of different ways. For example, a drug may be classified by its name, its action, or its method of legal purchase. When drugs are classified by name, it is important to know which kind of name is being used, since the same drug has at least three different names: a chemical name, a generic name, and a trade name.

Classification by Name

The first name that is likely to be applied to a drug is the *chemical name*, which identifies the actual chemical structure of the drug. The chemical name is often complex and is seldom of practical importance to the technologist.

The **generic name** is the name given to the drug when it becomes commercially available. The generic name is a simpler name derived from the more complex chemical name. It is usually easier to pronounce and is never capitalized. It is also called the *nonproprietary* name. Some drugs are best known by the generic name.

A *brand name* is the name given to a drug manufactured by a specific company. It is usually short and easy to remember. It may or may not reflect any characteristic of the chemical structure of the drug. Because the same drug is manufactured by more than one company, each company selects its own brand name or trademark for the drug. *Trademark, brand name, trade name,* and *proprietary name* are all terms used interchangeably to indicate a specific generic drug manufactured by a number of different companies. An example of the names currently used for a single drug follows:

Chemical name: 7-chloro-1,3-dihydro-1-methyl-5-phenyl-2H-1,4-benzodiazepin-2-one
Generic name: diazepam
Brand name: Valium

Confusion occurs when some physicians use generic names and others use trade names when requesting drugs. Therefore, the radiologic technologist should be aware of drug information resources that are available. One such source is the *Physicians' Desk Reference,* or *PDR,* as it is frequently called. The *PDR* is an annual publication that contains current product information. The pages are color coded for easy reference, and drugs are listed by both generic and brand names. The *PDR* gives the accepted uses, side effects, **contraindications,** and dosages for available drugs. If a *PDR* is not readily available in the radiology department, the next best source of drug information is the hospital pharmacist.

Classification by Action

Another way in which drugs are classified is according to action or function. Drugs that have similar chemical actions are grouped into categories called *drug families*. For example, drugs that relieve pain are classified as analgesics, drugs used to treat high blood pressure are classified as antihypertensives, and drugs used to fight inflammation are classified as anti-inflammatories. Although this is a convenient way to classify drugs for study purposes, it is not totally reliable or exclusive since one drug may have several different physiologic effects on the body, which means it would be listed under more than one category.

Legal Classification

According to federal laws, drugs are classified legally as either prescription or nonprescription. Prescription drugs require an order by a legally authorized health practitioner who is usually, but not always, a physician. The prescription is the documentation that specifies precisely the name of the patient, the name of the drug, and the dosage regimen to be followed. Prescription drugs are usually dispensed by a licensed **pharmacist,** although some physicians supply prescription drugs to their patients. Nonprescription drugs, better known as over-the-counter drugs, may be legally obtained without a prescription. The radiologic technologist should be aware that many over-the-counter products are capable of producing toxic effects if they are misused or used in combination with other drugs.

DOSAGE FORMS

The dosage form of a drug refers to the type of preparation or the manner in which the chemical agent is transported into the human body. A single drug may be available in a number of different forms to facilitate the administration and action of the drug under a variety of conditions. The dosage form may determine the speed, or onset, of the drug's therapeutic effect. Some of the common dosage forms include tablets, capsules, suppositories, solutions, suspensions, and transdermal patches.

Tablet

Tablets are the most common oral dosage form and one of the easiest to administer. A tablet is a granulated drug that has been compressed into a solid hard disc. Tablets are single-dose units that may be scored to facilitate division into halves or quarters. Some tablets are coated with a substance that delays the dissolution of the tablet until it is in the small intestines rather than in the stomach, where it is normally dissolved. These so-called enteric-coated tablets are used for drugs that might irritate the stomach (such as aspirin) or for drugs destroyed by the acid in the stomach.

Capsule

A capsule is a dosage form in which a powdered or liquid drug is contained in a gelatin shell. The gelatin shell dissolves in the stomach and releases its contents.

Suppository

A suppository is a dosage form shaped for insertion into a body orifice such as the rectum, vagina, or urethra. Once inserted, the suppository dissolves and releases the drug. It may have a local or systemic effect.

Solution

A solution is a dosage form in which one or more drugs are dissolved in a liquid carrier. Solutions are usually rapidly absorbed and may be administered orally or parenterally. **Parenteral** administration includes any injection of the drug with a needle and syringe beneath the surface of the skin.

Suspension

A suspension is a dosage form in which one or more drugs in small particles are suspended in a liquid carrier. Most suspensions are administered orally and should be shaken thoroughly just before administration. Suspensions should never be administered intravenously.

Transdermal Patch

A transdermal patch is a dosage form that permits a drug to be applied onto the skin surface, where it is absorbed into the bloodstream.

The patch-like device containing the drug is applied to the skin with a water-resistant covering. The patch releases the drug gradually over time.

Classification of Drugs

For easy reference, Table 18–1 lists commonly used drugs alphabetically by the trade name. Table 18–2 provides a cross-reference by generic name, and Table 18–3 provides a classification by drug action. The drugs commonly found on a crash cart for emergency situations are listed alphabetically by trade name in Box 18–1.

ACTIONS, INDICATIONS, AND PRECAUTIONS

Analgesics

Analgesics are drugs that relieve pain without causing loss of consciousness. Analgesics may be narcotic or nonnarcotic. Narcotic analgesics are derived from opium, such as *morphine* and *Demerol* (meperidine hydrochloride). They are used in the treatment of moderate to severe

BOX 18–1

> **Emergency Drugs Commonly Found on a Crash Cart**
>
> Adrenalin—bronchodilator
> Atropine—anticholinergic
> Benadryl—antihistamine
> Bretylol—antiarrhythmic
> Dilantin—anticonvulsant
> Dobutrex—stimulant
> Inderal—antiarrhythmic
> Intropin—stimulant
> Isoptin—vasodilator
> Isuprel—bronchodilator
> Lanoxin—antiarrhythmic
> Lasix—diuretic
> Levophed—vasoconstrictor
> Nitroglycerin—vasodilator
> Nitropress—vasodilator
> Pronestyl—antiarrhythmic
> Sodium bicarbonate—fluid replacement
> Xylocaine—antiarrhythmic

pain. Narcotics are capable of causing **physiologic dependency** with regular use. Adverse side effects such as nausea and vomiting are frequently associated with the administration of narcotic analgesics. Nonnarcotic analgesics such as *Tylenol* (acetaminophen) are relatively safe drugs used in the treatment of mild to moderate pain. They do not cause physiologic dependency but may be habit forming.

Anesthetics

Anesthetics are agents that act on the central nervous system (CNS) to produce a loss of sensation. There are two types of anesthetic agents: general anesthetics and local anesthetics. General anesthetics, such as *Pentothal* (thiopental sodium) act as CNS depressants by producing muscle relaxation and loss of consciousness. General anesthesia is commonly used on patients undergoing major surgical procedures. Local anesthetics, such as *Novocain* (procaine hydrochloride), block nerve conduction from an area of the body to the CNS. The extent of their action depends on the area to which they are applied.

Antianxiety Agents

Antianxiety agents or mild tranquilizers are drugs used in the treatment of anxiety. They act either to calm the patient without depressing the CNS or to elevate the patient's mood without stimulating the CNS. *Equanil* (meprobamate) is a nonbarbiturate drug that has an anxiety-reducing effect. It may cause physiologic dependency with prolonged use and has been associated with severe withdrawal reactions. *Valium* (diazepam) is one of the most widely prescribed drugs for the treatment of anxiety. It is also used to alleviate muscle spasms and is often used as a preoperative drug for various procedures performed in the radiology department.

Antiarrhythmics

Antiarrhythmics are drugs used to treat **arrhythmias,** which are any variation from the normal rhythm of the heart beat. The abnormal rhythm may occur in the atria, the upper chambers of the heart, or in the ventricles, the lower chambers of the heart. The antiarrhythmic agent used depends on the type of arrhythmia

Text continued on page 289

TABLE 18–1. Commonly Used Drugs by Brand Name

Brand Name	Generic Name	Route(s)	Classification
Adrenalin	epinephrine	Parenteral	Bronchodilator
Aminophylline	theophylline ethylenediamine	Oral/parenteral	Bronchodilator
Amoxil	amoxicillin	Oral	Antibiotic
Amphojel	aluminum hydroxide	Oral	Antiulcer
Amytal	amobarbital	Oral	Sedative
Antivert	meclizine	Oral	Antihistamine
Apomorphine	apomorphine HCl	Oral	Emetic
Aramine	metaraminol	Parenteral	Vasoconstrictor
Aspirin	aspirin	Oral	Analgesic
Ativan	lorazepam	Oral/parenteral	Antianxiety
Atropine	atropine	Oral/parenteral	Anticholinergic
Baking soda	sodium bicarbonate	Oral/parenteral	Antiulcer
Benadryl	diphenhydramine HCl	Oral/parenteral	Antihistamine
Bretylol	bretylium	Parenteral	Antiarrhythmic
Bumex	bumetanide	Oral/parenteral	Diuretic
Carafate	sucralfate	Oral	Antiulcer
Catapres	clonidine HCl	Oral/transdermal	Antihypertensive
Ceclor	cefaclor	Oral	Antibiotic
Cerespan	papaverine HCl	Oral/parenteral	Vasodilator
Chloral Hydrate	chloral hydrate	Oral	Sedative
Chloromycetin	chloramphenicol	Parenteral	Antibiotic
Chlor-Trimeton	chlorpheniramine	Oral	Antihistamine
Clozaril	clozapine	Oral	Antipsychotic
Codeine	codeine	Oral/parenteral	Analgesic
Compazine	prochlorperazine	Oral	Antiemetic
Coumadin	warfarin	Oral	Anticoagulant
Dalmane	flurazepam	Oral	Sedative
Darvon	propoxyphene HCl	Oral	Analgesic
Decadron	dexamethasone	Oral/parenteral	Corticosteroid
Deltasone	prednisone	Oral	Corticosteroid
Demerol	meperidine HCl	Oral/parenteral	Analgesic
Depo-Medrol	methylprednisolone	Parenteral	Corticosteroid
Dexedrine	dextroamphetamine	Oral	Stimulant
Diamox	acetazolamide	Oral/parenteral	Diuretic
Dicumarol	bishydroxycoumarin	Oral	Anticoagulant
Dilantin	phenytoin	Oral/parenteral	Anticonvulsant
Dimetane	brompheniramine	Oral	Antihistamine
Diuril	chlorothiazide	Oral	Diuretic
Dobutrex	dobutamine HCl	Parenteral	Stimulant
Dopram	doxapram HCl	Parenteral	Stimulant
Dramamine	dimenhydrinate	Oral	Antiemetic
Dulcolax	bisacodyl	Oral/rectal	Laxative
Elavil	amitriptyline HCl	Oral/parenteral	Antidepressant
Ephedrine	ephedrine sulfate	Oral/parenteral	Bronchodilator
Equanil	meprobamate	Oral	Antianxiety
Erythrocin	erythromycin	Oral/parenteral	Antibiotic
Esidrix	hydrochlorothiazide	Oral	Diuretic
Eskalith	lithium carbonate	Oral	Antianxiety
Feldene	piroxicam	Oral	Anti-inflammatory
Gantrisin	sulfisoxazole	Oral	Antibiotic
Geocillin	carbenicillin	Parenteral	Antibiotic
Hyperstat	diazoxide	Parenteral	Antihypertensive
Inderal	propranolol HCl	Oral/parenteral	Antiarrhythmic
Indocin	indomethacin	Oral/parenteral	Anti-inflammatory
Intropin	dopamine HCl	Parenteral	Stimulant
Ipecac	ipecac syrup	Oral	Emetic
Isoptin	verapamil HCl	Oral/parenteral	Vasodilator
Isuprel	isoproterenol HCl	Oral/parenteral	Bronchodilator
Klonopin	clonazepam	Oral	Anticonvulsant

Table continued on following page

TABLE 18–1. **Commonly Used Drugs by Brand Name** *Continued*

Brand Name	Generic Name	Route(s)	Classification
Lanoxin	digoxin	Oral/parenteral	Antiarrhythmic
Lasix	furosemide	Oral/parenteral	Diuretic
Levophed	norepinephrine	Parenteral	Vasoconstrictor
Librium	chlordiazepoxide	Oral/parenteral	Antianxiety
Liquaemin	heparin sodium	Parenteral	Anticoagulant
Lopressor	metoprolol	Oral	Antihypertensive
Luminal	phenobarbital	Oral	Sedative
Mellaril	thioridazine	Oral	Antipsychotic
Mephyton	phytonadione	Oral/parenteral	Coagulant
Metamucil	psyllium	Oral	Laxative
Milk of Magnesia	magnesium hydroxide	Oral	Laxative
Minipress	prazosin HCl	Oral	Antihypertensive
Morphine	morphine sulfate	Oral/parenteral	Analgesic
Motrin	ibuprofen	Oral	Anti-inflammatory
Naprosyn	naproxen	Oral	Anti-inflammatory
Nardil	phenelzine sulfate	Oral	Antidepressant
Nembutal	pentobarbital	Oral	Sedative
Neoloid	castor oil	Oral	Laxative
Nitrogard	nitroglycerin	Oral/parenteral	Vasodilator
Nitropress	nitroprusside	Parenteral	Vasodilator
Norpace	disopyramide	Oral	Antiarrhythmic
Novocain	procaine HCl	Parenteral	Anesthetic
Nubain	nalbuphine	Oral/parenteral	Analgesic
Omnipen	ampicillin	Oral/parenteral	Antibiotic
Pentids	penicillin	Oral/parenteral	Antibiotic
Pentothal	thiopental sodium	Parenteral	Anesthetic
Percodan	oxycodone/aspirin	Oral	Analgesic
Phenergan	promethazine HCl	Oral/parenteral	Antihistamine
Placidyl	ethchlorvynol	Oral	Sedative
Premarin	conjugated estrogens	Oral/parenteral	Female hormone
Pro-Banthine	propantheline bromide	Oral	Anticholinergic
Pronestyl	procainamide HCl	Oral/parenteral	Antiarrhythmic
Reglan	metoclopramide	Oral/parenteral	Antiulcer
Ritalin	methylphenidate	Oral	Stimulant
Scopolamine	scopolamine	Transdermal/parenteral	Anticholinergic
Seconal	secobarbital	Oral/parenteral	Sedative
Serpasil	reserpine	Oral	Antihypertensive
Sinequan	doxepin HCl	Oral	Antidepressant
Solu-Cortef	hydrocortisone	Parenteral	Corticosteroid
Sorbitrate	isosorbide dinitrate	Oral	Vasodilator
Streptase	streptokinase	Parenteral	Anticoagulant
Tagamet	cimetidine HCl	Oral/parenteral	Antiulcer
Talwin	pentazocine HCl	Oral/parenteral	Analgesic
Tenormin	atenolol	Oral	Antihypertensive
Tenuate	diethylpropion HCl	Oral	Stimulant
Terramycin	oxytetracycline	Oral/parenteral	Antibiotic
Thorazine	chlorpromazine	Oral/parenteral	Antipsychotic
Tigan	trimethobenzamide	Oral	Antiemetic
Tofranil	imipramine HCl	Oral/parenteral	Antidepressant
Tranxene	clorazepate dipotassium	Oral	Antianxiety
Tylenol	acetaminophen	Oral	Analgesic
Valium	diazepam	Oral/parenteral	Antianxiety
Vistaril	hydroxyzine HCl	Oral/parenteral	Antianxiety
Xanax	alprazolam	Oral	Antianxiety
Xylocaine	lidocaine HCl	Parenteral	Antiarrhythmic
Zantac	ranitidine HCl	Oral/parenteral	Antiulcer

TABLE 18–2. **Commonly Used Drugs by Generic Name**

Generic Name	Brand Name	Route(s)	Classification
acetaminophen	Tylenol	Oral	Analgesic
acetazolamide	Diamox	Oral/parenteral	Diuretic
alprazolam	Xanax	Oral	Antianxiety
aluminum hydroxide	Amphojel	Oral	Antiulcer
amitriptyline HCl	Elavil	Oral/parenteral	Antidepressant
amobarbital	Amytal	Oral	Sedative
amoxicillin	Amoxil	Oral	Antibiotic
ampicillin	Omnipen	Oral/parenteral	Antibiotic
apomorphine HCl	Apomorphine	Oral	Emetic
aspirin	Aspirin	Oral	Analgesic
atenolol	Tenormin	Oral	Antihypertensive
atropine	Atropine	Oral/parenteral	Anticholinergic
bisacodyl	Dulcolax	Oral/rectal	Laxative
bishydroxycoumarin	Dicumarol	Oral	Anticoagulant
bretylium	Bretylol	Parenteral	Antiarrhythmic
brompheniramine	Dimetane	Oral	Antihistamine
bumetanide	Bumex	Oral/parenteral	Diuretic
carbenicillin	Geocillin	Parenteral	Antibiotic
castor oil	Neoloid	Oral	Laxative
cefaclor	Ceclor	Oral	Antibiotic
chloral hydrate	Chloral Hydrate	Oral	Sedative
chloramphenicol	Chloromycetin	Parenteral	Antibiotic
chlordiazepoxide	Librium	Oral/parenteral	Antianxiety
chlorothiazide	Diuril	Oral	Diuretic
chlorpheniramine	Chlor-Trimeton	Oral	Antihistamine
chlorpromazine	Thorazine	Oral/parenteral	Antipsychotic
clozapine	Clozaril	Oral	Antipsychotic
clorazepate dipotassium	Tranxene	Oral	Antianxiety
cimetidine HCl	Tagamet	Oral/parenteral	Antiulcer
clonazepam	Klonopin	Oral	Anticonvulsant
clonidine HCl	Catapres	Oral/transdermal	Antihypertensive
codeine	Codeine	Oral/parenteral	Analgesic
conjugated estrogens	Premarin	Oral/parenteral	Female hormone
dexamethasone	Decadron	Oral/parenteral	Corticosteroid
dextroamphetamine	Dexedrine	Oral	Stimulant
diazepam	Valium	Oral/parenteral	Antianxiety
diazoxide	Hyperstat	Parenteral	Antihypertensive
diethylpropion HCl	Tenuate	Oral	Stimulant
digoxin	Lanoxin	Oral/parenteral	Antiarrhythmic
dimenhydrinate	Dramamine	Oral	Antiemetic
diphenhydramine HCl	Benadryl	Oral/parenteral	Antihistamine
disopyramide	Norpace	Oral	Antiarrhythmic
dobutamine HCl	Dobutrex	Parenteral	Stimulant
dopamine HCl	Intropin	Parenteral	Stimulant
doxapram HCl	Dopram	Oral/parenteral	Stimulant
doxepin HCl	Sinequan	Oral	Antidepressant
ephedrine sulfate	Ephedrine	Oral/parenteral	Bronchodilator
epinephrine	Adrenalin	Parenteral	Bronchodilator
erythromycin	Erythrocin	Oral/parenteral	Antibiotic
ethchlorvynol	Placidyl	Oral	Sedative
flurazepam HCl	Dalmane	Oral	Sedative
furosemide	Lasix	Oral/parenteral	Diuretic
heparin sodium	Liquaemin	Parenteral	Anticoagulant
hydrochlorothiazide	Esidrix	Oral	Diuretic
hydrocortisone	Solu-Cortef	Parenteral	Corticosteroid
hydroxyzine HCl	Vistaril	Oral/parenteral	Antianxiety
ibuprofen	Motrin	Oral	Anti-inflammatory
imipramine HCl	Tofranil	Oral/parenteral	Antidepressant
indomethacin	Indocin	Oral/parenteral	Anti-inflammatory
ipecac syrup	Ipecac	Oral	Emetic

Table continued on following page

TABLE 18–2. **Commonly Used Drugs by Generic Name** *Continued*

Generic Name	Brand Name	Route(s)	Classification
isoproterenol HCl	Isuprel	Oral/parenteral	Bronchodilator
isosorbide dinitrate	Sorbitrate	Oral	Vasodilator
lidocaine HCl	Xylocaine	Parenteral	Antiarrhythmic
lithium carbonate	Eskalith	Oral	Antianxiety
lorazepam	Ativan	Oral/parenteral	Antianxiety
magnesium hydroxide	Milk of Magnesia	Oral	Laxative
meclizine	Antivert	Oral	Antihistamine
menadione	Synkayvite	Oral/parenteral	Coagulant
meperidine HCl	Demerol	Oral/parenteral	Analgesic
meprobamate	Equanil	Oral	Antianxiety
metaraminol	Aramine	Parenteral	Vasoconstrictor
methylprednisolone	Depo-Medrol	Parenteral	Corticosteroid
methylphenidate	Ritalin	Oral	Stimulant
metoclopramide	Reglan	Oral/parenteral	Antiulcer
metoprolol	Lopressor	Oral	Antihypertensive
morphine sulfate	Morphine	Oral/parenteral	Analgesic
nalbuphine	Nubain	Oral/parenteral	Analgesic
naproxen	Naprosyn	Oral	Anti-inflammatory
nitroglycerin	Nitrogard	Oral/parenteral	Vasodilator
nitroprusside	Nitropress	Parenteral	Vasodilator
norepinephrine	Levophed	Parenteral	Vasoconstrictor
oxycodone/aspirin	Percodan	Oral	Analgesic
oxytetracycline	Terramycin	Oral/parenteral	Antibiotic
papaverine HCl	Cerespan	Oral/parenteral	Vasodilator
penicillin	Pentids	Oral/parenteral	Antibiotic
pentazocine HCl	Talwin	Oral/parenteral	Analgesic
pentobarbital	Nembutal	Oral	Sedative
phenelzine sulfate	Nardil	Oral	Antidepressant
phenobarbital	Luminal	Oral/parenteral	Sedative
phenytoin	Dilantin	Oral/parenteral	Anticonvulsant
phytonadione	Mephyton	Oral/parenteral	Coagulant
piroxicam	Feldene	Oral	Anti-inflammatory
prazosin HCl	Minipress	Oral	Antihypertensive
prednisone	Deltasone	Oral	Corticosteroid
procainamide HCl	Pronestyl	Oral/parenteral	Antiarrhythmic
procaine HCl	Novocain	Parenteral	Anesthetic
prochlorperazine	Compazine	Oral/parenteral	Antiemetic
promethazine HCl	Phenergan	Oral/parenteral	Antihistamine
propantheline bromide	Pro-Banthine	Oral	Anticholinergic
propoxyphene HCl	Darvon	Oral	Analgesic
propranolol HCl	Inderal	Oral/parenteral	Antiarrhythmic
psyllium	Metamucil	Oral	Laxative
ranitidine HCl	Zantac	Oral/parenteral	Antiulcer
reserpine	Serpasil	Oral	Antihypertensive
scopolamine	Scopolamine	Transdermal/parenteral	Anticholinergic
secobarbital	Seconal	Oral/parenteral	Sedative
sodium bicarbonate	Baking soda	Oral/parenteral	Antiulcer
streptokinase	Streptase	Parenteral	Anticoagulant
sucralfate	Carafate	Oral	Antiulcer
sulfisoxazole	Gantrisin	Oral	Antibiotic
theophylline ethylenediamine	Aminophylline	Oral/parenteral	Bronchodilator
thiopental sodium	Pentothal	Parenteral	Anesthetic
thioridazine	Mellaril	Oral	Antipsychotic
trimethobenzamide	Tigan	Oral/parenteral	Antiemetic
verapamil HCl	Isoptin	Oral/parenteral	Vasodilator
warfarin	Coumadin	Oral	Anticoagulant

TABLE 18–3. Commonly Used Drugs by Classification

Classification/ Brand Name	Generic Name	Route(s)
Analgesics		
Aspirin	aspirin	Oral
Codeine	codeine	Oral/parenteral
Darvon	propoxyphene HCl	Oral
Demerol	meperidine HCl	Oral/parenteral
Morphine	morphine	Oral/parenteral
Nubain	nalbuphine	Oral/parenteral
Percodan	oxycodone/aspirin	Oral
Talwin	pentazocine HCl	Oral/parenteral
Tylenol	acetaminophen	Oral
Anesthetics		
Novocain	procaine HCl	Parenteral
Pentothal	thiopental sodium	Parenteral
Antiarrhythmics		
Bretylol	bretylium	Parenteral
Inderal	propranolol HCl	Oral/parenteral
Lanoxin	digoxin	Oral/parenteral
Norpace	disopyramide	Oral
Pronestyl	procainamide HCl	Oral/parenteral
Antianxiety Agents		
Ativan	lorazepam	Oral/parenteral
Equanil	meprobamate	Oral
Eskalith	lithium carbonate	Oral
Librium	chlordiazepoxide	Oral/parenteral
Tranxene	clorazepate dipotassium	Oral
Valium	diazepam	Oral/parenteral
Vistaril	hydroxyzine HCl	Oral/parenteral
Xanax	alprazolam	
Antibiotics		
Amoxil	amoxicillin	Oral
Ceclor	cefaclor	Oral
Chloromycetin	chloramphenicol	Oral/parenteral
Erythrocin	erythromycin	Oral/parenteral
Gantrisin	sulfisoxazole	Oral
Geocillin	carbenicillin	Parenteral
Omnipen	ampicillin	Oral/parenteral
Pentids	penicillin	Oral/parenteral
Terramycin	oxytetracycline	Oral/parenteral
Anticholinergic Agents		
Atropine	atropine	Oral/parenteral
Pro-Banthine	propantheline bromide	Oral
Scopolamine	scopolamine	Transdermal/parenteral
Anticoagulants		
Coumadin	warfarin	Oral
Dicumarol	bishydroxycoumarin	Oral
Liquaemin	heparin sodium	Parenteral
Streptase	streptokinase	Parenteral
Anticonvulsants		
Dilantin	phenytoin	Oral/parenteral
Klonopin	clonazepam	Oral
Antidepressants		
Elavil	amitriptyline HCl	Oral/parenteral
Nardil	phenelzine sulfate	Oral
Sinequan	doxepin HCl	Oral
Tofranil	imipramine HCl	Oral/parenteral
Antiemetics		
Compazine	prochlorperazine	Oral/parenteral
Dramamine	dimenhydrinate	Oral
Tigan	trimethobenzamide	Oral/parenteral

Table continued on following page

TABLE 18–3. **Commonly Used Drugs by Classification** *Continued*

Classification/ Brand Name	Generic Name	Route(s)
Antihistamines		
Antivert	meclizine	Oral
Benadryl	diphenhydramine HCl	Oral/parenteral
Chlor-Trimeton	chlorpheniramine	Oral
Dimetane	brompheniramine	Oral
Phenergan	promethazine HCl	Oral/parenteral
Antihypertensives		
Catapres	clonidine HCl	Oral/transdermal
Hyperstat	diazoxide	Parenteral
Lopressor	metoprolol	Oral
Minipress	prazosin HCl	Oral
Serpasil	reserpine	Oral
Tenormin	atenolol	Oral
Anti-inflammatory Agents		
Feldene	piroxicam	Oral
Indocin	indomethacin	Oral/parenteral
Motrin	ibuprofen	Oral
Naprosyn	naproxen	Oral
Antipsychotic Agents		
Clozaril	clozapine	Oral
Mellaril	thioridazine	Oral
Thorazine	chlorpromazine	Oral/parenteral
Antiulcer Agents		
Amphojel	aluminum hydroxide	Oral
Baking soda	sodium bicarbonate	Oral/parenteral
Carafate	sucralfate	Oral
Reglan	metoclopramide	Oral/parenteral
Tagamet	cimetidine HCl	Oral/parenteral
Zantac	ranitidine HCl	Oral/parenteral
Bronchodilators		
Adrenalin	epinephrine	Parenteral
Aminophylline	theophylline	Oral/parenteral
Ephedrine	ephedrine sulfate	Oral
Isuprel	isoproterenol HCl	Oral/parenteral
Coagulants		
Mephyton	phytonadione	Oral/parenteral
Synkayvite	menadione	Oral/parenteral
Corticosteroids		
Decadron	dexamethasone	Oral
Deltasone	prednisone	Oral
Depo-Medrol	methylprednisolone	Parenteral
Solu-Cortef	hydrocortisone	Parenteral
Diuretics		
Bumex	bumetanide	Oral/parenteral
Diamox	acetazolamide	Oral/parenteral
Diuril	chlorothiazide	Oral
Esidrix	hydrochlorothiazide	Oral
Lasix	furosemide	Oral/parenteral
Emetic Agents		
Apomorphine	apomorphine HCl	Oral
Ipecac	ipecac syrup	Oral
Hormones		
Premarin	conjugated estrogens	Oral/parenteral
Laxatives		
Dulcolax	bisacodyl	Oral/rectal
Metamucil	psyllium	Oral
Milk of Magnesia	magnesium hydroxide	Oral
Neoloid	castor oil	Oral

TABLE 18–3. **Commonly Used Drugs by Classification** *Continued*

Classification/ Brand Name	Generic Name	Route(s)
Sedatives		
Amytal	amobarbital	Oral
Chloral Hydrate	chloral hydrate	Oral
Dalmane	flurazepam	Oral
Luminal	phenobarbital	Oral
Nembutal	pentobarbital	Oral
Placidyl	ethchlorvynol	Oral
Seconal	secobarbital	Oral/parenteral
Stimulants		
Dexedrine	dextroamphetamine	Oral
Dobutrex	dobutamine HCl	Parenteral
Dopram	doxapram HCl	Parenteral
Intropin	dopamine HCl	Parenteral
Ritalin	methylphenidate	Oral
Tenuate	diethylpropion	Oral
Vasoconstrictors		
Aramine	metaraminol	Parenteral
Levophed	norepinephrine	Parenteral
Vasodilators		
Cerespan	papaverine HCl	Oral/parenteral
Isoptin	verapamil	Oral/parenteral
Nitrogard	nitroglycerin	Oral/parenteral
Nitropress	nitroprusside	Parenteral
Sorbitrate	isosorbide dinitrate	Oral

to be treated. *Bretylol* (bretylium) is used for ventricular arrhythmias.

Antibiotics

Antibiotics or antimicrobials are drugs used to destroy or inhibit the growth of microorganisms. If the antibiotic is effective against a large number of microorganisms, it is termed a *broad-spectrum antibiotic*; if it is effective against only a few, it is termed a *narrow-spectrum antibiotic*. *Terramycin* (oxytetracycline) is a broad-spectrum antibiotic, and *Erythrocin* (erythromycin) is a narrow-spectrum antibiotic used primarily for respiratory tract infections. Allergic reactions to antibiotics are common and may range from mild to severe or even fatal.

Anticholinergics

Anticholinergics, or antispasmodics, are drugs that reduce smooth muscle tone, motility of the gastrointestinal tract, and secretions from respiratory tract and secretory glands. Patients taking anticholinergics perspire less and often complain of dry mouth. *Atropine* and *scopolamine* are drugs that are naturally derived from the plant *Atropa belladonna*, whereas *Pro-Banthine* (propantheline bromide) is a synthetically produced anticholinergic. High doses of these drugs may produce serious side effects such as delirium, rapid heart beat, and coma.

Anticoagulants

Anticoagulants are drugs that inhibit clotting of the blood or increase the coagulation time. They are used primarily to prevent or treat **thromboembolic disorders.** *Heparin* is the most commonly used parenteral anticoagulant. It produces effects immediately and is extremely effective when administered intravenously. Heparin is not effective when administered orally because it is not absorbed from the gastrointestinal tract, and it should not be administered intramuscularly because it may cause a **hematoma.** *Coumadin* (warfarin) and *dicumarol* (bishydroxycoumarin) are both examples of oral anticoagulants. Patients undergoing interventional procedures in the radiology department are often receiving these drugs and should be monitored closely to prevent massive hemorrhage, which may occur with overdosage.

Anticonvulsants

Anticonvulsants are drugs used to prevent or control the occurrence of seizures. Although these drugs do not treat the cause of seizures, they do reduce or eliminate seizure activity. *Klonopin* (clonazepam) is an effective oral anticonvulsant used to control **petit mal** (mild) **seizures.** *Dilantin* (phenytoin), which is available in oral or parenteral form, is effective in the treatment of **grand mal** (severe) **seizures.**

Antidepressants

Antidepressants are drugs used in the treatment of depression. These drugs often require several weeks of administration to achieve their maximal **therapeutic** effect. When administered for an extended period, antidepressants may cause dependency. *Elavil* (amitriptyline hydrochloride) and *Tofranil* (imipramine hydrochloride) are considered the drugs of first choice in treating clinical depression. Drug interactions are common in patients receiving other drugs in combination with antidepressants.

Antiemetics

Antiemetics are drugs used to prevent and treat nausea and vomiting. In general, these agents are more effective in preventing nausea and vomiting than they are in treating the symptoms once they have developed. Thus, they are most effective when given before the onset of symptoms. *Compazine* (prochlorperazine) and *Dramamine* (dimenhydrinate) are two of the most commonly used antiemetic agents and are available in both oral and parenteral forms.

Antihistamines

Antihistamines are drugs used primarily to treat allergic disorders, both acute and chronic. They are also used to treat upper respiratory tract infections and the common cold, both of which are viral infections. Drowsiness is a common side effect, and it may be greatly increased when the drug is combined with other CNS depressants such as alcohol or narcotics. *Phenergan* (promethazine hydrochloride) is an antihis-

tamine often used in preoperative patients. *Benadryl* (diphenhydramine), which is generally administered intramuscularly, is commonly used for moderately severe allergic reactions.

Antihypertensives

Antihypertensives are drugs used to treat moderate or severe **hypertension,** or high blood pressure. Because high blood pressure may be caused by a number of factors, a variety of drugs are included in this category. These drugs are commonly used in combination with other drugs such as diuretics in the treatment of hypertension. *Tenormin* (atenolol) and *Lopressor* (metoprolol) are two of the most frequently used oral antihypertensives. *Hyperstat* (diazoxide) is an effective drug administered intravenously for treating hypertension.

Anti-inflammatory Agents

Anti-inflammatory agents are drugs used to treat inflammation. The specific drugs included in this category are nonsteroidal anti-inflammatory drugs often referred to by the acronym NSAID. *Motrin* (ibuprofen) and *Feldene* (piroxicam) are two examples of oral NSAIDs commonly used to treat inflammatory conditions. The therapeutic effects of NSAIDs may not be evident for 1 to 2 weeks after the initial administration.

Antipsychotics

Antipsychotic drugs, also called major tranquilizers, are used to treat psychiatric disorders such as **schizophrenia.** A well-known and commonly used antipsychotic is *Thorazine* (chlorpromazine). It is available in both oral and parenteral forms. There are a wide variety of adverse side effects associated with antipsychotic drugs, including sedation, which may occur initially, and physiologic dependency, which may occur with extended use.

Antiulcer Agents

Antiulcer agents are used to treat peptic ulcers, both gastric and duodenal, and other gastric disorders that cause the excessive or prolonged secretion of hydrochloric acid within the stomach. *Tagamet* (cimetidine) and *Zantac* (ranitidine hydrochloride) are both effective antiulcer drugs that work by reducing acid secretion. *Reglan* (metoclopramide), available in oral and parenteral forms, increases **peristalsis** and accelerates gastric emptying without increasing gastric secretions. *Carafate* (sucralfate) does little to neutralize gastric acid; instead, it covers or coats the ulcer and protects it from the action of the stomach acids.

Bronchodilators

Bronchodilators are drugs used in the treatment of asthma and chronic obstructive pulmonary disease. These drugs work to dilate the size of the bronchioles by relaxing spasm in the bronchial walls. *Adrenalin* (epinephrine) is the most commonly used fast-acting bronchodilator. It is generally administered intravenously, but in an emergency situation, it may be injected directly into the heart for its adrenergic effect.

Coagulants

Coagulants are drugs used to control hemorrhage or speed up **coagulation.** Most coagulants are commercial preparations of vitamin K, a fat-soluble vitamin needed for normal blood coagulation. *Mephyton* (phytonadione) is a coagulant available in both oral and parenteral forms.

Corticosteroids

Corticosteroids are drugs used to reduce the symptoms associated with chronic inflammatory disorders or for the short-term treatment of acute inflammatory conditions. *Decadron* (dexamethasone) and *Solu-Cortef* (hydrocortisone) are steroid drugs employed for systemic use, whereas *Depo-Medrol* (methylprednisolone) is generally injected locally at the inflammatory site such as a joint or bursa. Prolonged use of corticosteroids may cause a variety of adverse side effects.

Diuretics

Diuretics are drugs that increase the amount of urine excreted by the kidneys, thus removing sodium and water from the body. *Lasix* (furosemide) is a potent diuretic often used to treat the **edema** associated with congestive heart failure. Diuretics are often used in conjunction with antihypertensive drugs for the treatment of high blood pressure. Patients receiving diuretics should be monitored for excessive fluid loss, which could result in an electrolyte imbalance.

Emetics

Emetics are drugs used to produce emesis or vomiting. *Ipecac* is an emetic drug that is administered orally. It is used primarily to empty the stomach of a patient who has ingested a toxic amount of a drug or noncorrosive poison. It usually produces vomiting within 30 minutes. *Apomorphine* is a fast-acting emetic that is injected subcutaneously to produce vomiting within a few minutes.

Hormones

Hormones are drugs that act as stimulants to increase the functional activity of a particular organ or gland. Sex hormones stimulate the development and maintenance of sexual characteristics. *Premarin* (conjugated estrogens) is a female sex hormone used in a wide variety of therapeutic applications. Interestingly, female sex hormones are sometimes used in male patients to treat **neoplastic** disorders involving the male sex organs, and male sex hormones are sometimes used in female patients to treat neoplastic disorders involving the female reproductive organs.

Laxatives

Laxatives are drugs that act to promote the passage and elimination of feces from the large intestines. Laxatives are frequently used in radiology to prepare patients for both gastrointestinal procedures and urinary tract procedures. *Dulcolax* (bisacodyl) is a stimulant laxative that increases the motility of the gastrointestinal tract and tends to produce a loose, watery stool.

Sedatives

Sedatives, or hypnotics, are drugs used to depress the CNS. The effect produced may range from a mild sedation to a deep loss of consciousness. *Seconal* (secobarbital) and *Nembutal* (pentobarbital) are two examples of commonly used sedatives. Extended use of these drugs may lead to addiction. Chloral hydrate syrup is often used as an effective sedative for children undergoing difficult procedures.

Stimulants

Stimulants are drugs that increase activity. CNS stimulants increase the activity of the brain and spinal cord. *Dexedrine* (dextroamphetamine) is an example of a CNS stimulant used primarily in the treatment of obesity. *Dopram* (doxapram hydrochloride) is used primarily as a respiratory stimulant. *Dobutrex* (dobutamine hydrochloride) and *Intropin* (dopamine hydrochloride) stimulate the myocardium of the heart and are administered parenterally to treat conditions such as hypotension and shock.

Vasoconstrictors

Vasoconstrictors are drugs that cause blood vessels to constrict, thus increasing heart action and raising blood pressure. *Levophed* (norepinephrine) is a potent vasoconstrictor administered parenterally in the treatment of shock. This drug should only be injected intravenously since **infiltration** may cause tissue necrosis. *Aramine* (metaraminol) is the vasoconstrictor of choice for intramuscular or subcutaneous administration.

Vasodilators

Vasodilators are drugs that cause blood vessels to dilate. They are useful in the treatment of vascular disease, particularly **atherosclerosis.** *Nitrogard* (nitroglycerin) is an effective coronary vasodilator used primarily in the treatment of angina. *Nitropress* (nitroprusside) is a peripheral vasodilator effective when used in a hypertensive crisis or in treating heart failure.

RESPONSE FACTORS

Drugs are intended to exert a variety of effects in the human body, but a specific drug is usually classified according to its most prominent effect. In addition to the intended effects, each drug is also capable of producing unintended and undesirable effects. These adverse drug effects include side effects, toxic effects, allergic reactions, and idiosyncratic reactions. **Side effects** result from the drug acting on tissues other than those intended, which causes a response unrelated to the intended action.

For example, an antihistamine is intended to counteract an allergic condition, but one of the side effects commonly produced by the drug is drowsiness, which is caused by the drug's unintended effect on the CNS. Toxic effects are adverse drug effects related to the dose of drug administered. Most drugs are capable of producing toxic effects if the therapeutic dosage is greatly exceeded. Allergic reactions occur when the body's immunologic system is hypersensitive to the presence of the drug. Allergic reactions can occur only after repeated exposure to the specific drug or a chemically related compound. However, it is important for the radiologic technologist to remember that prior sensitization to the drug may have taken place without the knowledge of the patient. An allergic reaction may take one of two forms: immediate or delayed. Immediate reactions may range from a mild response such as hives to a severe life-threatening response such as **anaphylaxis**, which may include respiratory or circulatory collapse. Delayed reactions are usually less severe and may not become evident for hours or even days after the drug is administered. **Idiosyncratic reactions** are abnormal responses to a drug caused by individual genetic differences. Unlike an allergic reaction, an idiosyncratic reaction may occur the first time the drug is administered to an individual. Drugs are used to obtain a desired systemic effect, but there is considerable variation in the way any two individuals respond to a specific drug. A number of factors may affect the intended drug response: age, sex, body weight, body surface area, metabolic rate, genetic factors, route of administration, and tolerance. Because of the variability of response, the technologist should monitor each patient closely after the administration of any drug. Unexpected signs or symptoms should be reported to the physician and treated promptly.

Principles of Administration

In preparing to administer drugs, the radiologic technologist should always follow the golden rules of drug administration, or what are commonly referred to as the "five rights" of drug administration (Box 18–2).

The *right drug* must be given. To ensure that the right drug is administered, always check the label on the container three times: once when the container is removed from the shelf, again

BOX 18–2

Five Rights of Drug Administration	
Right drug	Right time
Right amount	Right route
Right patient	

when the drug is removed from the container, and a third time when the container is replaced. Remember that the names of different drugs may sound similar. *Check the name carefully.* Never use a drug that is unlabeled, and always check labels for the expiration date. It is good practice never to administer a drug someone else has prepared. If you are asked to prepare a drug for another health professional to administer, always show the container to the individual who will administer the drug before you give him or her the dose.

The *right amount* of the drug must be used. To ensure that the right amount of the drug is used, it must be measured carefully and accurately. When preparing to administer an injectable drug, it is important to select the right size and type of syringe and needle.

The *right patient* must be given the drug. To ensure that you are administering the drug to the right patient, check the patient's arm band for proper identification and ask the patient to state his or her name. If the patient is too young to speak or is unable to speak, ask a parent or someone else present to identify the patient. Last, address the patient by name before administering the drug.

It must be the *right time.* The right time for the administration of the drug usually is indicated by the physician or practitioner responsible for ordering the drug. As a general rule, the radiologic technologist does not determine the time but should administer the drug at the time specified.

The *right route* must be used. Make certain that the drug is administered by the correct route. The physician usually specifies the route by which the drug should be administered. The radiologic technologist must be familiar with the terminology associated with the most common routes.

ROUTES

Drugs may be administered in a variety of ways including oral, sublingual, topical, and par-

enteral. General principles associated with each route of administration are discussed.

Oral

The oral route is the most common method of drug administration. The drug is taken by mouth and swallowed; it is absorbed from the gastrointestinal tract. When receiving drugs by the oral route, the patient must be conscious and the head should be elevated to aid in swallowing.

Sublingual

Administration by the **sublingual** route means that the drug is placed under the tongue and allowed to dissolve. Drugs that are intended to be administered sublingually should not be swallowed. One drug commonly given by the sublingual route is nitroglycerin.

Topical

The **topical** route of drug administration involves the application of a drug directly onto the skin. The drug is diffused through the skin and absorbed into the bloodstream. Topical drugs can be applied as cremes or ointments. Recently, drugs for topical application became available in a unit-dose device called a **transdermal** patch. The patch is applied to the skin and provides a precise dose of drug released over a specified time.

Parenteral

The term parenteral means administered by injection or by a route other than the gastrointestinal tract. Strict aseptic technique and standard precautions should always be used when drugs are administered with a needle. If a drug is injected incorrectly, it may cause nerve or tissue damage, or it may introduce **microorganisms** into the patient's system. The three most common routes by which drugs are administered parenterally are **intramuscular, subcutaneous,** and **intravenous.**

SUPPLIES

Drugs are injected into the body with a glass or plastic syringe. Plastic syringes are disposed of after being used only once, but glass syringes

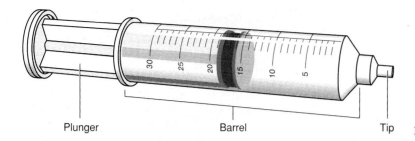

FIGURE 18–1. Parts of a syringe.

Plunger   Barrel   Tip

are resterilized for repeated use. The use of resterilizable glass syringes and needles violates current standard precautions. A syringe has three parts: the tip, where the needle attaches; the barrel, where the calibration scales are printed; and the plunger, which is the inside part that fits into the barrel. The parts of a syringe are shown in Figure 18–1. There are several different kinds of syringes, varying in size and shape. The tuberculin syringe and insulin syringe are designed for situations that require the precise measurement of a small volume of drug. The general purpose syringe comes in a variety of sizes including 2, 2.5, 3, 5, 10, 20, and 50 mL. Some syringes, called Luer-Lok, have a locking device on the tip that holds the needle firmly in place. An eccentric tip syringe is one that has the tip located to the side rather than in the center.

Needles used for injection are made of stainless steel and may or may not be disposable. The needle has three parts: the hub, which is the part that attaches to the syringe; the cannula or shaft, which is the length of the metal part; and the bevel, which is the slanted part at the tip of the needle. The parts of a needle are shown in Figure 18–2. Needles are sized according to length and gauge. The gauge refers to the thickness or diameter of the needle. The length refers to the measurement in inches of the shaft portion. The length may vary from ¼ to 5 inches, and the gauge may vary from 14 to 28. As a general rule, shorter needles are used for subcutaneous injections and longer needles are used for intramuscular injections. Needles in the 1- to 1½-inch length are most commonly used for intravenous injections. The smaller the

diameter of the shaft or the finer the needle, the larger the gauge number. For example, a 25-gauge needle has a very small diameter, and an 18-gauge needle has a large diameter. Subcutaneous injections often use a 25-gauge needle, and an intravenous injection generally uses a 20- or 21-gauge needle. A large-diameter needle such as an 18-gauge is often used to draw a drug or solution into the syringe but is seldom used to inject the drug into the patient. The package label indicates both the length and gauge of the needle. Two examples of prepackaged needles are shown in Figure 18–3. Thus, a package labeled "20 g/1½" indicates that the needle is 20 gauge and 1½ inches in length. The bevel of the needle may also vary from long to short. Figure 18–4 illustrates the difference between a long-bevel needle and a short-bevel needle. Long bevels are generally used for subcutaneous and intramuscular injections, and short bevels are used for intravenous injections.

An angiocath is a safer device to use when performing venipuncture (Fig. 18–5). An angiocath is used like any other needle to puncture the vein. It differs from other systems in that after venipuncture, the user pulls on a sheath, which extracts the needle up through a catheter and into the protective sheath where it cannot accidentally puncture anyone (Fig. 18–6).

Drugs intended for use by parenteral administration are packaged in two different kinds of containers: ampules and vials. An **ampule** is a sealed glass container designed to hold a single dose of a drug and intended for use only once. It is made of clear glass and has a shape with a scored constricted neck that is weakened so that it breaks more easily than other parts of the glass structure. If the neck is not scored, it must be filed with a small metal file before it is broken. To prepare the ampule, hold it upright and flick the top of the neck with your finger until all the drug is in the bottom part of the ampule (Fig. 18–7). Take a dry gauze pad, wrap it around the neck of the ampule and snap off

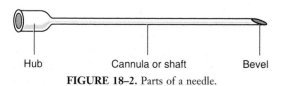

Hub   Cannula or shaft   Bevel

FIGURE 18–2. Parts of a needle.

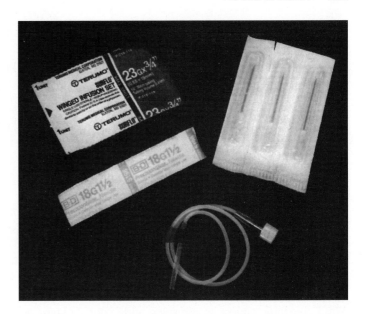

FIGURE 18–3. Prepacked needles and winged/butterfly infusion sets showing the gauge and length of needle.

the top (Fig. 18–7*B* and *C*). Care should be taken to avoid contaminating the needle by touching the outer broken edge of the ampule with the shaft of the needle when inserting it to draw out the contents. This is best accomplished by letting the tip of the needle rest on the inside of the ampule (Fig. 18–7*D*). The procedure is most easily performed when one person opens and holds the ampule while a second person withdraws the drug.

A **vial** is a small glass bottle with a sealed rubber cap. Vials come in different sizes and may contain multiple doses of a drug. To prepare the vial, remove the metal cap without breaking the outside metal seal, and wipe the exposed rubber stopper with an alcohol sponge. Open a syringe package and pull back the syringe plunger to pull air into the syringe equal to the amount of drug that will be withdrawn

from the vial. Open a needle package, and insert the needle on the end of the syringe without letting the end of the syringe or the end of the needle touch anything but each other. Hold the vial securely in the nondominant hand. Invert the vial and, with the dominant hand, insert the needle without letting the tip of the needle touch anything but the rubber stopper of the vial. With the tip of the needle in the fluid, inject the air equal to the volume of drug to be removed. If the needle is above the fluid level in the vial, air, instead of solution, will be drawn into the syringe. Pull back on the plunger until the correct amount of drug has been drawn into the syringe. Remove the needle and hold the syringe with the needle pointing up while you tap it with your finger to move any air bubble toward the hub, where it can be expelled by gently pushing on the plunger of the syringe. After use, the entire syringe and needle *must* be discarded into an acceptable "sharps" biohazard container. Figure 18–8 illustrates the entire procedure.

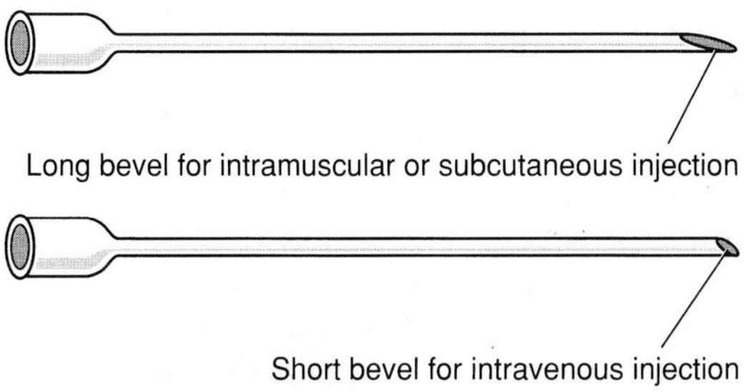

Methods of Administration

ORAL ADMINISTRATION

Oral administration is a safe and convenient method of drug administration if a few simple rules are followed (Box 18–3). Remember to always wash your hands thoroughly before pre-

Long bevel for intramuscular or subcutaneous injection

Short bevel for intravenous injection

FIGURE 18–4. Needle bevels. Long or regular bevels are usually used for intramuscular or subcutaneous injections. Short bevels are commonly used for intravenous injections.

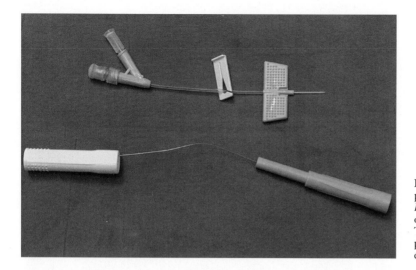

FIGURE 18–5. Angiocath veni-puncture set. *Top,* Set ready for use. *Bottom,* Set after use with catheter on left and needle sheath on right. The needle is pulled inside the protective sheath at the top so it cannot accidentally stick anyone.

paring or administering an oral medication. Avoid touching tablets or capsules with your hands. Transfer tablets, capsules, or liquid from the container directly into a medication cup or onto a clean paper towel. When pouring liquids, pour away from the label, and wipe the neck of the bottle with a clean damp cloth before replacing the cap. Always follow the golden rules of medication administration. At the completion of the procedure, chart the drug and all pertinent information with regard to the administration. In preparing a drug for the sublingual route of administration, follow the same rules as indicated for oral administration.

TOPICAL ADMINISTRATION

Drugs applied topically include tinctures, ointments, lotions, and sprays. To properly ad-minister a topical drug to the skin, follow the steps outlined in Box 18–4. Drugs administered by this route should not be applied with the bare hand. Following topical administration, monitor the skin area for any signs of local irritation.

PARENTERAL ADMINISTRATION

Drugs that are injected have a more rapid onset of action because they are absorbed directly into the bloodstream. All forms of parenteral administration require the use of a needle, syringe, and container. Because this method of administration involves the penetration of the protective layer of the skin, strict aseptic technique and standard precautions should be followed when preparing and administering the drug. Selecting the proper equipment and supplies for parenteral administration depends on the specific injection route, as well as the kind and amount of drug to be administered. Each

BOX 18–3

Rules for Oral Drug Administration

1. Wash hands thoroughly.
2. Place drug directly into medicine cup or on a clean paper towel. Do not touch the drug with your hands.
3. Read the label three times.
4. Check the patient's identification.
5. Explain the procedure to the patient.
6. Elevate the patient's head.
7. Provide water or liquid to aid in swallowing.
8. Chart all relevant information.

BOX 18–4

Rules for Topical Drug Administration

1. Wash hands thoroughly.
2. Put on disposable gloves.
3. Read the label three times.
4. Check the patient's identification.
5. Explain the procedure to the patient.
6. Apply the amount of drug prescribed.
7. Chart all relevant information.

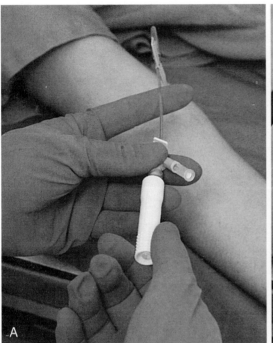

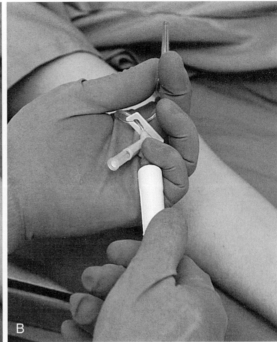

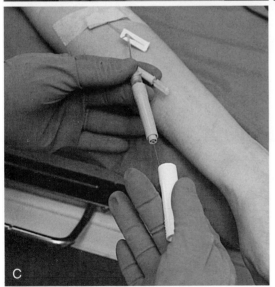

FIGURE 18–6. Using an angiocath venipuncture set. *A,* Perform normal venipuncture. *B,* After successful venipuncture, pull sheath away gently. This pulls the needle up the catheter and into the protective sheath. *C,* Continue pulling the sheath until it separates from the catheter, leaving the catheter in place inside the vein while the needle is safely encased in the protective sheath.

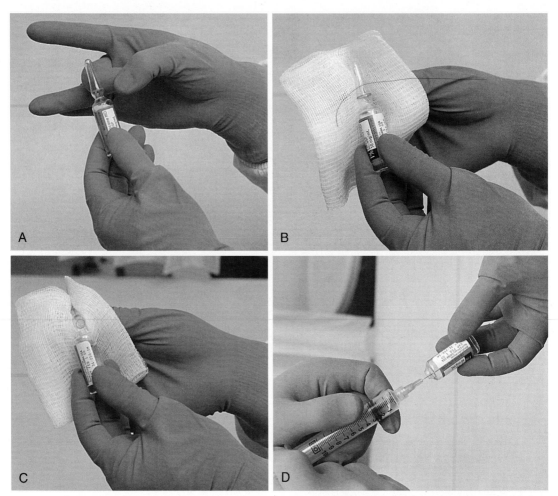

FIGURE 18–7. Withdrawing a drug from a glass ampule. *A,* Flick the top of the neck until all liquid is in the bottom of the container. *B* and *C,* With a gauze pad, snap off the top. *D,* Withdraw the contents, being careful not to let the shaft of the needle touch the broken edge of the ampule. One person opens and holds the ampule while a second person withdraws the drug.

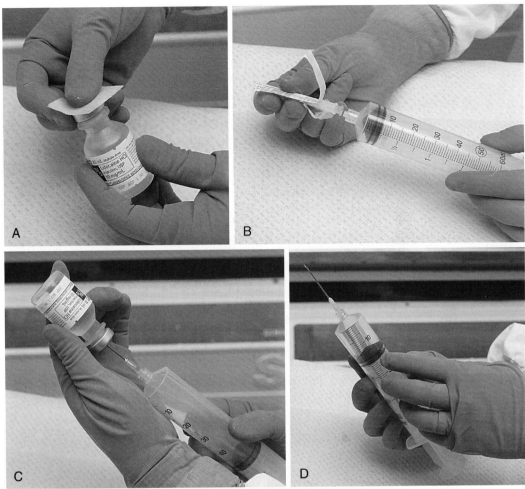

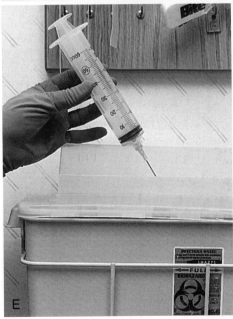

FIGURE 18–8. Withdrawing a drug from a vial. *A,* Break the seal, expose the rubber stopper, and wipe the stopper with an alcohol swab. *B,* Open a syringe package and pull back the syringe plunger to pull air into the syringe equal to the amount of drug that will be withdrawn from the vial. Open a needle package, and insert the needle on the end of the syringe without letting the end of the syringe or the end of the needle touch anything but each other. *C,* Invert the vial, and with the dominant hand, insert the needle without letting the tip of the needle touch anything but the rubber stopper of the vial. With the tip of the needle in the fluid, inject air equal to the volume of drug to be removed. Pull back on the plunger until the correct amount of drug has been drawn into the syringe. *D,* Remove the needle and hold the syringe with the needle pointing up while you tap it with your finger to move any air bubble toward the hub, where it can be expelled by gently pushing on the plunger of the syringe. *E,* After use, dispose of the entire syringe and needle into an acceptable "sharps" biohazard container.

parenteral route of injection will be discussed separately.

It is recommended that radiographic contrast media be stored in a warming unit to bring the drug to body temperature prior to injection (Fig. 18–9).

Subcutaneous Injection

When administering a subcutaneous injection, the drug is placed under the skin into the subcutaneous tissue that lies under the epidermal layers. The thickness of the subcutaneous tissue depends on the obesity of the patient. The most commonly used subcutaneous sites include the anterior thigh, upper back, outer surface of upper arm, and lower abdomen. The needle length and angle of insertion depend on the thickness of the subcutaneous tissue. Figure 18–10 illustrates the proper placement of the needle for a subcutaneous injection. For average-sized patients, a 25-gauge, ⅝-inch needle at a 45-degree angle of insertion is generally used. For above-average-sized patients, a 25-gauge, ½-inch needle at a 90-degree angle of insertion is generally used. Box 18–5 lists the steps involved in subcutaneous injection.

Intramuscular Injection

For an intramuscular injection, the drug is placed into muscle tissue that lies under the subcutaneous tissue layer. The most commonly used intramuscular injection sites include the deltoid muscle in the upper arm, the vastus lateralis muscle in the lateral thigh, and the gluteus maximus muscles in the buttocks. In general, use a needle length of 1 to 3 inches and 19 to 25 gauge, depending on the viscosity of the drug to be injected. Figure 18–11 demonstrates the proper placement of the needle for an intramuscular injection. A 90-degree angle of insertion is used for intramuscular injections. Box 18–6 lists the steps involved in intramuscular injection.

Intravenous Injection

When administering an intravenous injection, the drug is placed directly into a vein. The most commonly used intravenous injection sites include the cephalic vein on the lateral side and the basilic vein on the medial side of the anterior surface of the forearm and elbow, or the cephalic and basilic veins on the posterior sur-

BOX 18–5

Steps Involved in Subcutaneous Drug Injection

1. Wash hands thoroughly.
2. Put on disposable gloves.
3. Check the patient's identification.
4. Explain the procedure to the patient.
5. Prepare the site by cleansing it with an alcohol swab, using a circular motion and moving from the center to the outside.
6. With your free hand, pinch the skin gently together and insert the needle quickly at the appropriate angle for the patient's size.
7. Release the skin and pull back on the syringe plunger to make certain the needle is not in a blood vessel.
8. Inject drug slowly, and quickly withdraw the needle at the same angle used for insertion.
9. Massage the site with an alcohol swab while applying gentle pressure. If heparin is injected, do not massage the site.
10. Dispose of the syringe and needle properly.
11. Chart all relevant information.

face of the hand. Figure 18–12 shows the sites commonly used for **venipuncture.** The needle length and gauge depend on the viscosity of the drug, the site selected, and the specific method of injection.

One of the most commonly used intravenous needles is the winged tip or butterfly needle, which comes in lengths of ½ to 1¼ inch and 18 to 25 gauge. It has tubing 3 to 12 inches in length that extends from the needle to the hub. A butterfly needle is shown in Figure 18–3. Box 18–7 identifies the steps involved in venipuncture and intravenous injection. While injecting a drug into the vein, always observe the site closely for any signs of **extravasation** or infiltration. Should this occur, remove the needle, apply pressure to the injection site, and apply warm moist heat to relieve the discomfort. If the extravasation involves a corrosive drug, immediate attention is needed to prevent tissue necrosis. When a corrosive drug infiltrates the tissue, a cold compress rather than heat should be applied to the site.

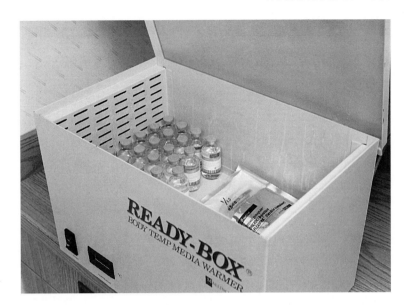

FIGURE 18–9. Contrast media warmer.

Drip Infusion

Drugs that are administered by the intravenous route may be injected using one of three methods. One involves a single administration in which the drug is injected slowly. A second method involves the administration of a drug by intravenous bolus or intravenous push. The term **bolus** refers to the amount of fluid injected, and *intravenous push* refers to a rapid injection. This method is generally used in an emergency when immediate drug action is required. The third method of administration involves the intravenous infusion of a large volume of fluid. This method is sometimes called drip infusion and requires some additional

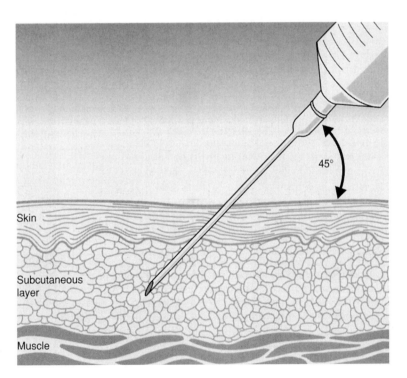

FIGURE 18–10. Proper needle placement for injection in the subcutaneous tissue. The needle is inserted at a 45-degree angle.

Skin

Subcutaneous layer

Muscle

45°

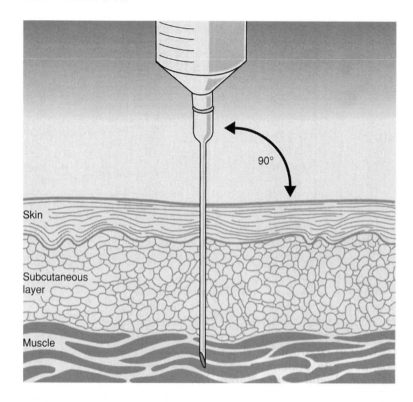

Skin

Subcutaneous
layer

Muscle

FIGURE 18–11. Proper needle placement for injection into the muscle tissue. The needle is inserted at a 90-degree angle.

equipment to ensure the accurate delivery of the intravenous solution.

An administration set for infusion of the solution and an intravenous pole are needed. Box 18–8 outlines the steps involved in preparing for drip infusion. The proper procedure for setting up drip infusion solutions is demonstrated in Figure 18–13.

When a standard administration set is used, the flow rate or drip rate is controlled by adjusting the clamp below the drip chamber. Unless otherwise instructed by a physician, 10 to 20 drops per minute is an acceptable flow rate. Patients receiving intravenous infusion should be monitored closely. If the flow stops, check the site of injection for signs of infiltration. If evidence such as swelling and pain around the injection site exists, stop the infusion immediately, remove the needle, and apply a warm cloth to the area.

Patients receiving medication by the intravenous infusion method may come to the radiology department with additional equipment attached to the administration set. An intravenous pump and controller are devices used to electronically regulate the flow rate (Fig. 18–14). A controller regulates the flow rate by counting the drops and compressing the intravenous tubing to adjust the flow. A pump propels the solution through the tubing at the desired rate under pressure. The pump is more accurate than the controller. Both devices have alarms that sound a beep or flash a light when the infusion fails to flow at the prescribed flow rate.

Charting Drug Information

Anytime a drug is administered to a patient, relevant information must be recorded on the patient's chart to document the event. The necessary information includes the name and dosage of the drug, the route of administration, the date, and the time. If the drug is administered parenterally, the site of injection should be included.

LEGAL CONSIDERATIONS

Increasingly, radiologic technologists are expected to chart a drug that they administered or helped to administer. It is important to follow the proper precautions and make certain that all information is documented on the patient's chart. If an error occurs in the adminis-

BOX 18–6

Steps Involved in Intramuscular Drug Injection

1. Wash hands thoroughly.
2. Put on disposable gloves.
3. Check the patient's identification.
4. Explain the procedure to the patient.
5. Prepare the site by cleansing the skin with an alcohol swab, using a circular motion and moving from the center to the outside.
6. With your free hand, retract the skin about 1 inch to either side of the site and hold it firmly.
7. Dart the needle in a 90-degree angle of insertion.
8. Continue to hold the skin while you gently pull back on the plunger to make certain it is not in a blood vessel.
9. If blood does appear in the syringe, remove the needle and prepare another site for injection. If no blood appears in the syringe, slowly inject the drug.
10. Withdraw the needle while releasing the tension on the skin.
11. Apply gentle pressure to the site with an alcohol swab.
12. Unless contraindicated, massage the injection site.
13. Dispose of the syringe and needle properly.
14. Chart all relevant information.

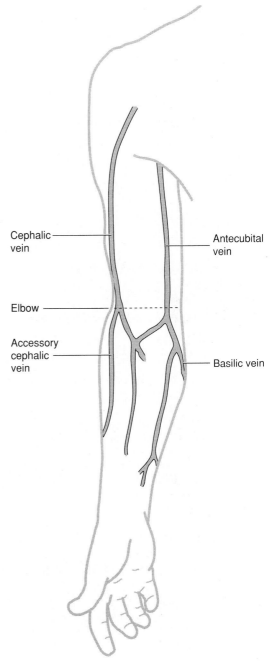

FIGURE 18–12. Sites commonly used for venipuncture.

tration of a drug, or if the patient experiences any adverse side effects to the drug, make certain to document the details of the incident thoroughly. Both students and radiologic technologists must follow these simple rules. Errors associated with drug administration are among the most common legal problems in which radiologic technologists are involved.

COMMON ABBREVIATIONS

Abbreviations are often used by health care professionals who order, dispense, or administer drugs. It is important to become thoroughly familiar with the common abbreviations that are used to ensure the safe and accurate administration of drugs. The list of abbreviations found in Table 18–4 include those most frequently encountered when administering drugs.

Summary

Pharmacology is the scientific study of drugs, including the origin, nature, effects, and uses of

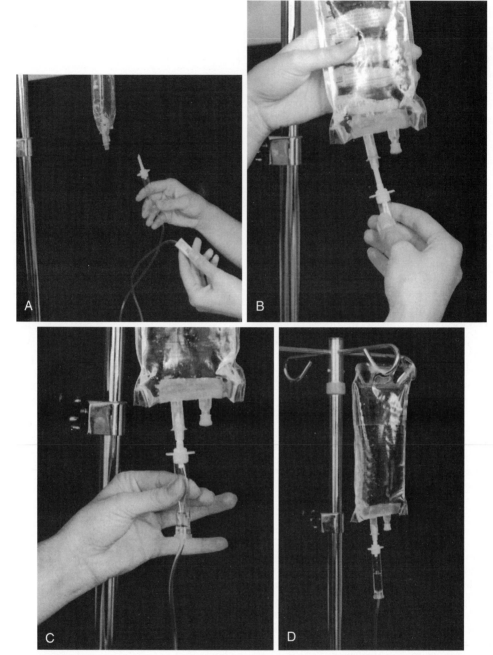

FIGURE 18–13. Drip infusion set-up. *A,* Remove the administration set from the box, straighten the tubing while checking for any cracks or holes, and slide the clamp up to the drip chamber and close it. *B,* Place the bag on a hard surface, remove the protective cap from the tubing insertion port on the bag, and wipe it with an alcohol sponge. Remove the protective cap from the spike on the drip chamber of the tubing and insert the spike into the port. *C,* Check again to make certain the clamp is closed, hang the bag on the IV pole, and squeeze the drip chamber until it is half full. *D,* Prime the IV set-up by removing the protective cap from the end of the tubing and holding it over a sink or wastebasket. Taking care to preserve the sterility of the cap and end of the tubing, release the clamp and allow the solution to run freely until all air bubbles are cleared from the tubing. Reclamp the tubing to stop the flow and replace the protective cap over the end of the tubing.

BOX 18–7

Steps Involved in Venipuncture and Intravenous Drug Injection

1. Wash hands thoroughly.
2. Check the patient's identification.
3. Explain the procedure to the patient.
4. Assemble all needed supplies and prepare the drug for administration.
5. Put on disposable gloves.
6. Once an appropriate site for venipuncture has been selected, clean it with an alcohol swab, using a circular motion while moving from the center to the outside.
7. Apply a tourniquet above the site, using sufficient tension to impede the flow of blood in the vein. Ask the patient to open and close the fist to distend the vein fully. When the vein has been identified, ask the patient to hold the fist in a clenched position.
8. To stabilize the vein, place your thumb on the tissue just below the site and gently pull the skin and vein toward the patient's hand.
9. Hold the needle with the bevel facing upward. When using a butterfly needle, pinch the wings together tightly.
10. Insert the needle next to the vein at a 15-degree angle and gently advance it into the vein. Blood flows back into the tubing when the needle is correctly positioned.
11. If the tubing of the butterfly needle has not previously been filled with solution, allow the blood to flow from the hub before attaching the syringe to ensure that no air bubbles are contained in the system.
12. Remove the tourniquet and inject the drug.
13. Unless otherwise instructed, remove the needle and apply gentle pressure to the site with an alcohol swab.
14. Dispose of the syringe and needle properly.
15. Chart all relevant information.

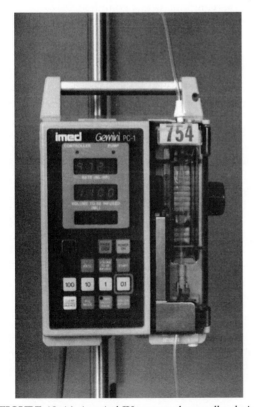

FIGURE 18–14. A typical IV pump and controller device.

TABLE 18–4. Common Abbreviations	
Abbreviation	**Meaning**
ac	Before meals
bid	Twice a day
c̄	With
cc	Cubic centimeter
et	And
g	Gram
gt(t)	Drop(s)
h	Hour
hs	At bedtime
hypo	Hypodermic(ally)
IM	Intramuscular(ly)
IV	Intravenous(ly)
mg	Milligram
mL	Milliliter
mm	Millimeter
OD	In the right eye
OS	In the left eye
pc	After meals
PO	By mouth
prn	As needed
qh	Every hour
q2h	Every 2 hours
q3h	Every 3 hours
qid	Four times a day
s	Without
SC	Subcutaneous
stat	Immediately
tid	Three times a day

BOX 18–8

Steps Involved in Intravenous or Drip Infusion Drug Administration

1. Wash hands thoroughly.
2. Check patient's identification.
3. Explain the procedure to the patient.
4. Assemble all needed supplies.
5. Remove the administration set from the box, and straighten the tubing while checking for any cracks or holes.
6. Slide the clamp up to the drip chamber and close it.
7. If the intravenous (IV) solution to be infused is contained in a bottle, place the bottle on a hard surface and remove the metal cap and rubber diaphragm that covers the rubber stopper. Wipe the rubber stopper with an alcohol sponge. Remove the protective cap from the spike on the drip chamber and firmly insert the spike into the center of the bottle's rubber stopper. Check to make certain the clamp is closed and invert the bottle. Hang the bottle on the IV pole, and squeeze the drip chamber until it is half full.
8. If the IV solution to be infused is contained in a plastic bag rather than a bottle, place the bag on a hard surface, re-move the protective cap from the tubing insertion port on the bag, and wipe it with an alcohol sponge. Remove the protective cap from the spike on the drip chamber of the tubing, and insert the spike into the port. Check again to make certain the clamp is closed, hang the bag on the IV pole, and squeeze the drip chamber until it is half full.
9. Prime all tubing before using the IV set-up by removing the protective cap from the end of the tubing and holding it over a sink or wastebasket. Take care to pre-serve the sterility of the cap and end of the tubing.
10. Release the clamp, and allow the solution to run freely until all air bubbles are cleared from the tubing.
11. Reclamp the tubing to stop the flow and replace the protective cap over the end of the tubing.
12. Loop the tubing over the IV pole until the injection site has been selected and the venipuncture is complete.

---

drugs. The radiologic technologist is expected to have a basic knowledge of pharmacology to prepare and administer drugs under the supervision of a licensed practitioner.

Drugs are classified in a variety of ways. A drug may be classified by name, action, or method of purchase. When drugs are classified by name, a single drug has a chemical name that represents its actual chemical structure; a generic name, which is a simplified version that reflects the chemical structure but is easier to pronounce; and the brand name, which is unique to the company that manufactures the drug. The *Physicians' Desk Reference* is an excellent reference, usually found in the radiology department, that contains up-to-date information on drugs, which are listed by both generic and trade names. Drugs may also be classified according to action, with drugs that have similar chemical actions grouped together. When drugs are classified according to the method of pur-chase, they are divided into two groups: prescription drugs and nonprescription drugs.

The dosage form indicates the type of prepa-ration for drug administration. Some common dosage forms include tablets, capsules, supposi-tories, solutions, suspensions, and transdermal patches.

The radiologic technologist should be famil-iar with the actions and precautions associated with commonly used drugs. A listing of com-monly used drugs arranged alphabetically by trade name and a list of drugs most often found on an emergency cart are provided in this chap-ter for easy reference. There is an additional list arranged alphabetically by generic name.

The golden rules of drug administration should always be followed when preparing to administer or when assisting with drug adminis-tration. Simply stated, the rules remind us to check for the right drug, right amount, right patient, right time, and right route. Drugs can be administered by the following routes: oral, sublingual, topical, and parenteral. When a drug is administered parenterally, it may be injected under the skin (subcutaneously), into the muscle (intramuscularly), or into the vein (intravenously). In all three methods of injection, strict aseptic technique should be followed when preparing and administering the drug.

Syringes and needles come in a variety of shapes and sizes. It is important to select the proper needle and syringe when preparing drugs. Angiocaths are recommended to avoid accidents. Drugs that are to be injected come in two different kinds of containers. One is an ampule, which usually holds a single dose, and the other is a vial, which is a small bottle holding multiple doses.

A number of factors affect the patient's response to a drug, which may be undesirable. Adverse effects include side effects, toxic effects, allergic reactions, and idiosyncratic reactions. Following drug administration by any route, the patient should be monitored closely for any signs of adverse effects.

Guidelines for oral, topical, and parenteral administration are included in this chapter. Detailed instructions are provided for subcutaneous injections, intramuscular injections, and intravenous injections. Following administration, relevant information should be recorded on the patient's chart.

◀R REVIEW QUESTIONS

1 Who is the person licensed to prepare and dispense drugs?
a) nurse
b) radiologist
c) physician
d) pharmacist

2 The name given to a drug manufactured by a specific company is the:
a) trade name
b) chemical name
c) generic name
d) nonproprietary name

3 A drug that relieves pain without causing a loss of consciousness is:
a) a sedative
b) an analgesic
c) an anesthetic
d) a hypnotic

4 A patient with an abnormal rhythm of the heart would most likely be receiving which of the following?
a) corticosteroids
b) anticholinergic agents
c) NSAIDs
d) antiarrhythmics

5 What class of drug is Benadryl?
a) diuretic
b) antibiotic
c) anticholinergic
d) antihistamine

6 In case of emergency, a patient with chronic obstructive pulmonary disease would most likely receive which of the following?
a) Adrenalin
b) Zantac
c) Dilantin
d) Elavil

7 Drugs placed under the tongue are said to be administered:
a) subcutaneously
b) sublingually
c) topically
d) parenterally

8 Which of the following statements expresses the correct relation between lumen diameter and gauge number?
a) As the diameter increases, the gauge number increases.
b) As the diameter decreases, the gauge number decreases.
c) As the diameter decreases, the gauge number increases.
d) As the diameter increases, the gauge number stays the same.

9 Long bevel needles are generally used for:
   1. subcutaneous injection
   2. intramuscular injection
   3. intravenous injection
a) 1 only
b) 3 only
c) 1 and 2 only
d) 1, 2, and 3

10 A severe life-threatening response to a drug is called:
a) idiosyncratic
b) anaphylaxis
c) palliative
d) pharmacognosy

BIBLIOGRAPHY

Asperheim MK: Pharmacology: An Introductory Text. 6th ed. Philadelphia, WB Saunders, 1987.

Carey KW, Goldberg KE: Medications and I.V.s: Clinical Pocket Manual. Springhouse, PA, Springhouse, 1987.

Dorland's Illustrated Medical Dictionary. 27th ed. Philadelphia, WB Saunders, 1988.

McKenry LM, Salerno E: Mosby's Pharmacology in Nursing. 17th ed. St. Louis, CV Mosby, 1989.

Miller BF, Keane CB: Encyclopedia and Dictionary of Medicine, Nursing, and Allied Health. 4th ed. Philadelphia, WB Saunders, 1987.

Pagliaro AM, Pagliaro LA: Pharmacologic Aspects of Nursing. St. Louis, CV Mosby, 1986.

Physicians' Desk Reference. Oradell, NJ, Medical Economics, 1997.

Reiss BS, Evans ME: Pharmacological Aspects of Nursing Care. 3rd ed. Albany, Delmar Publishing, 1990.

Shlafer M, Marieb EN: The Nurse, Pharmacology, and Drug Therapy. Redwood City, CA, Addison-Wesley, 1989.

Spencer RT, Nichols LW, Lipkin GB, Waterhouse HP, West FM, Bankert EG: Clinical Pharmacology and Nursing Management. 2nd ed. Philadelphia, JB Lippincott, 1986.

CHAPTER 19

CONTRAST MEDIA

Judith Baron, MS, RT(R)

The knowledge of our tools, their possibilities and limitations is essential in our work.

OVE MATTSSON

OBJECTIVES

On completion of this chapter, the student will be able to:

1 Discuss the factors of subject contrast.
2 Compare negative and positive contrast agents.
3 Match general types of contrast media to specific procedures performed.
4 State serious complications of the administration of barium sulfate.
5 Match specific procedures to particular patient instructions.
6 Locate various parts of iodinated contrast media molecules and state their functions if applicable.
7 Match the term *osmosis* to various effects of iodinated ionic contrast media.
8 Discuss the advantages of nonionic iodinated contrast media.

9 Differentiate between the major adverse effects of various contrast agents.
10 Match clinical symptoms of adverse reactions to iodinated contrast media to the level of treatment required.
11 Relate the patient history to the possibility of adverse reactions.

GLOSSARY

Acid Group: contains carbon double bonded to an oxygen, single bonded to another oxygen and has a negative charge at the pH of the body:

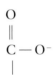

Amine Group: contains nitrogen bonded to two hydrogens:

$$H-N-H$$

Anaphylactoid: resembling an immune system response to foreign material (antigen)

Atomic Number: number of protons in the nuclei of the different elements

Bond: interactions between electrons of atoms that hold the atoms together in a stable group; a line drawn between atoms indicates a bond: H-O-H

Bronchospasm: involuntary constriction of the bronchial tubes usually resulting from an immune system reaction to a foreign particle or molecule

Contraindications: factors of a patient's history or present status that indicate that a medical procedure should not be performed or that a medication should not be given

Compound: substance composed of two or more elements combined in definite ratios that give the substance specific properties

Creatinine: nitrogen-containing waste products of metabolism excreted by the kidney's filtration system; high blood plasma levels indicate poor filtration by the kidney

Dimer: compound formed by bonding of two identical simpler molecules

Ester: group of organic compounds formed when alcohols and acids are combined chemically

Ethyl Group: two carbon atoms linked to each other and to hydrogen atoms

Extravasation: leakage from a vessel into the tissue

Fatty Acid: long chains of carbon atoms linked to each other and to hydrogen atoms; at one end of the chain is an acid group that contains two oxygen atoms and a hydrogen atom arranged in a particular way

Flocculation: formation of flaky masses resulting from precipitation or coming out of a suspension or solution

Histamine: molecular substance containing an amine group; it causes bronchial constriction and a decrease in blood pressure

Hydroxyl: common chemical group, part of the water molecule, containing one atom of hydrogen and one atom of oxygen; when not a part of a molecule, it carries a negative charge (anion)

Ion: atom or molecule having a negative charge (anion) or positive charge (cation)

Methyl: common biochemical group containing one carbon atom and three hydrogen atoms

Molecule: stable group of bonded atoms having specific chemical properties

Monomer: simple molecule of a compound of relatively low molecular weight

Osmolality: measurement of the number of particles (molecules or ions or cations) that can crowd out water molecules in a measured mass (kilogram) of water

Osmosis: movement of water from an area of high concentration to an area of lower concentration through a semipermeable membrane such as blood vessel walls and cell membranes

pH: relative acidity or basicity (alkalinity) of a solution; a pH below 7.0 is acidic and has more hydrogen cations than hydroxyl anions, whereas a pH above 7.0 is alkaline and has more hydroxyl anions than hydrogen cations

Shock: inadequate blood flow within the body with resulting loss of oxygen and, therefore, energy

Solution: uniform mixture of two or more substances composed of molecule-sized particles that do not react together chemically

Suspension: nonuniform mixture of two or more substances, one of which is composed of larger-than-molecule-sized particles that have a tendency to cluster together

Introduction to Contrast Media

PURPOSE OF CONTRAST MEDIA

Generally, the physical ability to see images is based on three factors:

- Magnification of an image until it is visible
- Resolution of the detail of an image to visualize the separate structures that make up the image
- Contrast of an image to distinguish different shades of density within it

Radiologic technologists have the conceptual knowledge and technical skills to enhance these factors so that diagnostic images are produced. Many methods are available to manipulate contrast, but the most difficult problem of contrast enhancement lies within the body. There is little contrast within the body aside from the bones. This lack of *subject contrast* is the reason for the use of different kilovoltage x-rays for different body parts. One reason computed tomography and magnetic resonance imaging have become so important is that these modalities greatly enhance subject contrast.

The body absorbs x-rays according to the various **atomic numbers** and densities (the amount of matter per volume of tissue). Higher atomic number elements absorb x-rays at a greater rate than low atomic number elements. For example, x-rays are absorbed by bone because calcium has a high atomic number; they are transmitted or scattered more easily through water, air, fat, and soft tissue.

If the muscle in the lower leg of a 20-year-old football player is compared with that of an 80-year-old man, it becomes apparent that there is less muscle fiber per volume in the 80-year-old man. This concept of density plays a role in subject contrast because the more tightly packed the tissue is within a given volume, the more it absorbs x-rays. The more x-rays are absorbed in the body, the less they reach the radiograph and the more light areas are seen. Without contrast, no image would be seen.

Contrast media are diagnostic agents that are introduced into body orifices or injected into the vascular system, joints, and ducts to enhance subject contrast in anatomic areas where there is insufficient natural contrast. The ability of the contrast media used in radiographic procedures to enhance subject contrast depends greatly on the atomic number of the element used in the particular medium and the concentration of atoms of the element per volume of the medium.

GENERAL TYPES OF CONTRAST AGENTS

Radiolucent (Negative)

X-rays are easily transmitted or scattered through radiolucent contrast media. As the name implies, these media are relatively lucent to x-rays. The anatomic areas filled by these agents appear dark on radiographs, so they are also called *negative contrast agents.* These media are composed of elements with low atomic numbers.

Radiopaque (Positive)

X-rays are absorbed by radiopaque contrast media because these media are opaque to x-rays. The anatomic areas filled by these agents appear light on radiographs, so they are also called *positive contrast agents.* These media are composed of elements with high atomic numbers.

Sometimes negative and positive agents are used together so that the lumen of organs, such as the colon (Fig. 19–1), can be visualized or so that anatomic structures within a space, such as the menisci of the knee, can be visualized.

HISTORIC ASPECTS OF CONTRAST AGENTS

Air, a negative contrast medium, was used initially in 1918 by Walter Dandy. Dandy, a neurosurgeon, did injections of air to study the cerebral ventricles of children with hydrocephalus. Dandy's published articles initiated the use of air to localize tumors within the brain and spinal cord. Later, carbon dioxide, nitrous oxide, and oxygen came into use.

Immediately after Röntgen's discovery of x-rays, physiologists realized that the functions of the digestive system could be followed by giving

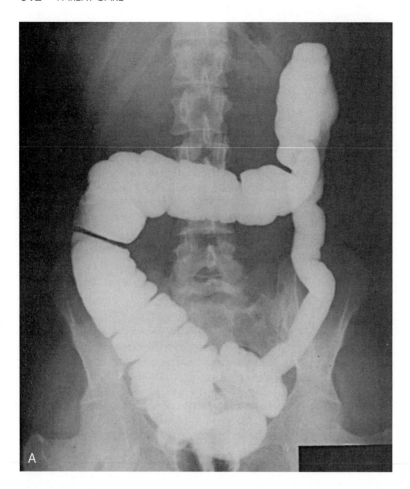

FIGURE 19–1. *A,* Radiopaque barium sulfate fills the colon in a lower gastrointestinal study.

animals food mixed with compounds of high atomic number and watching the mixture's passage by way of a fluorescent screen. In 1896, lead subacetate was used to study the digestive system of the guinea pig. Lead subacetate later proved to be toxic, however. In the same year, Walter Cannon, then a Harvard medical student, began a series of experiments to study the digestive system using bismuth subnitrate. His subjects included geese, cats, and a 7-year-old girl. Although bismuth subnitrate eventually proved to be toxic, Cannon is credited with awakening the medical profession to the realization that diseases of the gastrointestinal (GI) tract could be studied by watching the movement of radiopaque media through the tract.

Toxicity remained a problem with many of the high-atomic-number compounds in these early years. In fact, Thorotrast, which incorporated thorium, proved to be radioactive. By 1910, articles about the advantages of the inert and insoluble compound barium sulfate began to appear in the medical literature. Its use increased rapidly because of its lack of toxicity, its low cost, and its availability.

Water-soluble iodinated contrast media were introduced by Egas Moniz in 1927 when he injected sodium iodide into the cerebral vascular circulation by way of the carotid arteries. Sodium iodide proved to be a blood vessel irritant.

During the 1930s, chemical methods improved. Atoms with high atomic numbers such as iodine, could be placed on nontoxic water-soluble carrier **molecules.** Eventually, more iodine atoms per molecule were added, which increased visualization of the vascular and urinary systems. The 1950s saw the beginning of the use of three iodine atoms per carrier molecule. These tri-iodinated molecules are the basic chemical structures from which both ionic and nonionic water-soluble iodine contrast media originate.

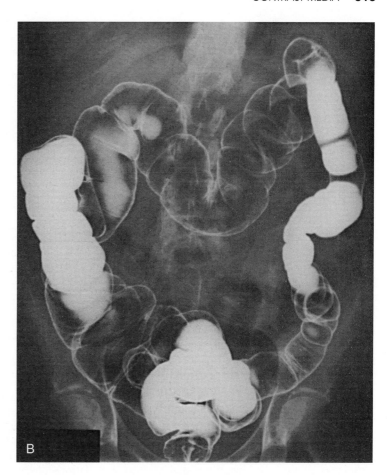

FIGURE 19–1 *Continued. B*, Barium sulfate and air are used together to visualize the lumen of the colon. (Courtesy of Margaret Weaver, RT(R).)

Negative Contrast Media

PHYSICAL PROPERTIES

Negative contrast media are composed of low-atomic-number elements and are administered as gas (air) or gas-producing tablets, crystals, or soda water (carbon dioxide). Because cells absorb oxygen quickly, this gas is rarely used as a contrast agent.

SPECIFIC PROCEDURES

Air alone provides negative contrast for laryngopharyngography. This is because upper respiratory structures contain air naturally. Otherwise, radiolucent contrast media are used in combination with radiopaque media to outline the lumens of, or spaces within, body structures. Table 19–1 lists common double contrast studies, contrast media used, patient preparations, patient care, and instructions.

ADVERSE REACTIONS

Generally, complications from administration of negative contrast agents are minimal, although air can cause emboli. These small air masses can enter the circulatory system and become lodged in blood vessels, causing pain and loss of oxygen to the area. Patients who receive barium sulfate with air should be instructed to drink plenty of fluids after the procedure to dilute and eliminate the barium sulfate. Administration of water-soluble iodine contrast media along with air in the joint spaces does not usually result in complications.

Barium Sulfate

PHYSICAL PROPERTIES

The element barium has an atomic number of 56; thus, it is radiopaque. Barium sulfate is an inert powder composed of crystals that is

TABLE 19–1. **Common Double Contrast Studies**

Area	Contrast Agent	Method of Administration	Patient Preparations	Patient Instructions/ Care During Procedure
Stomach	Barium sulfate Carbon dioxide as tablets, crystals, or soda water	Oral	Nothing to eat or drink after midnight before examination	Patient should not belch after carbon dioxide is given so that the lumen of the stomach can be seen
Large intestine	Barium sulfate Air	Rectal	Large amount of fluid before examination or fluid diet Nothing to eat or drink after midnight before examination Cleansing enema before examination	Supportive communication so that the patient does not lose control
Arthrography Shoulder Knee Wrist Hip	Water-soluble iodine media Air	Injection into joint space	None	Supportive communication, because stress views performed during procedure can be painful

used for examination of the digestive system. The chemical formula is $BaSO_4$, which indicates a ratio of one atom of barium to one atom of sulfur to four atoms of oxygen; thus, it is a **compound.** Barium sulfate is not soluble in water, so it must be mixed or shaken into a **suspension** in water. Depending on the environment of the barium sulfate, such as acid within the stomach, the powder has a tendency to clump and come out of suspension. This is called **flocculation.** Stabilizing agents such as sodium carbonate or sodium citrate are usually used to prevent flocculation. These ingredients are listed as suspending agents on the container labels. Other ingredients used in orally administered barium sulfate include vegetable gums, flavoring, and sweeteners to increase palatability. Barium sulfate suspensions must be concentrated enough so that x-rays are absorbed. These suspensions must flow easily yet coat the lining of organs.

Different concentrations of barium sulfate are used for different purposes. These concentrations are measured in weight percentage of barium sulfate. *Weight/weight ratio (W/W)* is the weight of barium sulfate divided by the weight of water to equal a total weight of 100 g of suspension. *Weight/volume ratio (W/V)* is the weight of barium sulfate divided by the total volume to equal the grams of barium sulfate in 100 mL of suspension. Barium sulfate preparations can be diluted to the required W/W or W/V percentages by using directions or graphs provided with these products (Fig. 19–2).

For studies of the small intestine, oral formulations of barium sulfate and methylcellulose, a nondigestible starch, have been introduced. These preparations are designed to give a "see-through" effect to better diagnose small lesions.

For lower GI studies, it is generally recommended that barium sulfate be mixed with *cold* tap water to reduce irritation to the colon and to aid the patient in holding the enema during the examination. The cold tap water reduces spasm and cramping.

A primary function of the colon is to absorb water from waste. However, increased water absorption by the colon can result in excess fluid entering the circulatory system (hypervolemia), a serious, sometimes fatal, complication. The addition of 2 teaspoons of table salt per liter of water used in the enema preparation reduces the risk of hypervolemia. It is critical to follow the manufacturer's directions when mixing barium sulfate suspensions so that diagnostic radiographs are obtained. Figure 19–3 shows various barium sulfate preparations, carbon dioxide crystals used for double contrast studies, and enema tips used for lower gastrointestinal studies.

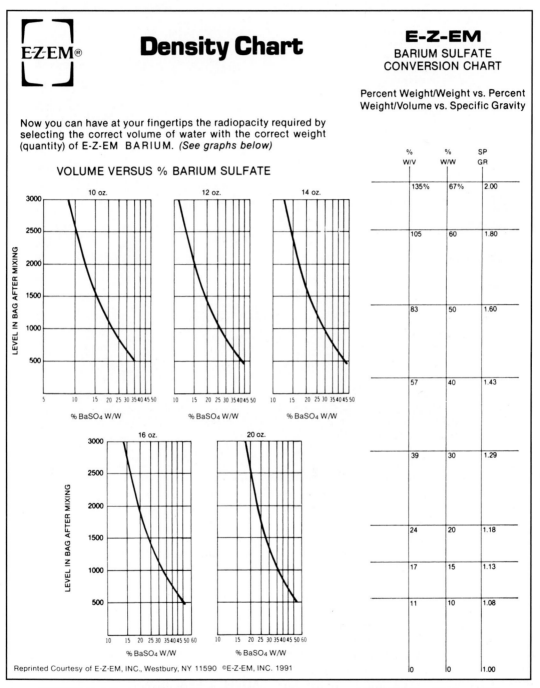

FIGURE 19–2. Barium sulfate density and conversion charts. (Courtesy of E-Z-EM, Inc., Westbury, NY.)

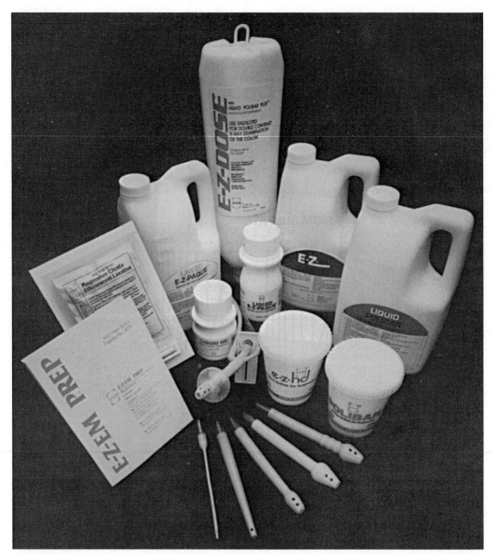

FIGURE 19–3. Various barium preparations and supplies. (Courtesy of E-Z-EM, Inc., Westbury, NY.)

SPECIFIC PROCEDURES

The administration of barium sulfate can result in complications, generally as a result of pre-existing patient disease or status. If a patient is suspected of having a perforation in the digestive tract, barium sulfate is contraindicated. This is because barium sulfate is not absorbed naturally by the body. If it enters the peritoneal or pelvic cavity, it can cause peritonitis and must be surgically removed. In place of barium sulfate, a water-soluble iodine contrast agent is recommended. The body is capable of absorbing these agents.

In certain patients, the administration of bar-ium sulfate can result in trauma such as perforation of the colon. The radiologic technologist must obtain a detailed patient history to give appropriate patient care. Table 19–2 outlines patient history factors that should be considered before administration of barium sulfate. Table 19–3 lists the specific procedures that use a barium sulfate suspension.

ADVERSE REACTIONS

As previously mentioned, patients should be instructed to drink plenty of fluids after receiving barium sulfate. All barium sulfate suspen-

TABLE 19-2. **Patient History Factors in Barium Sulfate Examinations**	
Factor	**Importance**
Age	Ability to communicate, hear, and follow directions
	Increased risk of colon perforation due to loss of tissue tone
Diverticulitis or ulcerative colitis	↑ difficulty in holding an enema
	↑ risk of colon perforation
Long-term steroid therapy	↑ risk of colon perforation
Colon biopsy within previous 2 weeks	Lower gastrointestinal series is contraindicated
Pregnancy	Inform radiologist before proceeding with examination
Mental retardation, confusion, or dizziness	↑ risk of aspiration during upper gastrointestinal series
Recent onset of constipation or diarrhea	↑ risk of colon perforation or tumor rupture
Nausea and vomiting	↑ risk of aspiration during upper gastrointestinal series

↑ = increased.

TABLE 19-3. **Common Procedures for Which Barium Sulfate Suspensions Are Used**				
Area	**Concentration (W/V%)**	**Method of Administration**	**Patient Preparation**	**Patient Instructions/Care During Procedure**
Esophagus: esophagram	30–50	Oral	None	Supportive communication For esophageal varices, the patient should exhale, swallow barium, and then hold his or her breath on that exhalation for that exposure.
Stomach: upper gastrointestinal series	30–50	Oral	Nothing to eat or drink after midnight before examination	Supportive communication Explanation of reasons for various positions
Small intestine: small bowel series	40–60 if included with stomach examination	Oral	If included with a stomach examination, a low-residue diet is eaten for 2 days before examination	Supportive communication Explanation for length of procedure *Note:* In most patients, the transit time of the barium sulfate suspension through the small intestine is about 1 hour.
Large intestine: colon or barium enema	12–25	Rectal	Large amount of fluid or fluid diet day before examination	Supportive communication so that the patient does not lose control
			Nothing to eat or drink after midnight before examination Cleansing enema before examination	Watch patient for changes in mental status that may indicate fluid overload
Stomach: computed tomography*	12–25	Oral	Nothing to eat or drink after midnight before the examination	Supportive communication: the patient should feel that the radiographer is constantly watching the procedure

*Generally used to accent contrast in the abdomen.

sions transit the colon. Because one function of the colon is to absorb water from waste, barium sulfate residue within the colon can dry and cause an obstruction. The major symptom of obstruction is constipation.

A complication related to the administration of barium sulfate during a lower GI examination is perforation of the colon with **extravasation** (leakage through a duct or vessel) into the abdominal cavity. Extravasation results in inflammation of the abdominal cavity, barium peritonitis. Elderly patients or those receiving long-term steroid medication are at increased risk for colon perforation because their tissues have become atrophic (lost elasticity and muscle tone). Also at risk are patients with diverticulitis and ulcerative colitis, because these diseases result in inflammation and degradation of the colon tissues. Patients with toxic megacolon should not have lower GI procedures because this serious complication of ulcerative colitis results in a dilated colon that can rupture. Recent biopsy of the colon is a contraindication to a lower GI series until the area heals. The barium retention catheter can be a source of colon perforation. The radiologic technologist should use one or two gentle squeezes to inflate the retention cuff.

Vaginal rupture, a rare complication of barium sulfate administration, is due to misplacement of the catheter before lower GI examinations. It is critical to know the anatomy of the female pelvis in the anteroposterior and lateral configurations. Female patients should be asked if they feel the enema tip in the rectum.

Water absorption from the colon is a serious complication of lower GI administration of barium sulfate suspensions. Water from the cleansing enema and the barium enema can be shifted from the colon into the circulatory system with a resulting increase in blood volume. Consequences of this fluid overload are pulmonary edema (fluid in the lungs), seizures, coma, and death. The table salt solution previously discussed reduces the possibility of hypervolemia. The radiologic technologist must observe patients for changes in mental status, such as apathy and drowsiness, that would indicate onset of hypervolemia. Symptoms of fluid overload are masked in sedated patients. Therefore, sedative premedication is contraindicated for lower GI examinations.

Sedated patients should not undergo upper GI examinations because the swallowing reflex is diminished. This greatly increases the risk of aspiration (inhalation) of the barium sulfate suspension with resultant barium pneumonia. Aspiration is also a risk for retarded patients and those with altered mental status because of age or disease.

A few allergic type reactions have been noted, but these may have been due to preservatives in the particular barium sulfate preparation or to latex used in barium enema retention catheters. Occasionally, barium sulfate has collected within the appendix. No directly related complications have resulted from this.

Oil-Based Iodine Contrast Media

PHYSICAL PROPERTIES

Oil-based iodine contrast media are made from **fatty acids** commonly found in plants and animals. A two–carbon atom chemical group called an **ethyl group** takes the place of the alcohol chemical group usually found in fatty acids. These chemical manipulations change the fatty acids into **esters.** Then, iodine atoms are added at certain areas of the ester molecules. The result is the description seen on the package inserts: iodinated ethyl esters of fatty acids.

Oil-based media are insoluble in water and do not flow easily because they are relatively viscous. When these esters are exposed to light, heat, or air, they decompose. Consequently, these media should be stored in a cool, dark area. Do not use any media that have darkened from their original pale yellow or pale amber color because the dark color indicates that they have decomposed. Plastic syringes should not be used for injection of oil-based iodine contrast media because toxic substances from the plastic can dissolve into the media. The main disadvantage of oil-based iodine contrast media is that they persist in the body because they are insoluble in water.

SPECIFIC PROCEDURES

Oil-based iodine contrast media are used for a select number of procedures, which are generally performed infrequently. These procedures include bronchography, dacryocystography, sialography, and lymphography and are outlined in Table 19–4. Before the introduction of non-

		Method of	Patient	Patient Instructions/
Area	**Contrast Agent**	**Administration**	**Preparation**	**Care During Procedure**
Lungs*: bronchography (usually imaged now by computed tomography or examined by bronchoscopy)	Iodine compounds suspended in oil such as propyliodine in peanut oil	Usually through catheter into the bronchus	Nothing to eat or drink after midnight before examination	Supportive communication: the patient should avoid coughing. Explain to the patient that he or she is tilted into various angles to spread the contrast throughout the bronchial tubes.
Tear ducts: dacryocystography	Iodinated ethyl esters; low viscosity such as Ethiodol	Usually through catheter into the duct	None	Supportive communication Advise patient that the contrast material will drain through the nose.
Salivary glands: sialography (suspected large masses are usually imaged by computed tomography)	Iodinated ethyl esters; low viscosity such as Ethiodol	Usually through catheter into the duct	None	Supportive communication After injection of contrast, the patient is given gum to chew to increase the flow of saliva; this should be explained to the patient.
Lymphatic system: lymphography	Iodinated ethyl esters; low viscosity such as Ethiodol	Through catheter into lymph vessel	None, although the patient should be advised that this procedure may take an hour or more to complete and that 24-hour follow-up films are done to image the lymph nodes.	Advise patient that he or she will have to remain relatively motionless on the x-ray table during the 30-minute contrast injection and for a time after the injection. A pad should be placed on the table for patient comfort. Constantly reassure the patient that the examination is going well. If patient complains of pain at or above injection site, inform the radiologist; injection pressure may be too high.

TABLE 19–4. **Some Procedures for Which Oil-Based Iodine Contrast Media Are Used**

*Some of these procedures have been superseded by other imaging methods.

ionic contrast media, myelography was a common procedure that used an oil-based medium.

As with all radiologic procedures, a complete patient history is important. In particular, the pre-existing patient history factors outlined in Table 19–5 may present complications during or after bronchography and lymphography.

ADVERSE REACTIONS

Any iodine-containing contrast agent may provoke an **anaphylactoid** (allergic-like) reaction, although this is rare with the use of oil-based media. The persistence of these media in the body generally does not pose problems unless pre-existing disease involves the areas examined.

Some adverse reactions are associated with specific examinations that use oil-based media. During bronchography, there is a temporary reduction in pulmonary function. Therefore, after the procedure, the patient should be encouraged to cough up the contrast media. Nausea, vomiting, and headache may also occur. During dacryocystography and sialography, very small ducts are dilated. Therefore, contrast media may be extravasated if an accidental tear occurs. In some patients, injection of iodine contrast into the parotid salivary gland causes

TABLE 19–5. **Patient History Factors in Bronchography and Lymphography**	
Factor	**Importance**
Age	Ability to communicate, hear, and follow instructions.
Lower back problems	Lymphography requires the patient to lie supine for a long period.
Chronic obstructive pulmonary disease	Procedures are contraindicated.
Radiation therapy to the lungs	Procedures are contraindicated.
Suspected spread of malignancy to the lymphatic system	Inform the radiologist before proceeding.
Surgery involving part of the lymphatic system (most common is breast cancer surgery)	Inform the radiologist before proceeding.

inflammation of the gland, iodine parotitis. During lymphography, extravasation may also occur. Itchy skin rashes, temporary lymphedema, and thrombophlebitis have been reported, although these reactions are infrequent.

Water-Soluble Iodine Contrast Media

PHYSICAL PROPERTIES

Ionic Iodine Contrast Media

The element iodine has an atomic number of 53, making it relatively radiopaque. Ionic media dissociate into two molecular particles in water or blood plasma just as table salt does. These media are **ionic** because one particle has a negative charge called an *anion*, and the other particle has a positive charge called a *cation*. The anion part of the molecule begins with a six-carbon bonded hexagon called *benzene*. A carbon atom is located at each corner of the hexagon but is not usually drawn because the molecular diagram would look cluttered. Every other carbon **bond** site of the benzene is bonded to an iodine atom, so each anion portion contains three iodine atoms: it is tri-iodinated. Of the three remaining carbon bond sites, one is occupied by an **acid group.** The acid group carries the negative charge at physiologic **pH.**

It is at the acid group

$$\begin{pmatrix} O \\ \parallel \\ C-O^- \\ \mid \end{pmatrix}$$

that the anion and cation dissociate on injection. The other two carbon bond sites are occupied by chemical structures that increase the solubility or the excretion rate of the contrast by the body. It is these two carbon bond sites that result in the different classes of ionic media: *diatrizoate*, *metrizoate*, and *iothalamate* (Fig. 19–4). The cation part of the molecule is either a sodium atom or a more complex structure, methylglucamine. Its rather long name describes its structure. The six carbons bonded to each other in a straight line and bonded to oxygens and hydrogens (**hydroxyl** groups) come from glucose, a common biologic sugar. The hydroxyl groups increase solubility. The nitrogen on the left is part of an **amine group.** (Amines are found in amino acids, and ammonia contains nitrogen.) Finally, a one-carbon, three-hydrogen group is attached to a nitrogen on the left. These one-carbon, three-hydrogen **methyl** groups are extremely common. Sometimes, methylglucamine is referred to as meglumine on package inserts.

Most ionic iodine contrast media are referred to as higher-osmolality contrast media because of their osmotic effects. **Osmolality** is a measure of the total number of particles in **solution** per kilogram of water. The osmolality of contrast media is of great biologic significance. Most adverse reactions to contrast media have been related to the osmolality of the media. This is because the osmolality of a solution determines osmotic pressure, which controls the movement of water in the body. Higher-osmolality contrast media have a larger number of particles in solution, such as blood plasma, which pull water toward them.

Nonionic Iodine Contrast Media

Efforts to decrease the many side effects of ionic iodine contrast media resulted in the development of molecules that do not dissociate into anions and cations (nonionics) or that are ionic but too big to have osmotic effects, such as ioxaglate (Hexabrix). These agents are referred to as lower-osmolality contrast media.

Ioxaglate is an ionic molecule composed of two connected benzene hexagons, one of which

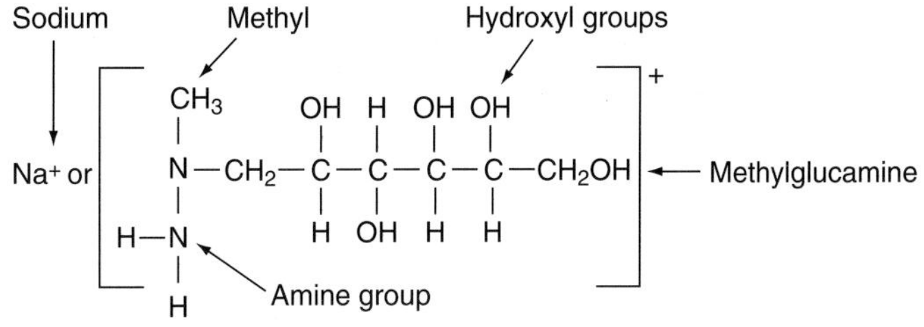

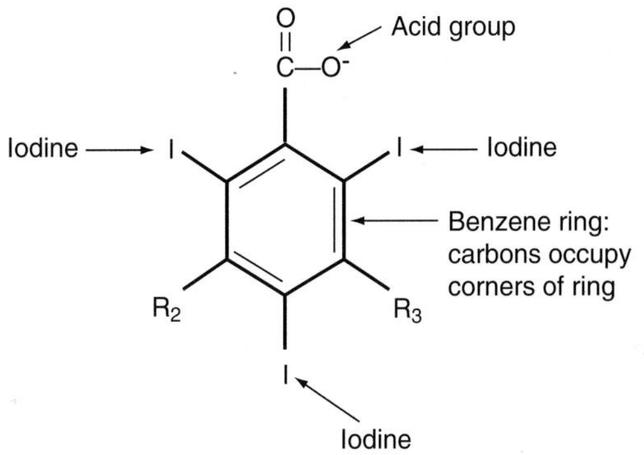

FIGURE 19–4. A typical ionic, water-soluble, tri-iodinated contrast molecule. The anion is the benzene ring with the negatively charged acid group attached. The groups R2 and R3 aid in solubility and excretion. The positively charged cations are sodium or methylglucamine. Some media contain both cations.

carries an acid group that dissociates on injection. This contrast agent is a **dimer** because it is composed of two identical simpler molecules. It carries six iodine atoms per molecule. It is ionic because it dissociates into two particles in blood plasma. Most ionic iodine contrast media are **monomers,** or simple molecules of relatively low molecular weight. Because dimers are large molecules, their osmotic effects are low. Because of their high molecular weights, they are viscous.

Recently a nonionic dimer, iodixanol (Visipaque), was introduced. Iodixanol is made to be isomolal (same number of particles) to blood plasma by the addition of electrolytes, small anions, and cations, which are normally present in blood plasma. Figure 19–5 is the molecular structure of the nonionic dimer iodixanol.

An additional advantage of the lower-osmolality contrast media is that they are more hydrophilic (water soluble) than the higher-osmolality contrast media. As a result, they may be less likely to be reactive with the cells that can trigger allergic effects. Figure 19–6 is the molecular structure of one of the water-soluble nonionic iodine contrast agents, ioversol (Optiray). It is a tri-iodinated benzene ring and does *not* carry an acid group. Many oxygen-hydrogen hydroxyl groups surround the benzene ring. These groups increase the solubility of the me-

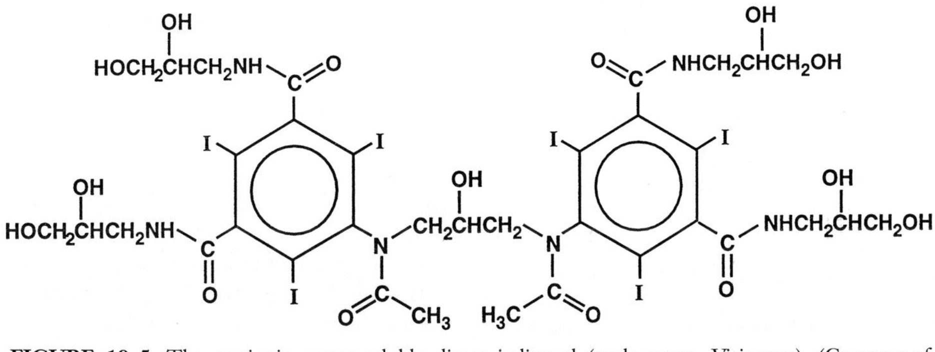

FIGURE 19–5. The nonionic, water-soluble dimer iodixanol (trade name, Visipaque). (Courtesy of Nycomed, Inc.)

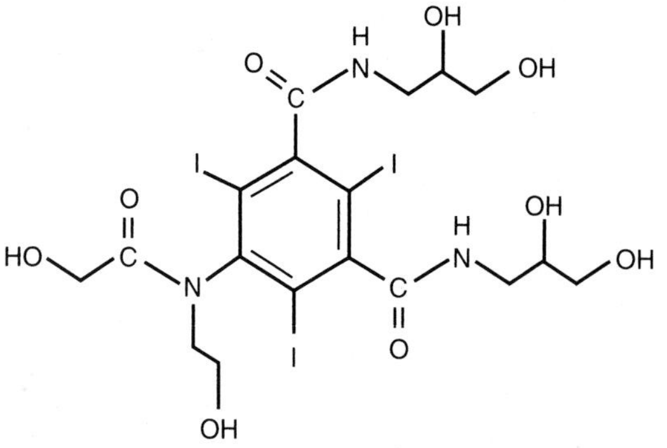

FIGURE 19–6. The nonionic, water-soluble, tri-iodinated contrast molecule ioversol (trade name, Optiray). (Courtesy of Mallinckrodt Medical, Inc., St. Louis, MO.)

dia in blood plasma. Figure 19–7 shows radiographs of some procedures performed using water-soluble nonionic iodine contrast agents.

Figure 19–8 is a photograph of another nonionic agent, iopamidol (Isovue). Iodine in its elemental form is chemically reactive and can be toxic in the body. Consequently, both ionic and nonionic agents contain additives such as citrate and calcium disodium edetate. These compounds prevent iodine atoms from being removed from the contrast molecules.

GENERAL EFFECTS

Water-soluble iodine contrast media have known physiologic effects. High osmolality and aspects of chemical structure are the major characteristics of the water-soluble media that are responsible for these effects. Although both ionic and nonionic iodine media have physiologic effects on the body, most ionic agents are higher-osmolality contrast media and have therefore shown greater effects and adverse reactions. Viscosity, or "friction," of the media is influenced by the concentration and size of the molecule. It affects the injectability, or delivery, of the media. Heating the media to body temperature significantly reduces the viscosity and facilitates the ability for rapid injection. This is commonly accomplished through the use of a *contrast warmer.*

Osmotic Effects

Because ionic media dissociate in water, their injection into the blood plasma results in a great increase in the number of particles present in

the plasma. This has the effect of displacing water. Water moves from an area of greater concentration to an area of lesser concentration; the process is called **osmosis.** When the plasma water is displaced by contrast particles, water from body cells moves into the vascular system. This results in hypervolemia and blood vessel dilatation, with pain and discomfort. Blood pressure may decrease because of vessel dilatation, or it may increase as a result of hypervolemia and the effects of hormones in the kidneys.

When higher-osmolality contrast media are given for imaging of the intestinal tract, fluid from cells is drawn into these areas. This osmotic effect can aid in reducing obstructions because the increase in fluid increases peristalsis. In dehydrated patients, however, the osmotic effect further reduces body cell volume and can result in **shock.** Consequently, it is important to obtain a patient history and to convey any **contraindications** to the radiologist or other physician. The number of molecular particles of a particular contrast medium is shown on the package insert in units of milliosmoles per kilogram of water at 37°C. The higher the number, the greater the number of particles that can produce osmotic effects. As an example, the osmolality of iodixanol at 300 mg of iodine per milliliter in milliosmoles per kilogram is 290, equal to that of blood plasma.

Allergic-Like Effects (Anaphylactoid)

Allergic reactions to water-soluble iodinated contrast media resemble allergic reactions to foreign substances such as pollen grains. Reactions of typical allergic patients may be minor, such as urticaria (hives). However, some patients experience wheezing and edema in the throat and lungs with accompanying **bronchospasm.** Other anaphylactoid effects of water-soluble iodinated contrast media are nausea and vomiting. These reactions are thought to be caused by the release of a substance called **histamine** from certain cells found in the lungs, stomach, and lining of blood vessels. Although some radiologists may believe that the allergic-like effects are due to extreme anxiety, they should be taken seriously by the radiologic technologist. Premedication with steroids and antihistamines (to prevent the release of histamine) can reduce or eliminate allergic effects.

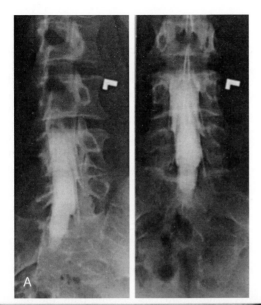

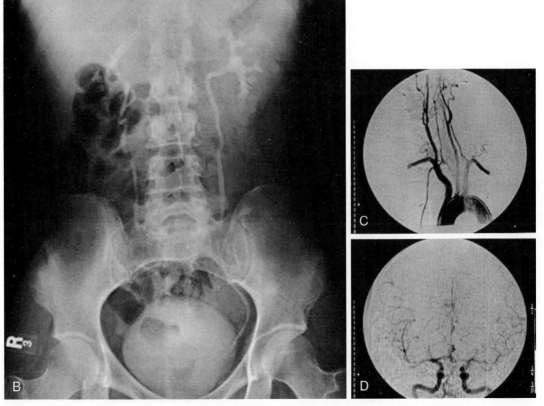

FIGURE 19–7. *A,* PA and oblique views of a lumbar myelogram. *B,* PA view of an excretory urogram. *C,* Digital cerebral angiogram. Vessels appear dark because of computer manipulation. *D,* Digital angiogram of the thoracic aorta and the main arteries it supplies (four-vessel study). Vessels appear dark because of computer manipulation. (*A* and *B* courtesy of Margaret Weaver, RT(R); *D* and *E* courtesy of David Skarbek, RT(R).)

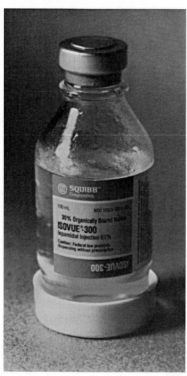

FIGURE 19–8. Iopamidol (trade name, Isovue) shown in the type of bottle used for injections into the arterial or venous system. (Courtesy of Bristol-Meyers Squibb, Princeton, NJ.)

Renal Effects

High-osmolality contrast media can cause the arteries of the kidneys to expand as a result of the osmotic effect. Arterial expansion results in the release of vasoconstrictors. These substances cause constriction of the renal arteries. Therefore, injection of the contrast media results in dilatation and then constriction of the renal arteries. The end result is diminished blood supply to the kidneys.

Osmotic effects are also presumed to cause an increase in the amount of molecular substances that cannot be reabsorbed by the renal tubules. This results in osmotic diuresis (increased secretion of urine) with dehydration. An increased **creatinine** (waste product of metabolism) level indicates that the patient may have renal disease and is a good indicator for possible contrast media-induced renal effects. Patients with renal disease or diabetes and those who are elderly are at increased risk for these complications. Intravenous fluid given before and during procedures can reduce the severity of renal effects. Theophylline, a substance found in tea, is currently being investigated as a preventative of toxic renal effects by increasing the filtering action of the kidneys.

Other Effects

Carotid artery injection of water-soluble iodine contrast media can alter the blood–brain barrier (separation between brain capillaries and support cells for the neurons) by causing the capillary cells to shrivel because of water loss. Some of these media can stimulate areas in the carotid artery that help to control heart rate and blood pressure. Clinical symptoms of these effects include increased blood pressure, bradycardia (slow heart beat), and tachycardia (fast heart beat).

In patients with sickle cell anemia and those who carry the trait but who are asymptomatic, injection of high-osmolality contrast media can cause the red blood cells to shrink and to sickle (assume an elongated shape). These sickled cells may be trapped in small-diameter blood vessels and capillaries, causing pain and blood clots. A common effect is a sensation of warmth and pain on injection into the arterial vessels. It is believed that this effect is due to dissociation of the contrast media into anions and cations.

In helical computed tomography procedures, a large amount of contrast material is injected at a rate of at least 2.5 mL per second. This increases the probability of nausea and vomiting and extravasation of the contrast with patient motion as a result.

Drug Interactions and Considerations

One class of drugs used to treat hypertension is the β-adrenergic blockers. These drugs reduce cardiac output but they also reduce dilatation of bronchial smooth muscle and block the effect of epinephrine. Patients who take these drugs are at an increased risk for anaphylactoid reactions during procedures in which water-soluble iodine contrast media are used.

Calcium channel blockers reduce hypertension by relaxing electrical conduction of cell membranes in arterioles (small arteries) and in heart muscle. Patients who take these drugs are at risk for heart block and abrupt decrease in blood pressure if ionic contrast media are used during cardiac catheterization.

Metformin (Glucophage) is a new type of drug used to treat non–insulin-dependent diabetes. Metformin should be discontinued for 48 hours before and 48 hours after the use of iodine contrast media. Although metformin does not interact with the iodine contrast agents, if renal failure should occur as an effect of iodine contrast administration, drug levels of metformin would accumulate in the patient and lactic acidosis could develop. (Metformin acts by increasing the uptake of glucose in body cells. One end product of glucose metabolism is lactic acid. Consequently, increased levels of metformin will increase lactic acid production and decrease the pH in body cells: acidosis.) See Table 19–7 for patient history factors.

CONSIDERATIONS IN THE USE OF NONIONIC MEDIA

Most of the adverse reactions associated with water-soluble ionic iodine contrast media are significantly decreased with the use of the nonionic media. This is attributed to the lower osmolality of the nonionic media. In addition, injection of nonionics during angiography is much less painful. However, kidney toxicity has not been reduced. It is important, therefore, to include the patient's creatinine level in the history. Nonionic iodine contrast media cost two to three times more than ionic media. Therefore, decisions about which patients will receive nonionic media are controversial. Some institutions have decided to use low-osmolality contrast media on all patients regardless of cost. Other institutions have established a selective use of these agents.

Sample criteria for the use of low-osmolality (nonionic) contrast media might include:

- patients with histories of adverse reactions to contrast media, excluding mild reactions such as the sensation of heat or flushing
- patients with histories of asthma or allergies
- patients with known cardiac problems
- patients with generalized severe debilitating conditions
- patients who will undergo helical computed tomography procedures

These criteria include such patients as those with diabetes mellitus, renal disease or elevated creatinine levels, or sickle cell disease.

SPECIFIC PROCEDURES

A wide variety of radiologic procedures use water-soluble iodine contrast media. These agents are important in visualizing the urinary and cardiovascular systems in particular. They are also commonly used in computed tomography studies of the brain, chest, and abdomen. Table 19–6 provides a list of the common procedures that use water-soluble iodine contrast agents.

The most important patient care aspect before administration of water-soluble iodine contrast media is the patient history. The possibility of patient reaction is closely related to the disease state or age of the patient. Moreover, the chemical nature of these contrast media can provoke severe reactions. The radiologic technologist is responsible for observation of patient well-being. Table 19–7 lists some patient history factors to consider before administering water-soluble iodine contrast media.

ADVERSE REACTIONS

As discussed in the section on the general effects of water-soluble iodine contrast media, these media have physiologic effects that may result in adverse reactions. The responsibility of the radiologic technologist in patient surveillance is critical in assessing the severity of these effects. Box 19–1 lists adverse reactions divided into three categories: mild, moderate, and severe. A discussion of treatment is also provided. Box 19–2 details the management of patients with acute reactions. Although adverse reactions can occur when using low-osmolality (nonionic) contrast media, they are most often associated with the higher-osmolality (ionic) contrast media.

Scheduling Contrast Media Procedures

Many contrast media procedures require fasting, laxatives, or cleansing enemas. For patients who are not debilitated, a single preparation may result in less patient discomfort. Another aspect to consider is that sedation is necessary for some examinations, but others require patient cooperation. The priority for scheduling contrast media examinations within the radiology department is generally as follows for fasting patients:

1 Elderly or debilitated patients
2 Diabetic patients
3 Children
4 Adults

TABLE 19–6. **Some Procedures for Which Water-Soluble Iodine Contrast Media Are Used**

Area	Contrast Agent	Method of Administration	Patient Preparation	Patient Instructions/ Care During Procedure
Brain: cerebral angiography computed tomography	Usually nonionic	Injection into vein or artery	Usually liquid diet to minimize nausea Premedication for sedation Intravenous fluids to aid hydration	Supportive communication Tell the patient that he or she may feel warm and sense a metallic taste on injection. Explain what is being done as it is being done. Watch patient for adverse reactions. Apply pressure to injection site after procedure is completed.
Thorax: thoracic angiography or four-vessel study	Usually nonionic	Injection into vein or artery	Usually liquid diet to minimize nausea Premedication for sedation Intravenous fluids to aid hydration	Supportive communication Tell the patient that he or she may feel warmth and sense a metallic taste on injection. Explain what is being done as it is being done. Watch patient for adverse reactions. Apply pressure to injection site after procedure is completed.
Lower limbs: venography	Usually nonionic	Injection into vein	Sometimes premedication for sedation Intravenous fluids for hydration	Supportive communication Tell the patient that he or she may feel warmth and sense a metallic taste on injection. Explain what is being done as it is being done; there may be some pain. Watch patient for adverse reactions. Apply pressure to injection site after procedure is completed.
Spinal canal: myelography	Only nonionic	Injection into subarachnoid space	Usually liquid diet Usually premedication for sedation	Supportive communication Explain the use of shoulder braces and that the table will be tilted but the patient's head must be kept in extension. Explain what is being done as it is being done. Watch the patient for adverse reactions. Advise nursing staff and patient that patient should remain in bed with the head up for 24 hours to prevent headache and nausea.

				Patient Instructions/ Care During Procedure
Area	**Contrast Agent**	**Method of Administration**	**Patient Preparation**	
Kidneys, ureters, and bladder: excretory urography, renal angiography, cystography	Usually nonionic	Injection into vein or artery For cystography, usually through catheter in urinary bladder	Liquid diet day before examination to reduce gas formation Laxatives or a cleansing enema may be given. Bladder should be emptied before the examination begins.	Supportive communication Tell the patient that he or she may feel warmth and sense a metallic taste during and just after injections; several injections may be done. Explain the timing of the radiographs and the x-ray tube movement if tomography is done. Watch the patient for adverse reactions. Angiography: apply pressure to the injection site after procedure is completed.
Heart and coronary arteries: cardiac catheterization	Usually nonionic	Usually through catheter	Liquid or low-residue diet usually is ordered the evening before the procedure. Antibiotics are usually ordered. Premedication for sedation Intravenous fluids for hydration Blood clotting (prothrombin) time must be within a range acceptable to the physician. Catheter may be inserted in femoral artery; therefore, strength of dorsal pedal pulses is evaluated.	Supportive communication Tell the patient that he or she may feel warmth and sense a metallic taste on injection. Explain what is being done as it is being done. The patient may be apprehensive about the movements of the x-ray tube around the body or the use of two x-ray tubes. Lead glass shielding should be explained. Nursing procedures: monitoring of peripheral pulses and blood pressure. Watch the patient for adverse reactions. Advise nursing staff that temperature may be elevated after procedure.

Controversy exists regarding preprocedure instructions for diabetic patients. Insulin, a pancreatic hormone, either is lacking in these patients or is not able to be used efficiently. Without insulin, diabetic patients suffer high blood sugar (hyperglycemia), in which there are too many sugar molecules in the blood plasma. Injection of water-soluble iodine contrast media increases the osmotic effect in these patients, thus increasing the risk of a diabetic coma. Conversely, injection of insulin in fasting diabetic patients results in low blood sugar (hypoglycemia). These patients must be observed for rapidly developing symptoms such as irritability, cold damp skin, and blurred vision. Generally, patients for whom no other contraindications exist are scheduled as shown in Table 19–8.

TABLE 19–7. **Patient History Factors in Water-Soluble Iodine Contrast Examinations**

Factors	Importance
Age	↑ Risk with increased age
Allergies or asthma	↑ Risk of allergic-like reactions
Diabetes	Insulin usually given before procedure; these patients should be scheduled before others.
Coronary artery disease	↑ Risk of tachycardia, bradycardia, hypertension, myocardial infarction (heart attack)
Hypertension	Hypertension with tachycardia
Renal disease	Inform radiologist if creatinine level is above 1.4 mg/dL.
Multiple myeloma	Abnormal protein binds with contrast and can cause renal failure. Patients must be hydrated.
Confusion or dizziness	Blood-brain barrier effects
Sickle cell anemia or family history of chronic obstructive pulmonary disease	↑ Risk of blood clots ↑ Risk of dyspnea (difficulty in breathing)
Previous iodine contrast examinations	Did the patient have difficulties with procedure?
Pregnancy	Inform radiologists before proceeding.
History of blood clots	↑ Risk of blood clots
Use of beta blockers	↑ Risk of anaphylactoid reactions
Use of calcium channel blockers	Risk of heart block
Use of metformin (Glucophage)	Risk of lactic acidosis if renal failure occurs

↑ = Increased

BOX 19–1

Categories of Reactions to Water-Soluble Iodine Contrast Media

MILD

Nausea and vomiting	Pallor
Cough	Flushing
Warmth (heat)	Chills
Headache	Shaking
Dizziness	Sweats
Anxiety	Rash (hives)
Altered taste	Nasal stuffiness
Itching	Swelling of eyes or face

Treatment

Requires observation and reassurance, but usually no treatment

MODERATE

Moderate degree of mild signs and symptoms* or systemic symptoms including:

Pulse change	Dyspnea-wheezing
Hypotension	Bronchospasm
Hypertension	Laryngospasm

Treatment

Requires close, careful observation and often treatment, but usually not hospitalization

SEVERE

Potentially life-threatening; moderate or severe signs and symptoms (e.g., laryngospasm) plus:

Unresponsiveness
Convulsions
Clinically manifest arrhythmias
Cardiopulmonary arrest

Treatment

Requires *prompt* recognition and treatment; almost always requires hospitalization

*Sufficient to be clinically evident.
Reprinted with permission from *Manual on Iodinated Contrast Media*, American College of Radiology, 1991.

BOX 19–2

Management of Acute Reactions

URTICARIA

1. No treatment needed in most cases
2. H₁-receptor blocker
      Diphenhydramine (Benadryl), PO, IM, IV 50 mg *or*
      Hydroxyzine (Vistaril), PO, IM, IV 25–50 mg
   H₂-receptor blocker may be added:
      Cimetidine (Tagamet), 300 mg PO, IV slowly, diluted in 10 mL D₅W solution *or*
      Ranitidine (Zantac), 50 mg PO, IV slowly, diluted in 10 mL D₅W solution

If severe or widely disseminated
      Alpha-agonist (arteriolar and venous constriction)
         Epinephrine (1:1000), 0.1–0.3 mL SC (if no cardiac contraindication)

FACIAL/LARYNGEAL EDEMA

1. Alpha-agonist (arteriolar and venous constriction)
      Epinephrine (1:1000), 0.1–0.3 mL SC; if SC route fails or peripheral vascular collapse
         occurs, epinephrine (1:10,000), 1–3 mL IV *slowly*
      May repeat 3 times as needed up to a maximum of 1 mg
2. Oxygen, 2–6 L/min

If not responsive to therapy or for obvious laryngeal edema (acute)
      Call anesthesiologist and CODE team
      Consider intubation

BRONCHOSPASM

1. Oxygen 2–6 L/min
2. Monitor ECG, oxygen saturation (pulse oximeter), blood pressure
      Epinephrine (1:1000), 0.1–0.3 mL SC or beta-agonist inhalers (bronchiolar
         dilators—i.e., metaproterenol [Alupent], terbutaline [Brethaire], or albuterol
         [Proventil]); if SC route fails or if peripheral vascular collapse occurs, epinephrine
         (1:10,000), 1–3 mL IV *slowly*
      May repeat 3 times as needed up to a maximum of 1 mg

Alternatively
1. Aminophylline, 6 mg/kg IV in D₅W over 10–20 minutes (loading dose); then 0.4–1.0
      mg/kg/hr as needed
         or
      Terbutaline, 0.25–0.5 mg IM, SC
2. Call CODE for severe bronchospasm (or if oxygen saturation is 88 or below)

Box continued on following page

BOX 19–2 *Continued*

Management of Acute Reactions

HYPOTENSION WITH TACHYCARDIA

1. Legs up; Trendelenburg position. Monitor ECG, pulse oximeter, blood pressure
2. Oxygen, 2–6 L/min
3. Rapid administration of large volumes of isotonic lactated
   Ringer's solution (Ringer's lactate > normal saline > D_5W)

If poorly responsive
   Epinephrine (1:1000), 0.1–0.3 mL SC; if SC route fails or if peripheral vascular collapse
   occurs, epinephrine (1:10,000), 1–3 mL IV *slowly*
   May repeat 3 times as needed up to a maximum of 1 mg

if still poorly responsive
   Transfer to ICU for further management

HYPOTENSION WITH BRADYCARDIA—VAGAL REACTION

1. Legs up; Trendelenburg position; secure airway; give oxygen
2. Secure IV access; give atropine, 0.6–1 mg IV slowly
3. Monitor vital signs, repeat atropine up to 2 mg total dose
4. Push fluid replenishment IV (Ringer's lactate > normal saline > D_5W)

HYPERTENSION, SEVERE

1. Monitors in place: ECG, pulse oximeter, blood pressure
2. Apresoline, 5 mg IV
3. Sodium nitroprusside—arterial line; infusion pump is necessary to titrate
4. For pheochromocytoma—phentolamine, 5 mg (1 mg in children) IV

SEIZURES/CONVULSIONS

1. Oxygen, 2–6 L/min
2. Consider diazepam (Valium), 5 mg or midazolam (Versed), 2.5 mg IV
3. If longer effect is needed, obtain consultation; consider phenytoin (Dilantin) infusion,
   15–18 mg/kg at 50 mg/min
4. Careful monitoring of vital signs is required

PULMONARY EDEMA

1. Elevate torso; rotate tourniquets (venous compression)
2. Oxygen, 2–6 L/min
3. Diuretics—furosemide (Lasix), 40 mg IV slowly
4. Consider morphine or meperidine (Demerol)
5. Corticosteroids optional

TABLE 19–8. Scheduling Protocol for Patients Having Multiple Procedures	
Procedure	**Determining Factor(s)**
Noncontrast radiography	Lingering contrast media are not seen if they are not given—lymphography, for example.
Any nuclear medicine imaging or function tests for which iodine is given	Iodine goes to the thyroid gland. Therefore, iodinated contrast media, if given before these studies, alter the results of these tests.
Urinary system radiography	Water-soluble iodinated contrast media are cleared by the kidneys.
Cholegraphy and other examination of the biliary system	Contrast media collect in the gallbladder or are rapidly excreted.
Colon examinations	Some barium sulfate may persist in patients for a day or two.
Studies of the esophagus, stomach, and small intestine	Barium sulfate is cleared from the upper gastrointestinal system rapidly; persistence in the colon for a day or two does not conflict with previous studies.
Bronchography and lymphography	Oily contrast media persist in body structures.

To summarize, scheduling protocol is as follows: noncontrast radiography, nuclear medicine imaging with iodine, water-soluble iodine contrast studies, barium sulfate procedures, and oil-based iodine contrast examinations.

Responsibilities of the Radiologic Technologist

SOURCES OF CONTRAST MEDIA INFORMATION

In almost no other medical specialty do practitioners inject, or have the patient ingest, such large amounts of nonbiologic substances over a short time as in radiology. It is obvious that the chemical structures of these agents greatly influence the (1) ability of the agents to enhance subject contrast, (2) types of agents used for specific procedures, and (3) reasons for adverse reactions that can occur in patients.

The discussion presented in this chapter about the physical properties of contrast media aids in reading the package inserts. It is important to look at the chemical structure presented and to locate the common chemical groups discussed. Then, the radiologic technologist can consider other information in the package inserts about specific procedures, dosage, and adverse reactions. Technical representatives from pharmaceutical companies that supply contrast agents can also supply journal articles as important sources of information. Problems arising from specific contrast media examinations should be discussed with the radiologist. Valuable insights for effective patient care are gained in this manner.

PATIENT SURVEILLANCE

The set-up for any contrast media procedure, patient positioning, and radiographic technique are important professional responsibilities. The patient must remain the focus of the procedure, however. The patient is usually anxious about the procedure and the reasons that made the procedure necessary. Often, the patient has an empty stomach, so he or she may be irritable. These feelings combined with the reasons for the adverse reactions from contrast media may result in an increased possibility of these reactions.

Owing to an increase in outpatient procedures that utilize water-soluble iodine contrast media, there are reported instances of adverse reactions that occur hours later. These reactions have been poorly communicated to radiologists due to lack of patient knowledge. The radiographer could develop an instruction sheet about mild adverse reactions and discuss these issues with the patient after the procedure is complete but before the patient leaves. Such instructions might include: Call the department (direct phone number) if you experience any of the following within 24 hours: hives, flushing, chills, nasal stuffiness, swelling of the eyes or face, or wheezing.

A calm, supportive manner on the part of the radiologic technologist is a necessity. Continued communication, with questions regarding patient comfort, allows observation of the patient's physical and emotional status. A professional demeanor can increase the well-being of the patient and thereby reduce the possibility of adverse reactions.

PATIENT CARE

Many procedures require patient preparation at home, such as enemas before lower GI procedures and fasting after midnight before some procedures. The diagnostic quality of procedures that require patient preparation is diminished by patient failure to follow instructions. Before beginning the examination, the radiologic technologist must ask the patient if he or she followed the instructions for it. Some patients comply with some but not all of the instructions. Therefore the radiologic technologist must also find out *to what extent* the patient complied. This information can usually be obtained by one question, "What did you do at home to prepare for your x-ray today?" If the patient forgets an aspect of the instructions, the radiologic technologist should use prompts such as, "What about the pills, Mr. Jones?"

Many referring physicians do not tell their patients what to expect during contrast media procedures. Also, many people have only a rudimentary knowledge of body functions. It is the radiologic technologist's responsibility to explain to the patients, in simple terms, what will be done. The radiologic technologist must also convey to the patient *a sense of being cared for* and *a sense of being safe* during the procedure. These subjective qualities can be communicated by addressing the patient by name (eg, Mr. Jones, Mrs. Green), using blankets or sheets for warmth and modesty, using pillows when possible, and asking questions such as, "Are you warm enough?" Many patients feel less anxious if the radiologic technologist explains the procedure as it is performed. Finally, a universal form of supportive communication is touch.

Summary

Radiographic contrast media are used to visualize areas within the body that otherwise could not be seen well. These agents are not drugs. However, they can affect the physiologic status of patients.

Radiolucent contrast media transmit x-rays and are usually used with radiopaque contrast media to visualize the lumens of organs and joint spaces. Radiopaque contrast media absorb x-rays and are used to demonstrate the gastrointestinal, biliary, urinary, circulatory, lymphatic, and respiratory systems.

Most adverse reactions encountered by patients are associated with the use of radiopaque contrast agents. Serious complications from the administration of barium sulfate include hypervolemia and colon and vaginal rupture. Water-soluble iodine contrast agents can cause allergic-like effects and can increase the severity of sickle cell anemia, renal disease, and diabetes. The patient history obtained by the radiologic technologist gives information about pre-existing disease that can increase the possibility of some adverse reactions. Appropriate patient preparation and care can then be given to eliminate or decrease these adverse reactions.

The radiologic technologist should be familiar with the general chemical structure of contrast media and the relation of the structure to the formal and trade names of the particular medium. It is critical that the radiologic technologist relate the various media to examinations for which they are best suited. Knowledge of specific patient preparations and adverse reactions associated with each agent is imperative.

The manner in which patient care is given can decrease the possibility of adverse reactions and can increase the diagnostic quality of the examination by increasing patient cooperation.

◀R REVIEW QUESTIONS

1 Subject contrast in radiographic imaging is difficult to obtain because:
   a) all of the x-rays are absorbed by body tissues
   b) most x-rays are scattered by body tissues
   c) most body tissues have similar atomic structure
   d) all body tissues contain hydrogen

2 An advantage of barium sulfate is that it:
   a) is not soluble in water
   b) can flocculate
   c) is relatively nontoxic
   d) is paramagnetic

3 Negative contrast agents:
   a) are composed of atoms with high atomic numbers
   b) absorb x-rays
   c) are radiopaque
   d) appear dark on film

4 Iodinated ethyl esters are found in:
   a) oily iodine contrast
   b) water-soluble ionic iodine contrast
   c) water-soluble nonionic iodine contrast
   d) iopamidol

5 Hydroxyl groups on nonionic water-soluble iodinated contrast media act to increase:
a) osmotic effects
b) solubility
c) blood pressure
d) bronchospasm

6 What type of patient reaction to injection of water-soluble iodine contrast usually does not require treatment?
a) metallic taste on injection
b) inability to maintain blood pressure within normal range
c) chest pain
d) dyspnea

7 When you schedule multiple procedures, what examination is usually done last?
a) thyroid function tests
b) lymphography
c) air contrast colon
d) laryngopharyngography

8 Which one of the following drugs should be discontinued 48 hours before and 48 hours after administration of water-soluble iodine contrast media?
a) insulin
b) glucagon
c) beta blockers
d) metformin

9 What can be done for a patient who will receive water-soluble iodine contrast media to reduce allergic-like effects?
a) premedicate with steroids and antihistamines
b) give intravenous fluids
c) instruct the patient to drink warm salt water before the procedure
d) give a negative contrast agent with the iodinated medium

10 Why should cold tap water be mixed with barium sulfate for lower gastrointestinal examinations?
a) It makes the suspension thicker.
b) It coats the colon.
c) It results in less cramping.
d) It reduces the possibility of flocculation.

BIBLIOGRAPHY

Ansell G, et al: Complications in Diagnostic Radiology. Philadelphia, JB Lippincott, 1976.
Ballinger P: Merrill's Atlas of Radiographic Positions and Radiologic Procedures. 7th ed., St. Louis, Mosby–Year Book, 1991.
Benison S, et al: Walter B. Cannon: The Life and Times of a Young Scientist. Cambridge, Harvard University Press, 1987.
Bettmann M: Ionic versus nonionic contrast agents for intravenous use: Are all the answers in? Radiology 175:616–618, 1990.
Curry N, et al: Fatal reactions to intravenous nonionic contrast media. Radiology 178:361–362, 1991.
Jacobson PD: Who decides who gets low-osmolar contrast? Diag Image April, 77–84, 1991.
Katayama H, et al: Adverse reactions to ionic and nonionic contrast media: A report from the Japanese committee on the safety of contrast media. Radiology 175:621–628, 1990.
Katzburg W (ed): The Contrast Media Manual. Baltimore, Williams & Wilkins, 1992.
Manual on Iodinated Contrast Media. Reston, VA, American College of Radiology, 1991.
Martin DW et al: Harper's Review of Biochemistry. 20th ed. East Norwalk, Appleton-Century-Crofts, 1985.
McClennan B: Ionic and nonionic iodinated contrast media: Evolution and strategies for use. AJR 155:225–233, 1990.
Package Insert: Metformin (Glucophage). Bristol-Myers Squibb Company, 1995.
Silverman P: Nonionic contrast use optimizes helical CT. Diagn Imag August, 67–69, 1996.
Skucas J: Radiographic Contrast Agents. 2nd ed. Rockville, MD, Aspen Publishers, 1989.
Torsten A: Relations between chemical structure, animal toxicity and clinical adverse effects of contrast media. In Enge I, Edgren J (ed): Patient Safety and Adverse Events in Contrast Medium Examinations. New York, Elsevier, 1989.

UNIT
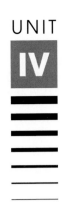

IV

Ethical and Legal Issues

CHAPTER 20

PROFESSIONAL ETHICS

Robert A. Buerki, PhD
Louis D. Vottero, MS

Knowing what's right doesn't mean much unless you do what's right.

ANONYMOUS

OBJECTIVES

On completion of this chapter, the student will be able to:

1 Explain the ethic of the radiologic technology profession.
2 Differentiate between the systems of ethics, law, and morals.
3 Explain the four-step problem-solving process of ethical analysis.
4 Explain two sources of moral judgment that underlie ethical decision making.

335

5 Identify moral dilemmas encountered in patient relationships.
6 Identify moral dilemmas encountered in physician relationships.
7 Identify moral dilemmas encountered in relationships with other health professionals.
8 Recognize values associated with ethical decision making in the practice of radiologic technology.
9 Apply critical analysis to ethical decision making.

GLOSSARY

Autonomy: a person's self-reliance, independence, liberty rights, privacy, individual choice, freedom of the will, and the self-contained ability to decide

Beneficence: doing of good; active promotion of good, kindness, and charity

Bioethics: the consideration of ethical issues in the full range of biologic sciences, including health care

Caring: to care for; an emotional commitment to, and a willingness to act on behalf of, a person with whom a caring relationship exists

Codes of Ethics: articulated statement of role morality as seen by the members of a profession

Common Morality: socially approved norms of human conduct that takes its basic premises from the morality shared in common by the members of a society; includes common sense and tradition

Confidentiality: belief that health-related information about individuals should not be revealed to others; maintaining privacy

Consequentialism: belief that the worth of actions is determined by their ends or consequences; actions are right or wrong according to the balance of their good and bad consequences

Duties: obligations placed on individuals, groups, and institutions by reason of the so-called "moral bond" of our interdependence with others

Ethical Dilemma: situation requiring moral judgment between two or more equally problem-fraught alternatives; there are two or more competing moral norms present, creating a challenge about what to do

Ethical Outrage: gross violation of commonly held standards of decency or human rights

Ethical Question: situation in which one or more moral norms are present and the correct action to take is apparent, but a barrier exists that prevents your taking that action

Ethical Theories: bodies of systematically related moral principles used to resolve ethical dilemmas

Ethics: the systematic study of rightness and wrongness of human conduct and character as known by natural reason

Ethics of Care: ethical reflections that emphasize an intimate personal relationship value system that includes such virtues as sympathy, compassion, fidelity, discernment, and love

Fidelity: strict observance of promises or duties; loyalty and faithfulness to others

Justice: equitable, fair, or just conduct in dealing with others

Laws: regulations established by government and applicable to people within a certain political subdivision

Language of Rights: supplies the basic terminology for expressing the moral point of view

Legal Rights: rights of individuals or groups that are established and guaranteed by law

Liberal Individualism: the basis for rights-based ethical theory; each individual is protected and allowed to pursue personal projects

Moral Philosophy: the original term for ethics; emphasizes the reasoning process inherent in the discipline of philosophy and its dependence on morals

Moral Principles: general, universal guides to action that are derived from so-called basic moral truths that should be respected unless there is a morally compelling reason not to do so; also referred to as *ethical principles*

Moral Rights: rights of individuals or groups that exist separately from governmental or institutional guarantees; usually asserted on the basis of moral principles or rules

Moral Rules: statements of right conduct governing individual actions

Moral Virtue: trait of character that is morally valued; a disposition to act—or a habit of acting—in accordance with moral principles, obligations, or ideals

Morality: widely shared social conventions about right and wrong human conduct including a conformity to the rules of right conduct; also see *Common Morality*

Morals: generally accepted customs, principles, or habits of right living and conduct in a society, and the individual's practice in relation to these

Nonconsequentialism: belief that actions themselves, rather than consequences, determine the worth of actions; actions are right or wrong according the morality of the acts themselves

Nonmaleficence: ethical principle that places high value on avoiding harm to others

Norm: standard set by individuals or groups of individuals

Principle-based Ethics: the use of moral principles as a basis for defending a chosen path of action in resolving an ethical dilemma; also see *Principlism*

Principlism: belief system based on a set of moral principles that are embedded in a common morality

Professional Disclosure Standard: standard for the disclosure of information to patients that is determined by a professional community's customary practices

Professional Ethic: publicly displayed ethical conduct of a profession, usually embedded in a code of ethics; affirms the professional as an independent, autonomous, responsible decision-maker

Professional Ethics: internal controls of a profession based on human values or moral principles

Professional Etiquette: manners and attitudes generally accepted by members of a profession

Rights: justified claims that an individual can make on individuals, groups, or society; divided into *Legal Rights* and *Moral Rights*

Rights-based Ethics: belief that individual rights provide the vital protection of life, liberty, expression, and property

Self-determination: right of individuals to decide their own course of action, especially in the context of medical care; codified by the 1991 Patient Self-Determination Act, which ensures that health-care institutions inform patients about their rights under state and federal law

Social Contract: exists when two mutually dependent groups in a society recognize certain expectations of one another and conduct their affairs accordingly

Values: ideals and customs of a society toward which the members of a group have an affective regard; a value may be a quality desirable as an end in itself

Value System: collection or set of values that an individual or group have as their personal guide

Veracity: duty to tell the truth and avoid deception

Virtue: trait of character that is socially valued, such as *courage*, also see *Moral Virtue*

Virtue-based Ethics: ethical theory that emphasizes the agents who perform actions and make choices; character and virtue form the framework of this ethical theory

The Importance of a Professional Ethic

Health-care professionals often encounter situations in their practices that they find deeply disturbing. These situations, which are usually unrelated to clinical procedures or medical intervention, may involve such basic human rights as the right to privacy and dignity or even the simple right to be told the truth. Professionals may encounter conflicting value or belief systems that can compromise patient care. They also must make hard choices that depend on their understanding of such moral principles as justice and beneficence, such virtues as compassion and caring, and such fundamental duties as honesty and loyalty to both patients and physicians.

All these situations are generally encompassed under the term **professional ethics.** Principles of professional ethics may be reduced to a written code, but professionals who attempt to apply such unyielding standards to their daily practice often become dismayed and frustrated because the code does not address their specific problems. When faced with an ethical problem or dilemma, many professionals simply follow the rules of their institution, the policies of their supervisor, or choose the least objectionable course of action among a bewildering array of choices, each of which may have profound consequences for patient care.

As emerging health care professionals in their own right, radiologic technologists play a critical supportive role between the physician and patient. They assist in providing valuable information that enables physicians to make accurate diagnoses and establish sound therapeutic plans.

As such, radiologic technologists must meet established standards of professional conduct as professional persons, standards that support the emotional and physical needs of the patients with whom they come in contact. Radiologic technologists, like all health care professionals, believe that their professional conduct is based on their complete, uncompromised devotion to patients as individuals, while providing them with the highest possible quality of medical care.

The public expects all professionals to exhibit self-discipline within a system of self-regulation. This sense of self-discipline is particularly important within the health care professions, where errors in judgment can have serious, even life-threatening, consequences. Furthermore, despite the increasing sophistication among segments of the American public, few individuals are able to judge the quality of the professional services they receive. Patients who submit to radiologic procedures, for example, have no way of determining whether the procedures have been performed properly or even whether they have been injured in the process. As a result, a **professional ethic** is one of several generally accepted criteria that serve to distinguish a profession from other occupations or trades.

State licensing laws reflect the public's demand that it be served by qualified health care practitioners. The professional licensing boards that enforce these and other professional practice laws provide one element of self-regulation. Professionals are given certain prerogatives by society, such as a quasimonopoly to operate in a certain professional arena. In return for granting these prerogatives, society expects professionals to be guided by a standard of conduct beyond mere conformity to law. This standard of conduct, this common concern for collective self-discipline, this control of the profession from within is known as **ethics.**

In philosophy, *ethics* is often defined as the science of rightness and wrongness of human conduct as known by natural reason. Professional ethics, however, may be defined as rules of conduct or standards by which a particular group regulates its actions and sets standards for its members. The system of ethics is closely related and overlaps two other systems designed to control society: law and morals. **Laws** refer to regulations established by a government applicable to people within a certain political subdivision; **morals** are generally accepted customs of right living and conduct and an individual's

practice in relation to these customs. Table 20–1 summarizes these distinctions.

At first glance, the system of laws, with its sanctions of fines and imprisonment for noncompliance, would seem to have the greatest payoff to society. Moreover, the system of laws is dynamic, subject to the ever-changing will of the people and their legislators. However, the system of laws does not cover all areas of professional conduct or potential risks a professional encounters. No matter how broadly laws and regulations are written or how detailed they may seem, there are still areas that must be covered by a system of voluntary self-discipline, the system of ethics.

Society expects a profession, through its collective members, to generate its own statement of acceptable and unacceptable behavior, usually in the form of a **code of ethics.** The Code of Ethics adopted by the American Registry of Radiologic Technologists is reproduced in Appendix E.

Ideally, all radiologic technologists subscribe to the ethical principles contained in these documents and apply them to problems in their professional practice. These codes serve the profession well by providing the practitioner with a detailed, explicit, operational blueprint of **norms** of professional conduct. Unfortunately, some of these principles are stated in abstract or idealized terms that provide little in the way of concrete guidance for young practitioners. For example, Principle 9 of the ARRT Code of Ethics states that the radiologic technologist "reveals confidential information only as required by law or to protect the welfare of the individual or the community." Under what circumstances, if any, could a patient's right to privacy be infringed on? What standards are used to determine when the welfare of the community supersedes the welfare of the individual? What information can be released, to whom, and under what circumstances? The answers to these questions, of course, are not usually found in codes of ethics. Furthermore, you may encounter situations that are not even remotely related to the statements in the codes, reflecting the static nature of any professional code. Finally, do the principles that make up the code take into consideration the role of human values and virtues in deciding professional practice behavior? These questions suggest that a more serviceable method for determining right conduct in professional practice involves something beyond mere reflection on a code of ethics.

			Enabling	
System	**Application**	**Control**	**Source**	**Sanctions**
Ethics	Specific group	Within group	Codes of ethics	Expulsion
Laws	Political subdivision	Outside group	Legislation	Fines, prison
Morals	Individuals	Conscience	Religious writing	Shame, guilt

TABLE 20–1. **Comparison of Systems of Ethics, Law, and Morals**

Ethical Evaluations

Before we can develop our own personal set of internal guidelines for determining what constitutes right conduct in our professional practice, we must clarify a few additional concepts. **Professional etiquette,** the manners and attitudes toward patients generally accepted by practitioners, should not be confused with professional ethics. For example, while being rude toward patients or being insensitive to their need for preserving their modesty may violate our sense of professional propriety, these actions are not considered breaches in professional ethics. We will consider professional ethics as rules of conduct or standards beyond conformance to either law or etiquette, the internal controls of a profession based on human values or moral principles.

Next, we must develop some skill in both recognizing and analyzing **ethical dilemmas.** While we may all agree on what constitutes patently unethical conduct, the so-called **ethical outrage,** the true ethical dilemma invites a wide range of personal opinion among colleagues in a profession, each of which is based on a highly individualistic, strongly held **value system.** For example, while we might agree that it is unethical to refuse to provide services to dirty, unkempt patients or even those infected with the AIDS virus, we might hold a variety of opinions on what degree of loyalty we owe to our fellow workers on the health care team. When does our loyalty to physicians or administrators overshadow our loyalty to our patients? On the other hand, if our loyalty to our patient's autonomy interferes with his or her decision to accept needed medical treatment, we may wish to temporarily set aside this value so that a higher human value, the resulting benefit to these patients, may be served. To a greater or lesser extent, all professional decisions in radiologic technology and other health care practices involve a consideration of human values. By the same token, every ethical decision also involves

human values, values that may often conflict and compete for recognition and acceptance among our professional colleagues.

Once we have identified an ethical dilemma and the human values that may be associated with that dilemma, how should we proceed to analyze the situation? The process of ethical analysis generally contains the following four components:

- identifying the problem
- developing alternative solutions
- selecting the best solution
- defending your selection

Many students encounter difficulty in *identifying the problem* simply because they are eager to get on with the problem-solving process. Thoroughness in problem identification, looking at every possible twist or nuance in a given situation, is absolutely essential for successful resolution of any ethical dilemma. In *developing alternative solutions*, we attempt to exhaust all possible pathways to a resolution of the dilemma, taking care to view the dilemma from the perspective not only of the patient and the patient's family but also the health care professionals and administrators to whom they entrust their care. The most challenging step in the problem-solving process is *selecting the best solution*, a very personal activity that involves choosing an alternative not only based on widely held moral standards but one that is also in full accord with your own individual value system. Finally, by *defending your selection*, you can explain the basis for your ethical decision in terms that you can justify to colleagues and patients alike. Although this process may seem difficult or even impossible at first glance, we can approach it with confidence once we have considered the underlying sources of moral judgment that allow us to move beyond feelings, emotions, and intuition toward more structured foundations for our ethical decision making. These sources of moral judgment are discussed under the general headings of moral rules and ethical theories.

MORAL RULES

In making our ethical decisions, we could rely on widely held **moral rules**: The Bible admonishes us to abide by the "golden rule" and obey the Ten Commandments, our schools teach us it is wrong to cheat, our professional associations promulgate codes of ethics that encourage practitioners to "do no harm." Many individuals successfully use moral rules to guide their behavior, but this approach has its limitations. The most serious limitation to using moral rules as a primary guide to moral behavior is that most people lack access to a complete set of moral rules or that a complete set of moral rules just does not exist. As noted, most codes of ethics are incomplete and do not speak to all ethical issues faced by radiologic technologists and other health care professionals.

ETHICAL THEORIES

Another approach to establishing a foundation on which to base ethical decision making involves normative ethical systems, that is, sets of principles that tell us what actions are right or wrong, or **ethical theories.** These systems are usually divided into two groups: **consequentialism** evaluates the rightness or wrongness of ethical decisions by assessing the consequences of these decisions on the patient—that is, producing a good effect for the patient or at least avoiding some potential harm; **nonconsequentialism** holds that there are other right-making characteristics of our actions beyond consequences that are needed to determine whether a given behavior is right or wrong. For example, persons who use the consequentialist system for ethical decision making may lie to a patient if they believe that the lie might ultimately benefit the patient; persons using the nonconsequentialist system would caution against lying to a patient under any circumstances since the act of lying is generally accepted as morally wrong in our society.

More recently, modifications to these ethical theories have been developed, including such concepts as social contracts, the ethics of care, rights-based ethics, principle-based ethics, and virtue-based ethics. These refinements are increasingly being used in medical practices to analyze and defend actions and their outcomes, especially those practices that attempt to fulfill the ethical mandates of quality patient care.

Social contract theory attempts to describe the relationship that exists between two mutually dependent persons or groups of persons in a society. Under this theory, these persons or groups—radiologic technologists and patients, in our context—recognize certain expectations of one another and act accordingly. For example, patients expect their radiologic technologist to tell them the truth; by the same token, radiologic technologists expect their patients to tell them the truth. While social contract theory sounds simple and straightforward, social contracts can be perplexing. Unlike legal contracts with their precise language and implicit sanctions, social contracts are unwritten, leaving the specific duties and actions expected of health care practitioners and their patients to be resolved through a process of reasoning and discernment.

The **ethics of care** cautions that our actions should not be examined as isolated events; instead, our actions should be considered as an integral part of the context of specific situations. For example, lying to a patient is not an isolated event; rather, this act is surrounded by a welter of circumstances—who the patients are, what their particular ills might be, how they relate to us, what beliefs we have, and so on. Furthermore, a caring ethic requires us to make moral judgments that reflect the values of the communities within which we live. The ethics of care require the decision-maker to more clearly focus on such basic moral skills as kindness, sensitivity, attentiveness, tact, patience, and reliability. Indeed, the ethics of care emphasizes the need for an accurate understanding of moral competence, a clear vision of the meaning of a "virtuous person," and finely honed skills in human relations.

Rights-based ethics, one of the more popular approaches to ethical reasoning, is based on an understanding of *human rights.* Advocates often express their human rights openly and forcefully, claiming a "right to health care." Advocates who are medical practitioners often champion the "rights of the health professions." The importance of human rights is reflected in the tenets of **liberal individualism,** a belief that an individual in a democratic society is shielded from undue forces and allowed to enjoy and pursue personal projects; that is, the individual has certain "rights." **Rights** are justified claims that an individual can make on others (individuals or groups) or on society, and may be considered as either **legal rights** or **moral rights.** *Legal rights* are claims that have a foundation in legal principles and rules; *moral rights* are claims that are justified by moral principles and rules. Moreover, a right, whether legal or moral, carries with it a corresponding **duty** that is placed on someone. *Duties* may be thought of as obligations placed on individuals, groups, and institutions by reason of the so-called "moral bond" of our interdependence with others. We expect to receive positive responses to our own needs and to be treated humanely. In addition, we form special relationships with our parents, our children, our spouses, our teachers, and our health-care professionals. Realizing our duties as radiologic technologists helps us to know to whom and what we are accountable. For this reason, rights-based ethical reasoning can have great appeal to beginning practitioners. However, radiologic technologists who attempt to apply rights theory to ethical dilemmas must be cautious because they may encounter considerable tension between what they envision as professional duties and what their patients claim as human rights.

Principle-based ethics, or **principlism,** the use of moral principles as a basis for defending a chosen path of action in resolving an ethical dilemma, has been widely accepted by medical communities. **Moral principles** (also referred to as *ethical principles*) are general, universal guides to action that are derived from so-called basic moral truths that should be respected unless there is a morally compelling reason not to do so. Moral principles include not only the two principles traditionally associated with the health-care professions, **beneficence** and **nonmaleficence,** but several newer principles such as **justice, autonomy, veracity,** and **fidelity.** Most professional codes of ethics are based primarily on the principle of *beneficence*; that is, the codes encourage practitioners to engage in actions that ultimately benefit their patients. For example, the Code of Ethics for radiologic technologists states that the ethical radiologic technologist "acts in the best interest of the patient," a clear appeal to beneficence. While these principles seem forbidding and difficult to grasp, they can be understood with some careful reading and reflection. Box 20–1 provides some definitions and examples of ethical principles to help clarify these difficult concepts.

BOX 20–1

Selected Ethical Principles	
Beneficence	Actions to benefit others. Decide and act always to benefit the patient.
Nonmaleficence	Above all, do no harm. Never perform or allow acts that may harm the patient.
Autonomy	Actions that respect the independence of other persons. The patient must decide what is done to his or her person.
Veracity	Being truthful is right. To tell the truth is expected.
Fidelity	Acts that observe covenants or promises are right. Be faithful.
Justice	Acts that ensure the fair distribution of goods and harm are right. Be fair.

Living a good life, becoming a good person, and acquiring certain desirable characteristics (called **virtues**) has been the main goal of ethics during most of its long history. **Virtue-based ethics,** the use of virtues in establishing right reason in action, offers the opportunity to include the character of each participant involved in an ethical dilemma and is an especially important consideration when linked to principlism. Virtues include such character traits as caring, faith, trust, hope, compassion, courage, and fidelity. Principle 2 of the ARRT Code of Ethics emphasizes this call to virtue by pledging the intent of the profession "to provide services to humanity with full respect for the dignity of mankind."

Patient Care and Interprofessional Relationships

Like members of the other allied health professions, radiologic technologists place a high value on quality patient care and solid interprofessional relationships. This section will help you explore these relationships in the context of ethical dilemmas that you may face in your professional practice. We have also provided several case studies to help you work through the problem-solving approach outlined earlier. We have analyzed the first case for you by way of illustration; the other cases give you an opportunity to practice using the problem-solving approach.

PATIENT RELATIONSHIPS

Two of the most frequently encountered ethical issues that affect the relationship between radiologic technologists and their patients involve maintaining patient faithfulness (i.e., keeping faith with our patients) and especially maintaining patient confidentiality. The following cases illustrate the types of problems associated with these ethical issues.

Case 1: Maintaining Patient Faithfulness

Radiologic technologists are often confronted by situations that test their ability to deal with sensitive patient care information. In many instances, the duty to respect the patient's confidences is compromised by pressures from authority figures or other individuals who may not share the radiologic technologist's value system.

"Do You Think My Doctor is Doing the Right Thing?"

Mrs. Brown, a 27-year-old patient of Dr. Smith, looks apprehensive as you begin your radiologic procedure. Mrs. Brown has found a lump in her breast and is worried about the possibility of having to endure a mastectomy. Your mammographic examination reveals that Mrs. Brown probably is only suffering from a small fibroid cyst. Mrs. Brown confides to you that Dr. Smith has mentioned the possibility of surgery. You are also aware that, given a choice, Dr. Smith nearly always operates. As you conclude your procedure, Mrs. Brown asks you whether surgery is indicated, adding, "Do you think my doctor is doing the right thing?"

IDENTIFYING THE PROBLEM. In this case, Mrs. Brown is seeking information that you may or may not be at liberty to provide. On one hand, as a health care professional, you sense a duty to provide Mrs. Brown with all the information available to you at this point about her condition. On the other hand, you feel a professional loyalty toward Dr. Smith and all other health professionals involved with Mrs. Brown's case.

DEVELOPING ALTERNATIVE SOLUTIONS. You could respond to Mrs. Brown's question truthfully by revealing your understanding of her medical condition and your concerns about Dr. Smith's tendency to employ surgery as a primary treatment. Alternatively, you could try to avoid answering her questions directly. Finally, you could refer Mrs. Brown's questions to Dr. Smith or some other physician in whom you have more confidence.

SELECTING THE BEST SOLUTION. The first alternative forces you to choose between being truthful to Mrs. Brown (veracity), possibly saving her from some harm (nonmaleficence), or maintaining your loyal relationship with Dr. Smith. The second alternative forces you to be evasive (and possibly untruthful) with your answers, thereby compromising your respect for Mrs. Brown's right to make informed decisions about her care (autonomy). The final alternative seems to be the best solution because it not only allows you to include Dr. Smith (or another physician) in Mrs. Brown's decision-making process, but it also places a high value on actions that may ultimately benefit Mrs. Brown (beneficence).

DEFENDING YOUR SELECTION. Principle 5 of the Code of Ethics states that the radiologic technologist "assesses situations, exercises care, discretion and judgment, assumes responsibility for professional decisions, and acts in the best interest of the patient." In this particular case, being completely truthful to Mrs. Brown may create unnecessary anxiety or cause her to question Dr. Smith's competence. By referring Mrs. Brown's questions to Dr. Smith and tactfully suggesting that she may wish to seek a second opinion if she has lingering concerns, we support Dr. Smith's treatment plan while allowing Mrs. Brown to become more involved in making decisions affecting her personal health care.

Case 2: Maintaining Patient Confidentiality

Of all the values associated with radiologic practice, patient **confidentiality** is the most easily identified and the most prevalent. On the surface, it seems that the trust that patients place in their health care providers cannot be compromised. Information obtained directly from the patient, observed, or obtained from other sources should be kept strictly confidential. The radiologic technologist should be alert to situations that may compromise patient confidences.

"Does Mr. Gray Have Cancer?"

The films you took of Mr. Gray do not look good. As a matter of fact, you overheard Dr. Jones mutter about the "advanced stage" of Mr. Gray's condition. The transporting aide wheels Mr. Gray back to his room and returns with your next patient. The patient slips behind a screen to change into an examination gown and is out of earshot. "Mr. Gray seemed real depressed," the aide volunteers. "How did his film look? Does Mr. Gray have cancer?" The aide is a good friend of yours and has always seemed committed to good patient care. How do you respond?

IDENTIFYING THE PROBLEM. Is Mr. Gray's condition confidential? Is an aide considered a member of the health care team? Does your friendship with the aide (loyalty) play a role in this case?

DEVELOPING ALTERNATIVE SOLUTIONS. Would Mr. Gray's confidence be compromised by telling the aide the truth? Should you refer the aide to Mr. Gray or to Mr. Gray's physician? Or is Mr. Gray's condition none of the aide's business?

SELECTING THE BEST SOLUTION. What solution would satisfy your professional ethics, the aide's curiosity, and Mr. Gray's right to privacy? Is there any possible action that would benefit Mr. Gray?

DEFENDING YOUR SELECTION. What principles in the Code of Ethics apply to this case? Is it possible to take an action that will strike a balance between providing a benefit to Mr. Gray and protecting his right to privacy?

PHYSICIAN RELATIONSHIPS

As a radiologic technologist, your relationships with physicians will be one of the most important aspects of your professional practice. Loyalty, faithfulness, and fairness are virtues all health professionals need to share with one another. Observing professional discretion in your relationships with physicians and recognizing your professional limitations in practice will serve as a firm foundation for maintaining your ethical standards.

Case 3: Observing Professional Discretion

Radiologic technologists see, hear, and experience a wide variety of personal and sensitive patient care activities. Radiologic technologists must both respect the confidences of their patients and safeguard the knowledge they obtain through their everyday practice activities. Questions concerning the competency or professional judgment of the physicians working with you often raise serious ethical issues and should be handled with professional discretion.

"I Think Dr. Jones Misread the Film."

You have just finished a routine radiologic procedure on Mrs. Green. As you develop the film, it becomes clear that Mrs. Green is probably suffering from a rare form of bone disease. Dr. Jones, a young resident, glances at the film and smiles. "I didn't think Mrs. Green had anything to worry about," he says. "That joint pain she was complaining about must be all in her head." Later, you see Dr. Jones talking to Mrs. Green's family. He is smiling and joking with them as he signs Mrs. Green's discharge papers. Shaken, you mutter to yourself, "I think Dr. Jones misread the film." What action, if any, should you take?

IDENTIFYING THE PROBLEM. Do you have an equal degree of loyalty to both Mrs. Green and Dr. Jones? Are there conflicting professional duties present in this case?

DEVELOPING ALTERNATIVE SOLUTIONS. Is this a personal matter between you and Dr. Jones? Should you discuss the issue with Dr. Jones's chief resident? The medical board? Mrs. Green or her family?

SELECTING THE BEST SOLUTION. Does a radiologic technologist have a professional obligation to point out a physician's possible errors?

Does Mrs. Green have a right to know about her possible serious condition?

DEFENDING YOUR SELECTION. Principle 6 of the Code of Ethics states that "interpretation and diagnosis are outside the scope of practice" for radiologic technologists. Does this principle apply in this case?

Case 4: Recognizing Professional Limitations

Like other health professionals, radiologic technologists have a specific role to perform on the health care team. Teamwork implies cooperation as well as a sharing of professional functions. Radiologic technologists should be aware of the limitations of their professional practice.

"In My Opinion, You'll Be Just Fine."

You are assisting Dr. Roe with a particularly complicated radiation treatment. Mr. Black has been on the table for nearly an hour and is clearly exhausted. As Dr. Roe leaves the area to respond to a page, Mr. Black groans as you help him off the table into his wheelchair and begins asking questions about his condition. "Is Dr. Roe doing the right thing? I feel terrible. What do you think?" Mr. Black has acquired a reputation of being somewhat of a hypochondriac. You are aware that Mr. Black is being treated for cancer and has a 50/50 chance of remission. Your initial impulse is to reassure him with a smile and say something like, "In my opinion, you'll be just fine."

IDENTIFYING THE PROBLEM. How do radiologic technologists identify the boundaries of their professional practice? Does your compassion for Mr. Black supersede your duty to respect your boundary of professional practice?

DEVELOPING ALTERNATIVE SOLUTIONS. Do you have a duty to respond to Mr. Black's questions? Should you follow your first impulse and simply reassure Mr. Black? Should you alert Dr. Roe to Mr. Black's concerns?

SELECTING THE BEST SOLUTION. Does Mr. Black share your value system? Do all your alternative solutions respect the values of the individuals associated with this case?

DEFENDING YOUR SELECTION. Principle 5 of the Code of Ethics states that radiologic tech-

nologists should always act "in the best interest of the patient." Can your decision be justified by this principle?

RELATIONSHIPS WITH OTHER HEALTH PROFESSIONALS

Although your primary professional responsibilities are to the physicians with whom you work, the radiologic technologist also interacts with a wide range of other health professionals. These relationships often provide a source of satisfaction and support but can be marred by so-called turf battles or role conflicts and unrealistic practice expectations. While most of us have grown up with a sense of loyalty and a corresponding aversion to report bad behavior in others, health care professionals have a special obligation to place the interests of their patients before such personal loyalty.

Case 5: Reporting Unethical Conduct in Others

Radiologic technologists have an ethical obligation to provide "quality patient care" and act "in the best interest of the patient." Taken to its logical extension, this obligation includes the reporting of unethical conduct in other health professionals.

"Do You Think Nurse Smith is Abusing Drugs?"

During your lunch break on the night shift, you decide to visit with Miss White, a patient with whom you have struck up a friendship. Miss White's room is directly across from the nursing station and she tells you she has noticed Nurse Smith slipping medications from the drug cart into her pocket. You recall seeing Nurse Smith occasionally swallowing some pills while on duty, but you had thought little about it up to this point. Since Nurse Smith is the only nurse providing patient care during this shift, you are concerned about the quality of patient care as well as Nurse Smith's health. Miss White asks, "Do you think Nurse Smith is abusing drugs?" You answer, "I hope not," but feel you must confront Nurse Smith directly. Despite your best efforts to be tactful, Nurse Smith explodes, "What I do on this ward is none of your business!" What do you do next?

IDENTIFYING THE PROBLEM. You have met the initial obligation to identify unprofessional conduct. Do you have an obligation to carry your complaint to Nurse Smith's superiors? What competing loyalties are involved in this case?

DEVELOPING ALTERNATIVE SOLUTIONS. Once you have confronted Nurse Smith, can you let the matter rest? Should Miss White become involved as a witness or complainant? Should you tell Nurse Smith's supervisor? Someone in the hospital administration? Call the police?

SELECTING THE BEST SOLUTION. What solution would both best serve Nurse Smith and improve patient care on her ward? Can you choose between your ethical obligation to report unprofessional behavior and good patient care? What balance should exist between "doing no harm" to the patient and loyalty to your colleagues?

DEFENDING YOUR SELECTION. Principle 9 of the Code of Ethics states that the radiologic technologist "respects confidences entrusted in the course of professional practice." Does this principle apply in this case? Do other personal values that you hold apply?

DEALING WITH MISTAKES

All humans make mistakes, and health care professionals are no exception. Because of the life-and-death nature of medical practice, mistakes made by health care professionals can create considerable, though unintentional, harm to patients. A full response to the human dimensions of health care requires that all persons involved be prepared to act faithfully and honestly when a patient-care mistake has been made. Radiologic technologists will make mistakes, due to the lack of attention to detail, preoccupation with other matters, or even a lack of professional commitment. A mistake can place significant emotional, financial, and psychological burdens on everyone involved, in addition to the possible harm caused to the patient.

Case 6: Dealing With Mistakes

Including patients in the resolution of a practice error also presents an opportunity for them to practice the virtue of forgiveness. Nonetheless, it is far more desirable to develop safeguards in your practice that will prevent mistakes. Dealing with mistakes openly in such a way that the patient and others involved know all aspects, including your remorse and proposed outcome, tests the mettle of the most experienced radiologic technologist and will require virtuous action, as the following case demonstrates.

"Keep This Matter Between the Two of Us."

Your assigned duties in the radiology department of the 1000-bed medical center in which you are employed are far from routine. The operation of the department is complex and at times hectic. Recently, the department head authorized a "tech check tech" system of work management in response to a shortage of staff and a dwindling budget. This resulted in the shifting of greater responsibilities onto your shoulders, including random review of image quality. During a monthly review of patients' examinations you discover an error was made: A chest procedure was ordered for a patient, but the examination performed was an abdomen that was ordered for a different patient. You immediately pull both patients' records and request a meeting with the department head who, after closely examining both records cautions, "Look, there is no harm done. Keep this matter between the two of us."

DEVELOPING THE PROBLEM. A potentially serious error has been made, but by the time it is discovered it seems clear that no real harm has been done to either patient. The real benefit and harm in this case, however, may not be with the patients involved; rather, there are others who may gain or lose, including the radiologic technologist who made the mistake and even the department head who authorized the management shift. More importantly, future patients may receive greater benefits if a more rigorous set of controls were instituted.

DEVELOPING ALTERNATIVE SOLUTIONS. Agreeing to the suggested silence would be the easiest alternative to follow. Another approach might be to request the department head to expand the meeting to include both patients, their physicians, and the radiologists and fully discuss the situation. Finally, you could request that an "incident report" be completed and filed with the medical center administration.

SELECTING THE BEST SOLUTION. Following the advice of the department head seems to ignore certain rights of the patients while at the same time shielding both the radiologic technologist and the department head from possible censure. Informing the medical center administration through an incident report may prompt beneficial management changes. The inclusion of the patients' physicians in the full discussion of the regrettable incident allows for the participation of both the concerned physicians and the radiologic technologists in the resolution of the incident.

DEFENDING YOUR SOLUTION. As mentioned in an earlier case, Principle 5 of the ARRT Code of Ethics pledges the radiologic technologist to act "in the best interest of the patient." Cases dealing with mistakes will often require the balancing of patient interests with the interests of others involved. Patients' interest in this case include not only physical well-being, but certain rights that need to be addressed.

Summary

The profession of radiologic technology shares the ethical concerns of other health professionals toward promoting good patient care. Radiologic technologists have emerged as health care professionals in their own right, as witnessed by their educational programs, licensure requirements, professional associations, journals, and a unique code of ethics that reflects their professional function in the health care arena.

Beyond subscribing to the principles contained in a professional code of ethics, however, radiologic technologists need to reflect on a broader base of moral principles in their ethical decision making. Moreover, ethical radiologic technologists must possess a keen sense of the role that human values can play in resolving ethical dilemmas that arise in their professional practice, both in their dealings with patients and in their interactions with physicians and other health professionals. By practicing the ethical problem-solving technique of identifying the problem, developing alternative solutions, selecting the best solution, and defending that solution, radiologic technologists not only can improve their professional stature but also can enhance the health outcomes of the patients in their care.

◀R REVIEW QUESTIONS

1 A personal value system can be defined in terms of:
   a) virtues
   b) values
   c) ethical principles
   d) all of the above

2 Professional ethics can be best defined as:
   a) reflective decision making
   b) rules of right living
   c) the science of rightness and wrongness of human conduct
   d) a common concern for collective self-discipline
   e) rules promulgated by professional societies

3 Which of the following statements is *not* true?
   a) Ethics apply to specific groups.
   b) Laws apply to political subdivisions.
   c) Morals apply to individuals.
   d) Morals control individuals within a group.
   e) Ethics control a group from within.

4 Which of the following statements is true?
   a) Codes of ethics are usually written by individuals.
   b) Religious writings form the basis for ethical control.
   c) Codes of ethics are a form of legislation.
   d) Conscience controls individual morality.
   e) Laws provide an internal control for society.

5 Which of the following statements is *not* true?
   a) Ethical dilemmas may have competing moral principles.
   b) Ethical dilemmas involve decisions based on human values.
   c) Ethical dilemmas are easily solved by codes of ethics.
   d) Ethical dilemmas can be resolved by problem solving.
   e) Ethical dilemmas invite a wide range of personal opinions.

6 Moral rules are best applied to ethical dilemmas when:
a) religious beliefs are strongly held
b) religious beliefs are not strongly held
c) the ethical dilemma is very narrow in scope
d) the ethical dilemma is very wide in scope
e) all individuals agree to use moral rules

7 Actions to benefit others is defined as:
a) veracity
b) fidelity
c) beneficence
d) justice
e) autonomy

8 Which is *not* a step in the problem-solving process?
a) Identifying the problem.
b) Developing alternative solutions.
c) Selecting the best solution.
d) Defending your selection.
e) Determining ethical sanctions.

9 The strict observance of promises or duties is defined as:
a) fidelity

b) justice
c) autonomy
d) confidentiality
e) veracity

10 Generally accepted customs of right living and conduct are:
a) codes
b) morals
c) laws
d) ethics
e) rules

BIBLIOGRAPHY

Golden DG: Medical ethics courses for student technologists. Radiol Tech 62:452–457, 1991.
Haddad AM: Teaching ethical analysis in occupational therapy. Am J Occup Ther 42:300–304, 1988.
Maestri WF: Basic Ethics for the Health Care Professional. Lanham, MD, University Press of America, 1982.
Purtilo R: Ethical Dimensions in the Health Professions. 2nd ed. Philadelphia, WB Saunders, 1993.
Veatch RM, Flack HE: Case Studies in Allied Health Ethics. Upper Saddle River, NJ, Prentice-Hall, 1997.
Warner SL: Code of ethics: legal implications. Radiol Tech 52:485–494, 1981.
Wright RA: Human Values in Health Care: The Practice of Ethics. New York, McGraw-Hill, 1987.

CHAPTER 21

HEALTH RECORDS AND HEALTH INFORMATION MANAGEMENT

Margaret A. Skurka, MS, RRA, CCS

Health information is indeed a strategic resource crucial to the health of individual patients and the population, as well as to the success of the institution or enterprise.

MERVAT ABDELHAK
HEALTH INFORMATION: MANAGEMENT OF A STRATEGIC RESOURCE, 1996

OBJECTIVES

On completion of this chapter, the student will be able to:

1 Identify major health information management department functions.
2 List key components of a patient health record in acute care.
3 List key components of a patient health record in alternate health care settings including ambulatory care and long-term care.
4 Describe how health record documentation affects hospital and physician reimbursement.
5 Describe the prospective payment system including diagnosis-related groups and coding and classification systems.
6 Identify coding as it relates to radiologic procedures and the reimbursement impact for hospitals and ambulatory care.

7 Identify components of quality management and the relationship of quality management to all hospital departments.

8 Differentiate between confidential and nonconfidential information.

9 Discuss the procedure for correcting or amending documentation errors in a patient health record.

GLOSSARY

Accredited Record Technician (ART): professional skilled in the collection, analysis, and reporting of health care data and provision of support to health care

Current Procedural Terminology (CPT): comprehensive listing of medical terms and codes for the uniform designation of diagnostic and therapeutic procedures; used in the United States for coding for physician reimbursement

Diagnosis-Related Group (DRG): system that categorizes into payment groups patients who are medically related with respect to diagnosis and treatment and statistically similar with regard to length of stay

Health Information Management Practitioner: term used to encompass both the registered record administrator (RRA) and accredited record technician (ART), since individuals with either of these credentials hold a variety of positions within the health information management profession

Health Record: permanent or long-lasting document of all patient care information that applies to an individual

International Classification of Diseases, 9th Edition, Clinical Modification (ICD-9-CM): universal statistical classification system used throughout the United States and the world for coding and reporting diagnoses and procedures

Joint Commission on the Accreditation of Healthcare Organizations (JCAHO): organization that accredits hospitals and other health care institutions in the United States

Prospective Payment System (PPS): system for Medicare hospital inpatients whereby payment groups are established in advance

Quality Management: process that monitors and evaluates the quality of the care and services provided to patients within a health care facility

Registered Record Administrator (RRA): professional skilled in the interpretation and analysis of health care data, design of information systems, and management of health care information systems operations

Health Information Management and Technology

Hospitals, ambulatory care facilities, emergency and trauma centers, rehabilitation centers, long-term care facilities, and home care programs all maintain **health records** on all individuals receiving health care services. Although these facilities vary according to the type and range of medical and health-related services they provide, they all have a common need to concentrate, within a single record, either paper based or computer based, all patient care information that applies to an individual. Such a concentration promotes effective communication among all the health care professionals involved in the care of the patient as well as continuity of patient care.

Every health care institution needs a health information management department that has been organized and staffed to provide adequate record management systems and practices. These systems facilitate the use of health records and protect the content of the record against unauthorized disclosure.

The functions of the health information management department are service oriented and support the optimal standards set forth for quality of care and services in the health care institution. Although the functions of the health information management department and specific demands for its services vary according to the type of institution, the common function of all these departments is the maintenance of health information systems in one or more forms to provide storage and ready retrieval of clinical information by patient name or number, physician name or number, diagnosis, procedure, and other subject items deemed necessary.

Health records can be stored as hard copy or

in miniaturized (microfilmed) or computerized form. The health information department's functions support the current and continuing care of patients; the institution's administrative processes; patient billing and accounting processes; medical education programs; health services research; utilization management, risk management, and quality assurance programs; legal requirements; and extraneous patient services.

Because clinical decision making and financial reimbursement depend on the information contained in the health record, maintaining complete and accurate records is essential. An error in recording the medications administered to a patient, for example, could lead to a life-threatening situation. An error in data reporting could mean a sizable financial loss for the hospital.

Since the implementation by the federal government of the **Prospective Payment System (PPS)** and **diagnosis-related groups (DRGs)** in 1983, the importance of several health information management functions has grown significantly. The coding of inpatient and outpatient diagnoses and procedures is of highest priority. Coding involves converting diagnoses and procedures into a numerical classification system. The numbers are reported to Medicare and other third-party payers such as insurance companies. Coding must be complete and accurate so that claims can be processed within prescribed time frames. The record has to be designed so that it is easy for the physician to complete the list of patient diagnoses and procedures at discharge.

The health record must also be complete and readily accessible to anyone who has a right to the information and the need to use it. The record is used for patient care, for hospital statistics and research, and for activities such as quality assurance and risk and utilization management. **Health information management practitioners (ARTs** and **RRAs)** must communicate needed data to departments such as radiology.

The Patient Record in Acute Care

Standards for the maintenance and the adequacy of health records have been established by the **Joint Commission on Accreditation of Healthcare Organizations (JCAHO)** as a part of its information management standards for hospital operations. It is the responsibility of the health information management practitioner to keep abreast of the standards for information management published in the latest edition of the *Accreditation Manual for Healthcare Organizations.*

HEALTH RECORD CONTENT

Regardless of the method used to record health information, the content of each health record depends on which health care facility department is treating the patient and recording the information. All departments that take part in the care of a patient must document that care in the health record. Documenting in the patient's record, or "charting," should be done by radiologists and radiologic technologists when a patient receives either diagnostic or therapeutic radiologic services. It is appropriate to chart information about the procedure, particularly information about contrast media administration, along with the patient's condition during an examination. This is routinely done as a part of most special procedures, especially invasive procedures such as angiography and myelography. Anytime a patient has an unusual reaction during a procedure, this information should be charted.

Neither the JCAHO nor the American Hospital Association (AHA) recommends any specific format or forms for use in hospital health records. Hospitals use forms and establish computerized record systems that best fit their needs. However, the JCAHO has established standards for health record content. The health record must contain sufficient information to identify the patient, support the diagnoses, justify the treatment, document the course and results, and facilitate continuity of care. Briefly, the standards for inpatient records require that the records include the following information:

- patient identification data
- medical history of the patient, including chief complaint; present illness or injury; relevant past, family, and social histories; and inventory by body system
- report of relevant physical examination
- diagnostic and therapeutic orders
- clinical observations, including results of therapy
- reports of diagnostic and therapeutic procedures and tests as well as their results

- evidence of appropriate informed consent (when consent is not obtainable, the reason should be entered in the record)
- conclusions at termination of hospitalization or evaluation of treatment, including any pertinent instructions for follow-up care

Radiologic technologists should be familiar with the health record format at their place of employment. It is often necessary for radiologic technologists to review the chart or access a radiology information system (RIS) to gather information, such as laboratory results, on their patients. A radiology department, in addition to using the hospital mainframe system for the master patient index or billing information, may have a department film tracking system. A computerized system tracks film and folders with a bar code system. Film control is a key issue, as lost or missing film can have a negative impact on patient care.

The JCAHO standards require that the health record contain evidence of informed consent for procedures and treatment for which hospital policy requires informed consent. The policy on informed consent is developed by the medical staff and the hospital governing board, consistent with legal requirements for appropriate informed consent. The term *informed consent* implies that the patient has been informed of the procedures or operation to be performed, of the risks involved, and of the possible consequences. By signing the consent form, the patient or the patient's representative indicates that he or she has been informed of and consents to the procedure or treatment.

An authorization for treatment, signed at the time of admission, is not to be confused with an informed consent. If, for some reason, the informed consent is not filed with the record, the record must indicate that an informed consent was obtained for a given procedure or treatment and where the informed consent form is located.

THE HEALTH RECORD IN RADIOLOGY

Before a radiologic procedure is performed, a radiology order or request for service should be completed. This order includes the patient demographic information (name, health record number, other identifying information), along with the specific procedure being requested. The physician ordering the procedure should

also be identified. These orders are typically sent to the radiology department by means of the computerized information system within the hospital.

The results of the procedure are documented on a radiology report (diagnostic, therapeutic, and nuclear medicine). These reports are included in the patient record to describe the radiologic services received by the patient. A physician, usually a radiologist, writes or dictates and authenticates a description of what is seen on the radiograph and the implications for the patient (Fig. 21–1). With therapeutic radiology, required documentation includes the amount of the dose of the x-ray or radioactive material administered as well as the date and time. Again, authentication is required on the report before it becomes a part of the patient's permanent record.

Any special reports documenting evaluation or treatment of a patient must be made a part of the patient's permanent record. The radiology department usually maintains a copy of the information submitted to the patient record with the hard copy images. However, the original document should be placed in the patient's permanent health record.

REQUIREMENTS OF HEALTH RECORD ENTRIES

Federal requirements and the JCAHO require that the medical staff of an institution have bylaws, rules, and regulations that include a provision for accurate and complete medical records with the original copies of documents in the patient record. Medical records must incorporate all significant clinical information regarding a patient. The record is the means of communication between the attending physician and all others rendering patient care.

There are various requirements throughout federal, state, and JCAHO regulations and standards that address signatures in the patient record. The JCAHO, for example, requires that all health record entries be dated, authenticated, and their authors identified. The use of a rubber stamp or computer-generated signature is of significance to radiology departments, since many radiologists choose to use this method of authenticating radiology reports. If a hospital allows the radiologist the use of a rubber stamp or a computer signature, there must be a signed statement available in the hospital's administra-

---

The Community Hospital
Anytown, Indiana

Radiology Report

Patient: Michael Carlton   Date Performed: 2/10/98
Patient Number: 012345
Dr. Erik Skurka
Examination: Chest, PA and Left Lateral

**Examination of the chest, PA and left lateral projection, shows no
apparent abnormalities of heart size or contour. The great vessel
and superior mediastinal shadows are not remarkable. There are
multiple large healed hilar calcifications but no other apparent
pulmonary abnormalities are noted.**

_____
Meredith A. Adler, M.D.

FIGURE 21–1. Sample radiology report for a chest procedure.

tive offices indicating that only the radiologist is in possession of the stamp or computer access code and that he or she is the only one who will use the stamp or code. A stamp or computer signature authorized for one person cannot be used by anyone else.

Regulations also address other medical record issues such as abbreviations used in the record, timeliness of documentation, record legibility, and correction of errors or omissions. Basically, an abbreviation in the record can be used only if it has been approved by the medical staff and if there is an abbreviation list on file that explains the abbreviations. Federal requirements mandate that current and discharged patient records be completed promptly. Record reports such as x-rays should be documented and completed as soon as possible after the procedure takes place.

Errors made in documentation are corrected by the individual who made the error. The individual should draw a single line through the erroneous documentation, write an explanatory note such as "error" near it, and then document the current information. The note should be dated and signed.

Health Record and Radiology Implications in Ancillary Health Systems

Radiology reports generated by a patient's encounter with health services need to be maintained in the patient's record, whether that be a hospital-based ambulatory care record or a record utilized in a variety of free-standing facilities. Examples of other health care areas in which radiology reports are often generated include emergency department encounters, surgery centers, ambulatory care facilities, physician offices, and urgent care centers. Ambulatory care records have similar requirements to inpatient care records. Federal and state regulations need to be followed as well as those of the JCAHO if the facility has JCAHO accreditation. The JCAHO specifies that ambulatory records include items such as patient identification; relevant history of the illness or injury; physical findings; diagnostic and therapeutic orders; clinical observations; reports of tests, procedures, and results; diagnostic impression; patient disposition and pertinent follow-up instructions; immunization records; allergy history; growth charts for pediatric patients; and referral information to and from any other health care facilities.

A long-term care health record is similar to an inpatient record. The long-term care facility can be subject to state, federal, and JCAHO regulations. In a long-term care facility, radiology services may be provided through a contract with an outside provider. The record must contain a written order for the service, and the actual radiology report should be dated, authenticated, and placed in the patient record. The physician is notified of the results of the diagnostic service.

Health Records in Reimbursement

PROSPECTIVE PAYMENT SYSTEM

Health record data serve as the basis for hospital reimbursement in the PPS using the DRG system. The concept of the DRG is that patients fall into statistically similar, diagnostically related groups. Therefore, the hospital receives payments based on the group the patient is in. The health information professional uses the diagnoses and procedure terminology provided by the physician and codes this information into the numbering system of the **International Classification of Diseases, 9th edition, Clinical Modification (ICD-9-CM)** and **Current Procedural Terminology (CPT).** Using a computer software program called a grouper, the health information practitioner computes the patient's DRG. For a Medicare patient, the hospital hopes to receive, as payment for its services, this DRG amount. The numerical ICD-9-CM codes are the basis for the DRG to which the inpatient is classified. CPT codes are used for outpatient encounters and coding for ancillary services such as radiology and laboratory.

The coding and classification functions of the health information services department have become more complex and significantly increased in importance since the implementation of PPS-based DRGs. The DRG classification is based on an inpatient classification scheme that categorizes patients who are medically related with respect to diagnosis and treatment and who are statistically similar in their lengths of stay. The health information management professional must be knowledgeable in the various case-mix classification systems used to measure the categories of patients and the types of patients treated by a health care institution.

A criticism of DRGs has been that the system does not take into account the severity of a patient's disease. Existing and available severity of illness methodologies go beyond DRGs to classify how sick a patient is. Clinical differences in patients with the same diagnosis can account for varying levels of care rendered and varying amounts of resources used. DRG payment is not currently affected but may be in the future.

It is important for management personnel in a radiology department to understand communication through the diagnostic codes of ICD-9-CM and the procedure codes of CPT. The correct billing process in a major revenue-producing department of a hospital such as radiology can be critical to a hospital's financial solvency.

THE CODING FUNCTION

The ICD-9-CM classification system is used for inpatient reporting. For outpatients, hospitals must report the diagnosis using the ICD-9-CM system and, in some instances, both the CPT and ICD-9-CM codes for the procedures. The physician's office uses the ICD-9-CM coding system for the diagnosis and the CPT coding system for the procedures. Radiology codes in CPT include diagnostic and therapeutic radiology, nuclear medicine, and diagnostic ultrasonography. The code numbers range from 70010 to 79999. For example, a chest radiograph, single view, frontal, would be coded as 71010.

Radiology departments may use the Index of Radiologic Diagnoses (IRD) of the American College of Radiology to classify radiologic specimens. This information can be used for statistics, for follow-up, or for evaluation of patient care. The JCAHO requires that information about important aspects of diagnostic radiology or therapy services be collected.

The IRD consists of a listing of diagnostic code numbers and an alphabetic index. The code number signifies topography and the pathology.

For example:

Osteogenic Sarcoma of Proximal Tibia
Code Number: 45.321

40.	Indicates Extremities
45.	Indicates Knee and Leg
.300	Indicates Neoplasm
.320	Indicates Neoplasm, malignant, primary
.321	Indicates Osteogenic sarcoma

The health information department would use an ICD-9-CM code to report this same diagnosis for billing and information management purposes. In this system, the code assigned would be 170.7. This is the code for a malignant neoplasm of the long bones of the lower limb.

Quality Management

Quality management is a process that monitors and evaluates the quality of the care and services provided to patients within a health care facility. The terms *quality assurance* and *quality assessment* are used to encompass all activities related to quality management, including utilization and risk management, infection control, surgical case review, medication usage evaluation, health record review, blood usage review, and pharmacy and therapeutic review. Quality management activities include work performed by various hospital committees and the medical staff as well as other professional staff from various hospital departments. A separate quality management department exists in many hospitals. In others, a unit or section within the health information management department is responsible for quality management.

The JCAHO's standards require that hospitals have a planned, systematic, and hospital-wide approach for monitoring, evaluating, and improving the quality of care and of key governance, managerial, and support activities. The JCAHO's current standards emphasize the following points:

- The activities are collaborative and interdisciplinary.
- New processes are designed well.
- The data are systematically collected.
- The hospital collects data on important processes or outcomes related to patient care and organization functions.

Data must be collected in areas such as the following: operative; other invasive and noninvasive procedures that put the patient at risk; processes related to medication and use of blood; the needs, expectations, and satisfactions of patients; and the staff's views regarding performance and improvement opportunities.

The JCAHO's standards also encourage the use of multiple data sources to identify problems and discourage the use of quality management studies for the sole purpose of documenting high-quality care. Examples of quality assurance activities in radiology departments include studying patient waiting times, doing "timely reporting" reviews, and doing equipment quality control.

The JCAHO's key steps in the quality assessment process for monitoring and evaluation are as follows:

1 Assign responsibility for the department's or service's monitoring and evaluation activities.
2 Delineate the scope of care or service provided by the department.
3 Identify the most important aspects of that care or service.
4 Identify indicators of quality and appropriateness for the identified most important aspects of care.
5 Establish thresholds (levels, patterns, trends) for evaluation (maximum allowable error rates).
6 Collect and organize relevant data, compare the data with the pre-established criteria, and analyze the findings.
7 Evaluate care. Compare actual rate to thresholds.
8 Take action to improve care and services.
9 Assess the effectiveness of the actions and maintain the gain.
10 Communicate the results to relevant individuals, departments, and services, and to the organization-wide quality management program.

QUALITY MANAGEMENT PLAN COMPONENTS

The JCAHO standards suggest a written plan for the quality management program that describes the following facets of the program:

Objectives—what the program is intended to achieve, at what level, and under what circumstances
Organization—the chain of command and the responsibilities of various persons and groups within the organization (a quality assessment committee may be assigned various areas of responsibility)
Scope—the program's emphasis on hospital-wide participation
Monitoring—the program's mechanism for the repeated measurement of various aspects of clinical decision making and patient management
Evaluation—the program's procedure for assessment and documentation of its effectiveness in meeting established objectives
Efficacy—the degree to which the care of the

patient has been shown to accomplish the desired or projected outcome

OPERATION OF A QUALITY MANAGEMENT PROGRAM

Each department or service is responsible for documenting the effectiveness of its quality management activities and for reporting such activities to the hospital-wide program. The staff members who perform the quality management coordinating function should, in turn, be responsible for demonstrating that the overall hospital program is functional and effective. The data must be consolidated and reported to the medical staff and to the hospital's board of trustees. Such a report might include a description of a process identified for improvement, the method used to identify that process, the department or service involved, the person assigned to perform the study, the data sources used, the cause of any identified variation, any corrective action taken, the person who implemented the action, the time table for implementation, whether the process was improved, plans for a monitoring procedure, and plans for restudy. The persons involved must remember that quality management activities are confidential matters, and special procedures should be followed to avoid or minimize possible incrimination of the parties involved. The JCAHO uses the evaluation or clinical outcomes as part of the accreditation process. The hospital must work to systematically improve its performance and must take action if it has identified an individual with performance problems who is unable or unwilling to improve. This may mean a modification in an individual's clinical privileges.

Legal Aspects of Health Records

The patient record is an important legal document that is used by the health care institution to define what was or was not done to the patient. The record may be submitted as evidence in court cases and used in any litigation in which the institution is involved.

Principles of both common law and statutory law have an impact on the legal aspects of medical records. Federal regulations affect an institution's participation in Medicare and Medicaid programs. Radiologic technologists or students may be required to give depositions or testimony regarding information in the health record or, in the case of a radiograph, testimony regarding the procedures involved.

CORRECTING OR AMENDING THE HEALTH RECORD

The proper method for correcting an error made by an author, as mentioned earlier, is for the author to line out the error, write the word "error," and then record the correct information. The individual should then date and authenticate the entry. The patient has the right to amend a record, but the original entry is not altered. The amendment then becomes a permanent part of the patient health record.

CONFIDENTIALITY OF HEALTH RECORDS

Radiologic technologists and students bear the same responsibility as all other hospital personnel to safeguard the confidentiality of health record information. Computerized information systems are a significant part of these records. Some employers require that any employee or student who has access to the medical record sign a confidentiality statement (Fig. 21–2). Technologists may be asked to release information to patients concerning results of procedures. It is the physician's responsibility to inform patients of examination results, and the technologist should refer the patient to his or her physician.

PRIVILEGED COMMUNICATION

States can enact statutes specifically recognizing the physician–patient privilege. If this legislation exists, a physician cannot testify in court or in any legal proceeding without the consent of the patient. A patient can waive this privilege through specific actions, such as bringing the subject of the medical condition into evidence.

CONSENTS TO RELEASE INFORMATION

Consents to release information from the patient record must be in writing and should con-

---

SAMPLE CONFIDENTIALITY STATEMENT

I understand and agree that in the performance of my duties as an employee of

_____ , I

must hold medical information in confidence. I understand that any violation of

the confidentiality of medical information may result in punitive action.

_____   _____

     Date   Signature of Employee

(It is recommended that this form be completed by any employee having access to medical information. It should be used as a part of an institution's orientation to its policies on the confidentiality of medical information.)

FIGURE 21–2. Sample confidentiality statement. (Reprinted with permission from Confidentiality of Patient Health Information, a position statement of the American Health Information Management Association.)

tain items such as to whom the information is to be released; the patient's name, address, and birth date; the extent of the information to be released; the date; and the signature of the patient or legal representative. Figure 21–3 represents excerpted information from the American Health Information Management Association (AHIMA) regarding disclosure of health information.

A department needs to protect itself against redisclosure, or secondary disclosure, of information. For example, a patient was transferred from hospital A to hospital B and information was sent from hospital A to hospital B to become a part of the health record. The patient is then transferred to a long-term care facility. Hospital B can only release information that originated at that hospital for the future care of the patient. It cannot release to the long-term care facility information that was received from hospital A.

FACSIMILE TRANSMISSION OF HEALTH INFORMATION

The use of a facsimile (fax) machine is commonplace in health care communications today. The instant transmission of data enhances patient care but also presents confidentiality issues. The AHIMA has developed a "Practice Brief" detailing an appropriate procedure for faxing (Fig. 21–4).

INFORMATION SECURITY

The confidential nature of paper- or computer-based records is paramount in this information-driven age. Hospitals and other institutions must protect patient information in the health information system. Figure 21–5 summarizes key points of access to patient information.

Disclosure of Health Information

Background

Complete, accurate health information must be readily available for patient care, but patients must be assured that the information they share with healthcare professionals will remain confidential. Without such assurance, patients may withhold critical information that could affect the quality and outcome of care, as well as the reliability of the information.

Disclosure of Health Information

Health records (regardless of the media on which they are maintained) are the property of the healthcare provider, but the health information contained in the records belongs to the patient. Disclosure of health information must be done prudently to protect the patient's right to privacy.

Each healthcare facility must develop policies and procedures for disclosure of health information in accordance with federal and state laws. To assure consistent compliance with these policies and procedures, disclosure of health information should be made only by those appropriately trained and qualified to do so.

Patient Care

Complete, accurate health information must be readily available for patient care. Information may be disclosed without patient authorization as required for continued care.

Nonpatient Care

Careful consideration must be given to any other disclosure of any health information, even that information generally considered to be nonconfidential. Although healthcare providers have no obligation to disclose this information, it may be disclosed to legitimate requesters on a "need-to-know" basis without the patient's authorization unless otherwise requested by the patient or his legal representative or prohibited by law. When disclosing this information, there should be evidence that the requester has a legitimate right to the information which is not inconsistent with the patient's best interests.

Rediscloure of Health Information

A healthcare provider's records may contain information about a patient from another healthcare provider. Such information is sent with patients who are transferred or referred to a facility for definitive treatment or continuing care. At times, a patient hospitalized and treated in one facility may be referred to another facility for diagnostic testing or therapeutic treatment not available at the first facility. The resultant reports are sent to the referring facility to be incorporated into the patient's record.

A provider may redisclose health information from another provider facility without authorization from the patient or his legal representative if it is needed urgently for the patient's continuing care. If time permits, authorization from the patient or his legal representative should be obtained prior to redisclosure to a third party.

FIGURE 21–3. Excerpted information from a disclosure document.

PATIENT ACCESS TO THE HEALTH RECORD

Regulations regarding patient access to health records vary across the country. The Health Insurance Portability and Accountability Act (HIPAA) of 1996 mandates that, within 3½ years, federal laws or federal regulations ensure the confidentiality of medical records. A patient or patient representative should have access, the right of copy, and the right of rotation, amendment, or correction of health care information concerning the patient. However, a collection of health information should be restricted only to the extent necessary to carry out the legitimate purpose for which it was collected. The HIPAA contains penalties for wrongful disclosure of individually identifiable health information.

In many states, patients have a right to access their medical records. Hospitals have the right to charge a copy fee to the patient for this record. The hospital also has the right to require a properly completed and signed patient authorization. A hospital does have the right to prohibit patient access when the provider reasonably believes that it is not in the best interest of the patient's health to have access or if the knowledge of the health care information could cause danger to the life or safety of any person. Radiologic technologists are sometimes asked by patients if they can examine their

Facsimile Transmission of Health Information

Transmission of Health Information

The American Health Information Management Association (AHIMA) recommends facsimile transmission of health information only when the original record or mail-delivered copies will not meet the needs of immediate patient care. The sensitive information contained in health records should be transmitted via facsimile only when (1) urgently needed for patient care or (2) required by a third-party payer for ongoing certification of payment for a hospitalized patient. The information transmitted should be limited to that necessary to meet the requester's needs. Routine disclosure of information to insurance companies, attorneys, or other legitimate users should be made through regular mail or messenger service.

Except as required by law, a properly completed and signed authorization should be obtained prior to the release of patient information. An authorization transmitted via facsimile is acceptable. If authorization cannot be obtained in cases of explained medical emergency, information may be released for patient care without authorization from the patient or legal representative.

The cover page accompanying the facsimile transmission should include a confidentiality notice that indicates the information is confidential and limits its use. A sample statement is provided below:

Confidentiality Notice

The documents accompanying this telecopy transmission contain confidential information, belonging to the sender, that is legally privileged. This information is intended only for the use of the individual or entity named above. The authorized recipient of this information is prohibited from disclosing this information to any other party and is required to destroy the information after its stated need has been fulfilled.

If you are not the intended recipient, you are hereby notified that any disclosure, copying, distribution, or action taken in reliance on the contents of these documents is strictly prohibited. If you have received this telecopy in error, please notify the sender immediately to arrange for return of these documents.

Reasonable efforts should be made to assure the facsimile transmission is sent to the appropriate destination. Destination numbers should be pre-programmed into the machine, if possible, to eliminate errors in transmission from misdialing.

FIGURE 21–4. Sample facsimile transmission of health information.

records while in transit, waiting for a procedure, or undergoing an examination. The record information should not be shared with the patient in this fashion because misinterpretation of information could occur. The technologist should again refer the patient to the physician for discussion of record documentation.

THE HEALTH RECORD IN COURT

The health record is a legal document that is admissible as evidence in court. A health information manager may be required to honor a subpoena for the record and take the record to court. The original record is never left in court, but rather a photocopy is used. The original record is then retained in the hospital health information services department.

Summary

The health information department is a key hospital department that affects many other departments. Health information departments do not render patient care but rather are identified as a support service department. Because of the coding function, health information departments directly affect hospital revenue and therefore hospital operation. The health record is the document that communicates information pertaining to patient care. The record is also a valuable tool in preparing health service statistics; substantiating patient care services and treatment provided; supporting medical education, health services, and clinical research; maintaining quality assessment and risk management; and making financial planning decisions.

Information Security: A Checklist for Healthcare Professionals

Access Control

❏ The organization has written policies outlining who may access patient information.

❏ There are mechanisms in place to control access to both paper and computer-based patient records. These mechanisms apply to all settings where records are kept in the organization, including physician offices that may have access to the organization's information system.

❏ There is a written organizational policy prohibiting the disclosure or sharing of pass-words, access codes, key cards, or other user identifiers, and the policy is strictly enforced.

❏ Passwords contain at least seven alphanumeric characters to make them more difficult to guess.

❏ Passwords are changed frequently and users are limited to one log-on at a time.

❏ Each user's access is restricted to the information needed to do his/her job.

❏ If a user attempts to access information beyond his/her security clearance with repeated use of an improper code, the system locks the user out or sounds an alarm.

❏ When a user leaves the facility, his/her password and access codes are deactivated immediately.

❏ Access to computer-based records is tracked by individual user to discourage unauthorized viewing.

❏ The information system limits mass copying, printing, or downloading of patient records.

❏ Periodic audits are done to see if the organization's policies are being followed and are still effective.

❏ If inactive paper-based or computer-based records are archived, they are protected from loss, defacement, or unauthorized disclosure.

❏ Access controls are in place for clinical systems such as laboratory, radiology, and nuclear medicine.

❏ Appropriate protections are in place to protect the organization's computer system from remote access risks. (Dial-up access enables outsiders to make repeated attempts to gain access without being visible to the organization using the system.)

Financial Data

❏ There are adequate procedures to protect patient-related financial data that contain diagnostic or procedural codes and other information that may reveal the reason for a patient's treatment.

Information Services

❏ If confidential information is transmitted via the Internet, it is encrypted to protect it during transmission.

FIGURE 21–5. Key points of access to patient information.

The health record is the legal document that attests to the care that was rendered to the patient. The record is a recapitulation of all patient care events. The radiology department contributes to this complete record by thorough documentation of all cases.

◄R REVIEW QUESTIONS

1 Which of the following is not a function of a hospital health record or health information department?
a) coding of diagnoses and operative procedures

b) documenting relevant patient information in the medical record
c) quality management
d) release of medical information

2 The prospective payment system is a payment system based on which of the following?
a) the DRG
b) the ICD-9-CM coding system
c) the CPT coding system
d) the resource-based relative value system

3 Which organization accredits hospitals and other health care institutions in the United States?

a) American Hospital Association
b) American Medical Association
c) Joint Commission on Accreditation of Healthcare Organizations
d) American College of Radiology

4 The chief complaint, included in a patient's history, is a statement made by the:
a) physician
b) patient
c) admitting officer
d) admitting nurse

5 The HIPAA of 1996 affects radiology and other hospital departments by its focus on:
a) patient record confidentiality
b) facility reimbursement
c) quality management
d) risk management

6 Which of the following is *not* required to be included in a patient's health record?
a) medical history
b) radiology reports
c) patient's phone number
d) physical examination report

7 Criteria used in quality management activities must be all of the following except:
a) clinically valid
b) diagnosis or procedure oriented
c) generally acceptable to department staffs
d) written

8 Assessment of problems in quality management activities must be:
a) ongoing
b) physician directed
c) subjective
d) objective

9 In making a correction to an entry in the health record, the individual should:

a) line out the error, authenticate, and insert correct information
b) erase the incorrect information and insert correct information
c) leave the incorrect entry alone and add the new correct information
d) remove the incorrect page from the record and begin a new page of documentation

10 The organization (chart order, forms) of a hospital patient record is determined by:
a) the JCAHO's required format
b) Medicare regulations
c) the AHA-suggested format
d) the hospital's own preference

BIBLIOGRAPHY

Abdelhak M, Grostick S, Hanken ME, Jacobs E: Health Information: Management of a Strategic Resource. Philadelphia, WB Saunders, 1996.

American College of Radiology: Index for Radiologic Diagnoses. Revised, 4th ed. Chicago, American College of Radiology, 1992.

American Medical Association: Current Procedural Terminology. Chicago, American Medical Association, 1997.

Cofer J, et al: Information Management: The Compliance Guide to the JCAHO Standards. 2nd ed. Marblehead, MA, Opus Communications, 1996.

Department of Health and Human Services: International Classification of Diseases, 9th edition, Clinical Modification (ICD-9-CM). Department of Health and Human Services, 1997.

Glondys B: Documentation Requirements for the Acute Care Patient Record. 4th ed. Chicago, American Health Information Management Association, 1996.

Huffman E: Health Information Management. 10th ed. Berwyn, IL, Physicians' Record Company, 1994.

Joint Commission on Accreditation of Healthcare Organizations: Accreditation Manual for Hospitals 1997. Chicago, Joint Commission on Accreditation of Healthcare Organizations, 1996.

Skurka M: Health Information Management: Principles and Organization for Health Record Services. 4th ed. Chicago, American Hospital Publishing, 1998.

Stewart L: Applying HIM skills to radiology management. J Am Health Information Manag Assoc 67(1):30–31, 1996.

CHAPTER 22

MEDICAL LAW

Ann Obergfell, JD, RT(R)

The liability of the technologist is not the same as the radiologist involved, but the liability is potentially real.

ALBERT BUNDY, MD, JD, 1988

The Law	**Privacy of Records**
Types of Law	
	Negligence
Standard of Care	
	Other Legal Theories
Causes of Action	Res Ipsa Loquitur
Torts	Respondeat Superior
Assault	Corporate Liability
Battery	
False Imprisonment	**Informed Consent**
Defamation	**Summary**

OBJECTIVES

On completion of this chapter, the student will be able to:

1 Differentiate between the various types of law.
2 Outline how the standard of care is established for radiologic technologists.
3 Discuss the concept of tortious conduct and causes of action that may arise from the behavior of a health care practitioner.
4 Argue the importance of privacy of records and the relation between privacy of records and patient confidentiality issues.
5 Explain negligence and the four elements necessary to meet the burden of proof in a medical negligence claim.
6 Explain the legal theory of res ipsa loquitur and how it may be used by an attorney in a claim of medical negligence.
7 Illustrate how a hospital may be liable under the doctrine of respondeat superior.
8 Justify the need for informed consent.
9 Outline the information a patient must have before an informed consent may be given.

GLOSSARY

Assault: any willful attempt or threat to inflict injury on the person of another, when coupled with the apparent present ability to do so, and any intentional display of force such as would give the victim reason to fear or expect immediate bodily harm

Battery: any unlawful touching of another that is without justification or excuse

Defamation: holding up a person to ridicule, scorn, or contempt in a respectable and considerable part of the community

False Imprisonment: conscious restraint of the freedom of another without proper authorization, privilege, or consent

Informed Consent: person's agreement to allow something to happen (such as surgery) that is based on a full disclosure of facts needed to make the decision intelligently— that is, knowledge of risks involved, alternatives, and so forth

Negligence: failure to do something that a reasonable person guided by those ordinary considerations that ordinarily regulate human affairs would do, or the doing of something that a reasonable and prudent person would not do

Res Ipsa Loquitur: "the thing speaks for itself"; legal theory requiring three elements: (1) that the type of injury did not occur except for negligence; (2) that the activity was under the complete control of the defendant; and (3) that the plaintiff did not contribute to his or her own injury in any way

Respondeat Superior: "the master speaks for the servant"; master is liable in certain cases for the wrongful acts of his or her servants

Tort: private or civil wrong or injury, other than breach of contract, for which the court provides a remedy in the form of an action for damages

The Law

Today's litigious society requires that all health care professionals, including radiologic technologists, be aware of the areas of the law that may affect the delivery of health care services. A basic principle of the law was defined in Schloendorf v. Society of New York Hospital in 1914 and lays a foundation for the relation between patients and health care practitioners:

Every human being of adult years and sound mind has a right to determine what shall be done with his own body and a surgeon who performs an operation without his patient's consent commits an assault, for which he is liable in damages.

This doctrine serves six functions. It (1) protects individual autonomy, (2) protects the patient's status as a human being, (3) avoids fraud and duress, (4) encourages health care practitioners to carefully consider their decisions, (5) fosters rational decision making by the patient, and (6) involves the public in medicine. Despite this carefully formed doctrine and its well-articulated functions, many members of the health care team take a paternalistic role in their practice and forget the patient's right to be informed of and to make decisions about his or her own health care diagnosis and treatment. This violation of patient rights, as articulated in the American Hospital Association's Bill of Rights (Appendix F), not only is improper from a moral and ethical standpoint but may well be construed as improper from a legal perspective. While it is clear that health care practitioners need to inspire confidence in their patients, they must remember this fundamental principle underlying the delivery of health care in the United States.

Medicine and the law are sometimes in conflict because each looks at a situation from a different perspective. One is looking to see that the patient's physical needs are being met through diagnosis and treatment, whereas the other attempts to control the abuse of patients and to ensure that they are compensated for injuries suffered at the hands of negligent health practitioners. Both processes are necessary to ensure that the patient receives the best possible care. To gain a better understanding of the relation between law and the delivery of health care, it is helpful to look at the law and how it may be applied to everyday situations in radiology.

TYPES OF LAW

The law is multifaceted and draws its principles from several foundations. The first and probably most important is the Constitution of the United States. This document, considered supreme law of the land, was written to separate powers of the three branches of government, the Executive, or the Presidency, the Legislative, and the Judiciary. The separation offers a system of checks and balances that prohibits any one branch from becoming more powerful than another. The Constitution also protects the individual rights of all citizens of the United States. Each state has a constitution that defines its government and articulates the rights of its citizens.

The second form of law is that enacted by legislative bodies or administrative agencies. This system of statutes and regulations is written at local, state, and federal levels and runs the gamut from who will drive cars to how citizens will be taxed. Many areas of health care are defined and regulated by these statutes and regulations. For instance, state legislators may adopt a statute that defines radiation machine operators and may, through statutes, delegate power to an administrative agency, such as a board of health, to establish regulations and guidelines that more closely define the practice. Examples of such definitions may include restrictions on who may practice and how ionizing radiation equipment is registered. These statutes and regulations may change from time to time at the discretion of the legislature or agency as needs and scopes of practice change within the profession. Legislators and administrators may also be persuaded to make changes if the profession or others find that the statutes or regulations are too loose or restrictive as written.

The third area of the law is case law, which is derived from the Common Law of England. This type of law is decided on a case-by-case basis by either a judge or a jury. The decisions in these cases may be precedent setting for future cases, but if the fact situation varies enough, the controversy may be decided contrary to what has gone before.

While the Constitution defines individual rights and the statutes define the practice, it is the case law that will dictate the fate of the health care practitioner who has been sued for medical negligence or malpractice. The judge and jury hear the facts as presented by both parties, which includes testimony from expert witnesses who testify as to the appropriate standard of care. After careful deliberation, the judge or jury will determine whether the practitioner violated the standard of care by performing his or her duties in a negligent or offensive way.

Standard of Care

Each profession or area in the health care delivery system has a standard of care. The standard for radiologic technology is not written in stone and is constantly changing because of the dynamic structure of the technology. Regardless of the changing nature of the discipline, it is necessary for guidelines to be established to help define the standard of care.

The general definition of the standard of care is that degree of skill (proficiency), knowledge, and care ordinarily possessed and employed by members in good standing within the profession. The test of whether the standard of care has been met by an individual under certain circumstances is to determine what a reasonable, prudent practitioner would have done under the same or similar circumstances.

The court looks to the profession as it tries to establish the standard of care for a particular practice. The determinative areas include federal and state regulations, job descriptions, curriculum guides, course goals and objectives, and professional customs and standards of practice. These areas are defined by expert witnesses who are generally educators or long-term practitioners in the area under scrutiny.

The standard of care will change and grow as the profession grows; therefore, it is imperative that all radiologic technologists keep abreast of current trends in the profession, since these are likely to be the standards to which they will be held.

Causes of Action

Newspaper headlines often proclaim huge monetary awards given to an individual as a result of medical negligence. These headlines are followed by stories of horrendous injuries patients suffered at the hands of negligent doctors, nurses, or other health care professionals. These cases are quite disturbing, but they are generally found to be the exception instead of the rule. Even if these cases are the exception, it is clear that the general public will not tolerate actions by health care practitioners that are less than the generally accepted standard of care. It has been estimated that 10% of all medical negligence claims are somehow related to diagnostic imaging either by improper diagnosis or by injuries to patients suffered during diagnostic procedures. Therefore, any radiographer may be called to testify at any time either as a defendant or as a witness to the practice of another.

TORTS

A patient's claim that he or she has been wronged or has suffered some injury, other than a breach of contract, for which he or she believes there is cause for an action for damages is known as a **tort**. This type of claim arises from a violation of a duty imposed by general law on all persons involved in a transaction or situation. For a patient to have a claim there must be some breach of duty on the part of the health care practitioner.

In a case against a radiologic technologist, the patient contacts an attorney if he or she has suffered some injury or thinks he or she has been injured while in the radiology department. The patient may also look for legal guidance if he or she believes that the care received has been less than optimal or that he or she has been threatened in any way. Although these legal inquiries may not lead to lawsuits, many of the complaints are based on legitimate concerns of negligent care or claims of assault, battery, or false imprisonment.

Assault

An **assault** claim may arise when a patient believes he or she has been threatened in such a way that there is reason to fear or expect immediate bodily harm. This fear may arise from comments made by a technologist to the patient before or during the examination. For example, threatening to repeat a painful examination if the patient does not hold still may be construed as an assault. This type of threat may appear on the part of the technologist to be innocuous, but if the patient truly feels threatened, the claim may be valid.

Battery

Likewise, if a technologist performs an examination or touches a patient without that patient's permission, a **battery** may occur even if no injury arises from such contact. Any unlawful touching may constitute a battery if the patient thinks that the technologist has touched him or her in an offensive way. Such a touch may occur if an examination is performed on the wrong patient or if a patient is moved roughly about the radiographic table while being positioned for an examination.

False Imprisonment

The more common claim of **false imprisonment** arises when a person is restrained against his or her will. This phenomenon is most prevalent with patients who are unable to cooperate, such as inebriated, senile, or pediatric patients. Each of these types of patients poses an interesting and often confusing set of problems that must be handled without compromising the quality of medical care.

Inebriated patients pose a problem in that they are unable to consent to treatment and may oppose restraint. The general practice in such cases is to speak with the physician who has ordered the examination to determine whether the requested procedure is of the utmost importance and must be completed immediately or whether the examination may be delayed until the patient is coherent enough to make informed decisions. If the examination must be done immediately, or if the patient is in such a condition that he or she may bring harm to self or the technologist, appropriate restraints may be applied.

In the case of senile, pediatric, or other incompetent patients, it is important to obtain consent to restrain or immobilize from someone authorized to give consent. This person may be a parent or guardian who has the legal right to make decisions about the treatment and care of the patient. This person must be informed as to the reasons for the restraint and the possible risks that may occur if restraints are not used before any such devices may be applied.

These principles may sometimes be in opposition to the paternalistic attitude of health care professionals. However, it is important that patient rights and autonomy be safeguarded by all health care professionals.

Defamation

Health care professionals have an obligation to maintain patient confidentiality and are required to keep all information concerning the patient, the diagnosis, and the prognosis in strictest confidence. This information should be shared only with those who need to know and who have a relationship with the patient in subsequent diagnosis and treatment. If information concerning a patient were leaked to individuals who did not need to know, and if the information was disseminated in such a way that the patient was subject to ridicule, scorn, or contempt or was injured in some other way as through loss of job or home, an action for **defamation** could be brought against the individual responsible for the breach of patient confidence.

Privacy of Records

Privacy of records and confidentiality are two principles clearly articulated in the American Hospital Association's Patient's Bill of Rights. Although the patient's medical record belongs to the hospital, the information contained in the record belongs to the patient and therefore may not be distributed without the patient's consent. The records, which include radiographic films, should be kept in a secured area with access given only to those individuals who need to know what is contained in them. The patient generally has a right to see what is contained in his or her records. In some limited cases, however, the physician may determine that the patient should not have access to the files. Such a case may arise when a physician believes that a patient may not be emotionally stable enough to understand or handle what has been written in the chart.

The AIDS issue has brought to the attention of health care workers the sensitivity of the concept of confidentiality of records. Information disclosed from records of patients who are HIV-positive or who have AIDS may cause them to lose their jobs or to be discriminated against. Such a breach of confidentiality may place a health care practitioner at legal risk for defamation or for negligence in the breach of the duty to hold information confidential.

Negligence

Medical malpractice litigation is predominately founded in a **negligence** theory of liability. Negligence is a failure to use such care as a reasonably prudent person would use under like or similar circumstances. Medical negligence uses this theory, but instead of the prudent person, the reasonably prudent health care professional or, in the case of radiologic technology, the reasonably prudent technologist is used as a model.

For a patient (plaintiff) to recover damages for injuries suffered because of alleged negligence, four elements must be proved: (1) a duty to the patient by the health care practitioner (in medical-related cases this is defined as the standard of care), (2) breach of this duty by an act or by failing to perform some act (deviation from the standard of care), (3) a compensable injury, and (4) a causal relation between the injury and the breach of duty.

For example, a patient arrives in the radiology department on a cart. After the radiographer has completed the examination, the patient is transferred back to the cart, but the side rails are not raised. In moving about, the patient falls from the cart and fractures a hip. The radiographer has a duty to protect the patient from falls by raising the side rails on the cart, and this duty was breached by the radiographer's failure to lock the side rails in the raised position. The injury element is demonstrated by the fact that the patient has fractured a hip as a result of the fall. The causation factor is generally the most difficult to prove; however, it would appear that the fractured hip was a direct result of the fall from the cart, which, but for the failure of the radiographer to place the side rails in the raised position, would not have occurred.

Each of the four elements must be proved before the radiographer can be found to be negligent. The evidence requirements may vary from one jurisdiction to another, and other legal factors may affect the outcome. However, these same basic elements must be proved no matter where the case is filed.

Other Legal Theories

Whereas negligence is the primary theory of liability in medical malpractice claims, attorneys may employ other legal theories to switch the burden of proof from the plaintiff to the defendant or to bring additional parties into the litigation. Such theories include res ipsa loquitur, respondeat superior, and corporate liability.

RES IPSA LOQUITUR

The legal doctrine of **res ipsa loquitur** sometimes arises in cases of medical negligence and is used to switch the burden of proof from the plaintiff to the defendant. *Res ipsa loquitur* translates to "the thing speaks for itself" and describes how a patient is injured through no fault of his or her own while in the complete control of another. In these cases, the plaintiff must show that the action causing the injury was in the exclusive control of the defendant and that the injury is a type that would not have occurred but for the negligent activity of the defendant. This type of case occurs most often in the surgical setting in which a patient is anesthetized and suffers an injury that would not have happened in the ordinary course of the operation. Radiology may be involved in such a case—for example, when a patient suffers a burn from a portable machine when the field light remains on while in contact with the patient's skin.

In a case in which the theory of res ipsa loquitur is raised, the burden of proof shifts from the patient's proving the negligence to the defendant health care practitioner's proving that he or she was not negligent.

RESPONDEAT SUPERIOR

If the radiographer in the previous scenario were sued for negligence, more often than not the hospital and surgeon would also be named as defendants. This legal theory is known as **respondeat superior** or "the master speaks for the servant." In cases of medical negligence, it is a well-established theory that the physician or the health care facility is responsible for the negligent acts of its employees. Many critics of this theory claim that this is a "deep pocket" approach to legal recovery based primarily on the fact that a physician or health care facility has more money than an individual technologist. Although this may be true in many cases, there are other reasons and strategies used when determining who to name as defendants in a medical negligence complaint. Such a theory is that a lone technologist on the stand is a more sympathetic character than a wealthy physician or hospital corporation.

CORPORATE LIABILITY

The theory of corporate liability requires the hospital or health care entity to be responsible for the quality of care delivered to consumers. This liability extends not only to actual employees of the corporation but to independent contractors, such as physicians who practice within the facility.

Courts have in recent years expanded the concept of corporate liability to include the following:

1 Duty of reasonable care in the selection and retention of employees and medical staff
2 Duty of reasonable care in the maintenance and use of equipment
3 Availability of equipment and services

Under these guidelines, the health care corporation has the responsibility to assess and evaluate the quality of care delivered and must be prepared to make changes as needed to protect the consumer of health care services. The corporation may be required to intervene if suboptimal care is being provided by one of its independent contractors.

Informed Consent

When patients enter a health care facility for examination or treatment, they place their trust in the health care professionals. This trust includes an assumption that the correct procedures are being performed and that the professional is meeting the appropriate standard of care. This does not mean, however, that patients relinquish their right to make decisions about their own health care. They rely on the fact that health care professionals must give them all of the information necessary to make an informed decision.

Only when patients have all of the information that they need to make decisions about their health care will they be able to give an **informed consent** for examination and treatment. Informed consent is required when a patient is subjected to any type of invasive procedure. In radiology departments, this consent requirement runs the gamut from excretory urography to interventional vascular examinations.

When patients are informed that a particular procedure would assist the physician in making a diagnosis, they should also be informed of the techniques that will be used to complete the examination, the possible risks associated with it, the benefits, and any alternative procedures that could be performed. A good example may be the patient who is scheduled for a myelogram. The patient should receive a careful explanation of how the procedure is to be performed along with an enumeration of the benefits and risks that may be associated with it. The patient should also be informed of alternatives such as computed tomography or magnetic resonance imaging and should be informed of the risks and benefits of each. All of this information must be relayed to patients in language that they can understand. It is impossible for a patient to understand the explanation of a procedure if the health care practitioner uses medical terminology foreign to the patient. This is similar to explaining something to a Spanish-speaking individual in English and expecting him or her to understand.

After the patient has been given all of the information necessary to make an informed decision, a consent form should be signed that documents the information that has been given. These forms are usually prepared by the health care facility. As a general rule, a consent form should contain (1) an authorization clause, to permit the physician or other health care professional to perform the examination; (2) a disclosure clause, to explain the procedure, its risks and benefits, and possible alternatives to the procedure; (3) an anesthesia clause if required; (4) a no-guarantee clause for therapeutic procedures; (5) a tissue disposal clause, if the removal of tissue may be necessary; (6) a patient understanding clause, which usually states that all of the information contained in the consent form has been carefully explained to the patient; and (7) a signature clause, which calls for the signature of the patient as well as that of a witness. The witness should be a disinterested third party who will not be involved in the actual performance of the procedure.

The amount of information given to the patient must be evaluated on a case-by-case basis. Every individual is different, so the need for information differs from patient to patient. The health care professional who is obtaining the consent must assess the patient as the information is received and base the disclosure of information on the responses and history of the patient. The circumstances surrounding the signing of consent forms are also important, and the department should establish a policy as to how consent forms are to be signed. The evaluation process in determining the policy should include when the consent should be signed, who will be available to answer questions from the patient, who will obtain the signature, and how it will be determined whether the patient is mentally and physically able to make an informed consent.

The patient's autonomy should always be considered when performing diagnostic or therapeutic procedures. If the patient consents to a procedure and then revokes the consent, the health care practitioner must recognize the patient's right to revoke and must stop the procedure at a point where the patient will not be injured in any way. A case such as this may arise during a barium enema procedure when a patient suffering much discomfort determines that he or she does not want to proceed with the examination. The radiologist and radiographer must comply with the patient's wishes by stopping the flow of barium and allowing any barium already administered to flow back into the enema bag. Simply stopping the procedure without allowing the barium to flow back may cause a subsequent injury to the patient, since barium not evacuated in a timely fashion may cause a perforated colon or other injury.

Summary

Radiologic technologists are legally liable for their actions in the daily performance of diagnostic procedures. They must follow the appropriate standard of care and should be well versed in current practice and procedure. They should also understand the civil liability of such actions as assault, battery, and false imprisonment. Any information the technologist acquires during the course of an examination must be kept in strictest confidence. The basic right to determine the course of diagnosis and treatment must always be recognized. Therefore, the patient must be given information that allows for quality decision making and the ability to give informed consent.

Health care practitioners who do not remain current in the field or who do not follow the accepted standard may be liable under the legal theory of medical negligence. Likewise, the health care facility and the supervising physician may be liable under the theory of respondeat superior.

◀R REVIEW QUESTIONS

1 If a technologist threatens a patient during the course of a procedure and has an apparent immediate ability to perform the threatened act, which of the following torts may be claimed?

a) assault
b) battery
c) negligence
d) false imprisonment

2 The legal theory of respondeat superior requires that:
a) the employee is responsible for the actions of the employee
b) each person is responsible for his or her superior
c) the employer be responsible for the employee's actions
d) the employee is responsible for the employer's actions

3 A technologist who has completed a procedure on a patient leaves the area grumbling about how he hates to do AIDS patients because he is afraid of catching the disease. A member of the housekeeping staff hears the technologist and asks who has AIDS. The technologist responds by giving the patient's name and room number. After this, housekeeping personnel refuse to clean the room. One person from housekeeping tells the story to members of her church, where the patient is also a member. After learning of the patient's condition, the church asks the patient not to return. What type of complaint could possibly be brought against the technologist?
a) negligence
b) defamation
c) assault
d) false imprisonment

4 The claim of false imprisonment requires the patient to show proof that the technologist restrained his or her freedom without consent. The defenses a technologist may raise include all of the following except:
a) the risk that the patient was going to hurt himself or herself
b) the risk that the patient was going to hurt the technologist
c) the life-threatening condition of the patient's health
d) the need for motionless films

5 In a case in which the legal theory of res ipsa loquitur is being raised, the evidence presented must show all of the following elements except that:

a) the injury would not have occurred except for negligence
b) the patient contributed to his or her injury
c) the defendant was in complete control
d) the patient did not contribute to his or her injury in any way

6 A consent form has been signed by a patient who will be undergoing an excretory urogram. A witness should sign the form after the patient. Who is the best witness?
a) a member of the patient's family
b) the radiographer performing the procedure
c) a ward clerk who has no relationship with the patient or the procedure
d) the patient's physician

7 Informed consent requires that the patient be given enough information to make an educated decision about his or her health care. The information the patient needs to make this decision includes all of the following except:
a) how the procedure will be performed
b) the benefits of the procedure
c) the alternatives to the procedure
d) the cost of the procedure

8 What complaint may be brought against a technologist if he or she touches a patient in any way without the patient's permission?
a) assault
b) battery
c) false imprisonment
d) harassment

9 A radiographer is performing an abdominal series on a patient from the emergency department. To complete the examination, the patient must be moved from a supine to an upright position using the remote control on the table. During this movement, the patient falls from the table and suffers a fractured hip. A complaint of negligence is brought against both the radiographer and the hospital. The elements the patient (plaintiff) must prove include all the following except:
a) a breach of the duty to the patient
b) an injury
c) a direct causal relation between the breach of duty and the injury
d) that the radiographer acted outside of his or her scope of practice

10 A patient consents to a procedure in the radiology department, but after it has started he decides that he does not want the procedure completed. The technologist should:
a) stop immediately
b) complete the procedure because the patient may not revoke consent once it is given
c) stop the procedure as soon as it is safe to do so
d) none of the above

BIBLIOGRAPHY

Anderson GR, Glesnes-Anderson V: Health Care Ethics: A Guide for Decision Makers. Rockville, MD, Aspen Publishers, 1987.

Bundy AL: Radiology and the Law. Rockville, MD, Aspen Publishers, 1988.

Capron A: Informed consent in catastrophic disease research and treatment. PA Law Rev 123:365–376, 1974.

Furrow BR, et al: Health Law: Cases, Materials, and Problems. St. Paul, West Publishing, 1987.

Furrow BR, et al: Liability and Quality Issues in Health Care. St. Paul, West Publishing, 1991.

King JH: The Law of Medical Malpractice. St. Paul, West Publishing, 1977.

Miller RD: Problems in Hospital Law. Rockville, MD, Aspen Publishers, 1986.

Pozgar GD: Legal Aspects of Health Care Administration. Gaithersburg, MD, Aspen Publishers, 1993.

Sanbar SS, et al: Legal Medicine: American College of Legal Medicine. 3rd ed. St. Louis, MO, Mosby–Year Book, 1995.

Schloendorf v. Society of New York Hospital, 211 NY 125, 105 NE 92, 1914.

PRACTICE STANDARDS FOR MEDICAL IMAGING AND RADIATION THERAPY

Introduction to Radiography Practice Standards

The complex nature of disease processes involves multiple imaging modalities. Although an interdisciplinary team of radiologists, radiographers, and support staff plays a critical role in the delivery of health services, it is the radiographer who performs the radiographic examination that creates the images needed for diagnosis. Radiography integrates scientific knowledge and technical skills with effective patient interaction to provide quality patient care and useful diagnostic information.

RADIOGRAPHER

Radiographers must demonstrate an understanding of human anatomy, physiology, pathology, and medical terminology.

Radiographers must maintain a high degree of accuracy in radiographic positioning and exposure technique. They must maintain knowledge about radiation protection and safety. Radiographers prepare for and assist the radiologist in the completion of intricate radiographic examinations. They prepare and administer contrast media and medications in accordance with state and federal regulations.

Radiographers are the primary liaison between patients and radiologists and other members of the support team. They must remain sensitive to the physical and emotional needs of the patient through good communication, patient assessment, patient monitoring, and patient care skills.

Radiographers use professional and ethical judgment and critical thinking when performing their duties. Quality improvement and customer service allow the radiographer to be a responsible member of the health care team by continually assessing professional performance. Radiographers embrace continuing education for optimal patient care, public education, and enhanced knowledge and technical competence.

EDUCATION AND CERTIFICATION

Radiographers prepare for their role on the interdisciplinary team by satisfactorily completing an accredited educational program in radiologic technology. Two-year certificate, associate degree, and four-year baccalaureate degree programs exist throughout the United States.

Accredited programs must meet specific curricular and educational standards. The Joint Review Committee on Education in Radiologic Technology (JRCERT) is the accrediting agency for radiologic technology programs recognized by the U.S. Department of Education.

Upon completion of a course of study in radiologic technology, individuals may apply to take the national certification examination. The American Registry of Radiologic Technologists (ARRT) is the recognized certifying agency for radiographers and offers examinations three times per year. Those who successfully complete the certification examination in radiography may use the credential R.T.(R) following their name; the R.T. signifies registered technologist and the (R) indicates radiography.

To maintain ARRT certification, a level of expertise, and awareness of changes and advances in practice, radiographers must complete 24 hours of appropriate continuing education every two years.

PRACTICE STANDARDS

The practice standards define the practice and establish general criteria to determine compliance. Practice standards are authoritative statements enunciated and promulgated by the profession for judging the quality of practice, service, and education. They include desired and achievable levels of performance against which actual performance can be measured.

Professional practice constantly changes and actual practice varies from state to state as determined by local law and community custom. Recognizing this, the profession has adopted standards that are general in nature. The general format was favored over a "cookbook" style or "step-by-step" approach that would be difficult to maintain in a changing environment and confining for those practitioners with an expanded practice.

The standards focus on the dynamic nature of the health care delivery system. The standards are adaptable not only to the area of practice but also to the locality of practice and institutional needs. While a minimum standard of acceptable performance is appropriate and should be followed by all practitioners in a specific area, it is unrealistic and highly inappropriate to assume that professional practice is the same in all regions of the United States.[1] State statute or regulation may dictate practice parameters. To conduct an appropriate review of the standards, one must look to the professional standard as well as local or state law that may impact the nature and scope of practice.

---

[1]The term "practitioner" is used in all areas of the standards in place of the various names used in medical imaging and radiation therapy, such as radiologic technologist, sonographer, or radiation therapist. Practitioner is defined as any individual practicing in a specific area or discipline. The profession believes that any individual practicing in one of the defined disciplines or specialties should be held to a minimum standard of performance to protect the patients who receive professional services.

FORMAT

The cohesive nature and inherent differences of medical imaging and radiation therapy are recognized in the general format of the standards. The standards are divided into three sections: clinical performance, quality performance, and professional performance.

Clinical Performance Standards

The clinical performance standards define the activities of the practitioner in the care of patients and delivery of diagnostic or therapeutic procedures and treatments. The section incorporates patient assessment and management with procedural analysis, performance, and evaluation.

Quality Performance Standards

The quality performance standards define the activities of the practitioner in the technical areas of performance including equipment and material assessment, safety standards, and total quality management.

Professional Performance Standards

The professional performance standards define the activities of the practitioner in the areas of education, interpersonal relationships, personal and professional self-assessment, and ethical behavior.

Each section of the standards is subdivided into individual standards. The standards are numbered and followed by a term or set of terms that identify the standards, such as "assessment" or "analysis/determination." The next statement is the expected performance of the practitioner when performing the procedure or treatment. A rationale statement follows and explains why a practitioner should adhere to the particular standard of performance.

Criteria

Criteria are used in evaluating a practitioner's performance. Each set of criteria is divided into two parts, the general criteria and the specific criteria. Both the measurement and specific criteria should be used when evaluating performance.

General Criteria

General criteria are written in a general style that applies to either medical imaging or radiation therapy practitioners. These criteria are the same in all sections of the standards and should be used for the appropriate area of practice. For example, a radiographer should use good professional judgment to make decisions concerning the adaptation of equipment and technical variables for a diagnostic procedure. Under these circumstances, the evaluation of the decision-making process concerning radiation therapy procedures would not be appropriate and should not be applied unless the procedure is diagnostic in nature, such as simulation.

Specific Criteria

Specific criteria meet the needs of the practitioners in the various areas of professional performance. While many areas of performance within medical imaging and radiation therapy are similar, others are not. The specific criteria are drafted with these differences in mind. For example, a criterion that calls for daily review of patient treatment records and doses to ensure that treatment does not exceed prescribed dose or normal tissue tolerance is imperative for those who practice in radiation therapy yet is not applicable to those who practice in the imaging professions.

A profession's practice standards serve as a guide for appropriate practice. Standards provide role definition for practitioners that can be used by individual facilities to develop job descriptions and practice parameters. Those outside the medical imaging and radiation therapy community can use the standards as an overview of the role and responsibilities of the practitioner as defined by the profession.

Radiography Clinical Performance Standards

STANDARD ONE: ASSESSMENT

The practitioner collects pertinent data about the patient and about the procedure.

Rationale

Information about the patient's health status is essential in providing appropriate imaging and therapeutic services.

General Criteria

The practitioner:

1 Uses consistent and appropriate techniques to gather relevant information from the medical record, significant others, and health care providers. The collection of information is determined by the patient's needs or condition.
2 Reconfirms patient identification and verifies the procedure requested or prescribed.
3 Verifies the patient's pregnancy status when appropriate.
4 Determines whether the patient has been appropriately prepared for the procedure.
5 Assesses factors that may contraindicate the procedure, such as medications, insufficient patient preparation, or artifacts.

Specific Criteria

The practitioner:

1 Identifies artifact-producing objects such as dentures, chest leads, jewelry, and hearing aids.

STANDARD TWO: ANALYSIS/ DETERMINATION

The practitioner analyzes the information obtained during the assessment phase and develops an action plan for completing the procedure.

Rationale

Determining the most appropriate action plan enhances patient safety and comfort, optimizes diagnostic and therapeutic quality, and improves cost effectiveness.

General Criteria

The practitioner:

1 Selects the most appropriate and cost-effective action plan after reviewing all pertinent data and assessing the patient's abilities and condition.
2 Uses his or her professional judgment to adapt imaging and therapeutic procedures to improve diagnostic quality and therapeutic outcome.
3 Consults appropriate medical personnel to determine a modified action plan when necessary.
4 Determines the needs for accessory equipment.

Specific Criteria

The practitioner:

1 Evaluates laboratory values prior to administering contrast media and beginning interventional procedures.
2 Selects appropriate shielding devices.
3 Selects appropriate patient immobilization devices.
4 Determines appropriate type and dose of contrast agent to be administered, based on the patient's age, weight, and medical/physical status.
5 Reviews the patient's chart and the physician's request to determine optimal imaging procedure for suspected pathology.

STANDARD THREE: PATIENT EDUCATION

The practitioner provides information about the procedure to the patient, significant others, and health care providers.

Rationale

Communication and education are necessary to establish a positive relationship with the patient, significant others, and health care providers.

General Criteria

The practitioner:

1 Verifies that the patient has consented to the procedure and fully understands its risks, benefits, alternatives, and follow-up. Verifies that written consent has been obtained when appropriate.
2 Provides accurate explanations and instructions at an appropriate time and at a level the patient can understand. Addresses and documents patient questions and concerns regarding the procedure when appropriate.
3 Refers questions about diagnosis, treatment, or prognosis to the patient's physician.
4 Provides appropriate information to any individual involved in the patient's care.

Specific Criteria

The practitioner:

1 Consults with other departments, such as patient transportation and anesthesia, for patient services.
2 Instructs patients regarding preparation prior to imaging procedures, including providing information about oral or bowel preparation and allergy preparation.
3 Ensures that all procedural requirements are in place to achieve a quality diagnostic examination.
4 Explains precautions regarding administration of contrast agents to nursing mothers.

STANDARD FOUR: IMPLEMENTATION

The practitioner implements the action plan.

Rationale

Quality patient services are provided through the safe and accurate implementation of a deliberate plan of action.

General Criteria

The practitioner:

1 Implements an action plan that falls within established protocols and guidelines.
2 Elicits the cooperation of the patient to carry out the action plan.
3 Uses an integrated team approach as needed.
4 Modifies the action plan according to changes in the clinical situation.
5 Administers first aid or provides life support in emergency situations.
6 Uses accessory equipment when appropriate.
7 Assesses and monitors the patient's physical and mental state.

Specific Criteria

The practitioner:

1 Performs venipuncture, IV patency, and maintenance procedures according to established guidelines.
2 Administers contrast agents according to established guidelines.
3 Monitors the patient for reactions to contrast agent.
4 Uses appropriate radiation safety devices.
5 Monitors the patient's physical condition during the procedure.

6 Applies appropriate patient immobilization devices when necessary.

STANDARD FIVE: EVALUATION

The practitioner determines whether the goals of the action plan have been achieved.

Rationale

Careful examination of the procedure is necessary to determine that all goals have been met.

General Criteria

The practitioner:

1 Evaluates the patient and the procedure to identify variances that may affect patient outcome. The evaluation process should be timely, accurate, and comprehensive.
2 Measures the procedure against established protocols and guidelines.
3 Identifies any exceptions to the expected outcome.
4 Documents any exceptions clearly and completely.
5 Develops a revised action plan to achieve the intended outcome if necessary.
6 Disseminates reasons for revisions to all team members.

Specific Criteria

The practitioner:

1 Reviews images to determine if additional images will enhance the diagnostic value of the procedure.

STANDARD SIX: IMPLEMENTATION

The practitioner implements the revised action plan.

Rationale

It may be necessary to make changes to the action plan to achieve the intended outcome.

General Criteria

The practitioner:

1 Bases the revised action plan on the patient's condition and the most appropriate means of achieving the intended outcome.
2 Takes action based on patient and procedural variances.
3 Measures and evaluates the results of the revised action plan.
4 Notifies appropriate health provider when immediate clinical response is necessary based on procedural findings and patient condition.

Specific Criteria

None added.

STANDARD SEVEN: OUTCOMES MEASUREMENT

The practitioner reviews and evaluates the outcome of the procedure.

Rationale

To evaluate the quality of care, the practitioner compares the actual outcome with the intended outcome.

General Criteria

The practitioner:

1 Reviews all diagnostic or therapeutic data for completeness and accuracy.
2 Determines whether the actual outcome is within the established criteria.
3 Evaluates the process and recognizes opportunities for future changes.
4 Assesses the patient's physical and mental status prior to discharge from the practitioner's care.

Specific Criteria

None added.

STANDARD EIGHT: DOCUMENTATION

The practitioner documents information about patient care, the procedure, and the final outcome.

Rationale

Clear and precise documentation is essential for continuity of care, accuracy of care, and quality assurance.

General Criteria

The practitioner:

1 Documents diagnostic, treatment, and patient data in the appropriate record. Documentation must be timely, accurate, concise, and complete.
2 Documents any exceptions from the established criteria or procedures.
3 Records diagnostic or treatment data.

Specific Criteria

None added.

Quality Performance Standards

STANDARD ONE: ASSESSMENT

The practitioner collects pertinent information regarding equipment, the procedures, and the work environment.

Rationale

The planning and provision of safe and effective medical services rely on the collection of pertinent information about equipment, procedures, and the work environment.

General Criteria

The practitioner:

1 Ensures that services are performed in a safe environment in accordance with established guidelines.
2 Ensures that equipment maintenance and operation comply with established guidelines.
3 Assesses equipment to determine acceptable performance based on established guidelines.
4 Ensures that protocol and procedure manuals include recommended criteria and are reviewed and revised on a regular basis.

Specific Criteria

The practitioner:

1 Maintains controlled access to restricted area during radiation exposure to ensure safety of patients, visitors, and hospital personnel.

STANDARD TWO: ANALYSIS/DETERMINATION

The practitioner analyzes information collected during the assessment phase and determines whether changes need to be made to equipment, procedures, or the work environment.

Rationale

Determination of acceptable performance is necessary for the provision of safe and effective services.

General Criteria

The practitioner:

1 Assesses whether services, procedures, and the work environment meet or exceed established guidelines. If not, the practitioner develops an action plan.
2 Evaluates equipment to determine if it meets or exceeds established standards. If not, the practitioner develops an action plan.
3 Analyzes information collected during the assessment phase to determine whether optimal services are being provided. If not, the practitioner develops an action plan.

Specific Criteria

None added.

STANDARD THREE: EDUCATION

The practitioner informs patients, the public, and other health care providers about procedures, equipment, and facilities.

Rationale

Open communication promotes safe practices.

General Criteria

The practitioner:

1 Elicits confidence and cooperation from

the patient, the public, and health care providers by providing timely communication and effective instruction.

2 Presents explanations and instructions at the learner's level of understanding and learning style.

Specific Criteria

The practitioner:

1 Instructs health care providers and students regarding radiographic procedures and radiation safety.

2 Educates the public about radiographic procedures and radiation safety.

STANDARD FOUR: PERFORMANCE

The practitioner performs quality assurance activities or acquires information on equipment and materials.

Rationale

Quality assurance activities provide valid and reliable information regarding the performance of materials and equipment.

General Criteria

The practitioner:

1 Performs quality assurance activities based on established quality protocols.

2 Provides evidence of ongoing quality assurance activities.

Specific Criteria

The practitioner:

1 Monitors image production to determine variance from established quality standards.

STANDARD FIVE: EVALUATION

The practitioner evaluates quality assurance results and establishes an appropriate action plan.

Rationale

Materials, equipment, and procedure safety depend on ongoing quality assurance activities that evaluate performance based on established guidelines.

General Criteria

The practitioner:

1 Compares quality assurance results to established acceptable values.

2 Verifies quality assurance testing conditions and results.

3 Formulates an action plan following verification of testing.

Specific Criteria

None added.

STANDARD SIX: IMPLEMENTATION

The practitioner implements the quality assurance action plan.

Rationale

Implementation of a quality assurance action plan is imperative for quality diagnostic and therapeutic procedures and patient care.

General Criteria

The practitioner:

1 Obtains assistance from appropriate personnel to implement the quality assurance action plan.

2 Implements the quality assurance action plan.

Specific Criteria

None added.

STANDARD SEVEN: OUTCOMES MEASUREMENT

The practitioner assesses the outcome of the quality assurance action plan in accordance with established guidelines.

Rationale

Outcomes assessment is an integral part of the ongoing quality assurance plan to enhance diagnostic and therapeutic services.

General Criteria

The practitioner:

1 Reviews the implementation process for accuracy and validity.
2 Determines whether the performance of equipment and materials is safe for practice based on outcomes assessment.
3 Develops and implements a modified action plan when testing results are not in compliance with guidelines.

Specific Criteria

None added.

STANDARD EIGHT: DOCUMENTATION

The practitioner documents quality assurance activities and results.

Rationale

Documentation provides evidence of quality assurance activities designed to enhance the safety of patients, the public, and health care providers during diagnostic and therapeutic services.

General Criteria

The practitioner:

1 Maintains documentation of quality assurance activities, procedures, and results in accordance with established guidelines.
2 Provides timely, concise, accurate, and complete documentation.
3 Provides documentation that adheres to current protocol, policy, and procedures.

Specific Criteria

None added.

Professional Performance Standards

STANDARD ONE: QUALITY

The practitioner strives to provide optimal care to all patients.

Rationale

All patients expect and deserve optimal care during diagnosis and treatment.

General Criteria

The practitioner:

1 Works with others to elevate the quality of care.
2 Participates in quality assurance programs.
3 Adheres to the accepted standards, policies, and procedures adopted by the profession and regulated by law.
4 Provides the best possible diagnostic study or therapeutic treatment for each patient by applying professional judgment and discretion.
5 Anticipates and responds to the needs of the patient.

Specific Criteria

None added.

STANDARD TWO: SELF-ASSESSMENT

The practitioner evaluates personal performance, knowledge, and skills.

Rationale

Self-assessment is an important tool in professional growth and development.

General Criteria

The practitioner:

1 Monitors personal work ethics, behaviors, and attitudes.
2 Monitors and evaluates orientation guidelines and recommends improvements or changes as needed.
3 Evaluates performance and recognizes opportunities for improvement.
4 Recognizes his or her strengths and uses them to benefit patients, coworkers, and the profession.
5 Performs procedures only after receiving appropriate education and training.
6 Recognizes and takes advantage of opportunities for educational growth and improvement in technical and problem-solving skills.

7 Actively participates in professional societies and organizations.

Specific Criteria

None added.

STANDARD THREE: EDUCATION

The practitioner acquires and maintains current knowledge in clinical practice.

Rationale

Advancements in medical science require enhancement of knowledge and skills through education.

General Criteria

The practitioner:

1 Maintains appropriate credentials and certification related to clinical practice.
2 Demonstrates completion of the appropriate education related to clinical practice.
3 Participates in educational activities to enhance knowledge, skills, and performance.
4 Shares knowledge and expertise with others.

Specific Criteria

None added.

STANDARD FOUR: COLLABORATION AND COLLEGIALITY

The practitioner promotes a positive, collaborative practice atmosphere with other members of the health care team.

Rationale

To provide quality patient care, all members of the health care team must communicate effectively and work together efficiently.

General Criteria

The practitioner:

1. Shares knowledge and expertise with colleagues, peers, students, and all members of the health care team.
2 Develops collaborative partnerships with other health care providers in the interest of diagnostic and therapeutic quality and cost effectiveness and safety.

Specific Criteria

None added.

STANDARD FIVE: ETHICS

The practitioner adheres to the profession's accepted Code of Ethics.

Rationale

All decisions and actions made on behalf of the patient are based on a sound ethical foundation.

General Criteria

The practitioner:

1 Provides health care services with respect for the patient's dignity and age-specific needs.
2 Acts as a patient advocate to support patients' rights.
3 Takes responsibility for professional decisions.
4 Delivers patient care and service without bias based on personal attributes, nature of the disease, sex, race, creed, religion, or socioeconomic status.
5 Respects the patient's right to privacy and confidentiality.
6 Adheres to the established practice standards of the profession.

Specific Criteria

None added.

STANDARD SIX: EXPLORATION AND INVESTIGATION

The practitioner participates in the acquisition, dissemination, and advancement of the professional knowledge base.

Rationale

Scholarly activities such as research, scientific investigation, presentation, and publication advance the profession and thereby improve the quality and efficiency of patient services.

General Criteria

The practitioner:

1 Reads and critically evaluates research in diagnostic and therapeutic services.
2 Investigates new, innovative methods and applies them in practice.
3 Shares information with colleagues through publication, presentation, and collaboration.
4 Pursues lifelong learning.
5 Participates in data collection.

Specific Criteria

None added.

Radiography Glossary

Artifact: False feature in the image produced by patient instability or equipment deficiencies.

Assess: To determine the significance, importance, or value.

Clinical: Pertaining to or found on actual observation and treatment of patients.

Competency: Having the ability to perform a task.

Contrast medium: Substance administered to subject being imaged to alter selectively the image intensity of a particular anatomical or functional region.

Contraindicate: To make the indicated or expected treatment or drug inadvisable.

Disease: A disorder or abnormal condition having a characteristic train of symptoms that may affect the whole body or any of its parts. Its etiology, pathology, and prognosis may be known or unknown.

Ethical: Conforming to the standards of conduct of a given profession or group.

Interpret: To understand and explain an image to provide a diagnostic report.

Interventional procedure: Percutaneous catheterization for diagnostic and therapeutic purposes.

Quality assurance: A comprehensive set of policies and procedures designed to optimize the performance of personnel and equipment.

Radiation protection: Procedures followed to prevent inappropriate or accidental irradiation of patient, public, and health care professionals.

Radiography: An image produced on a sensitized film by x-rays.

Venipuncture: The puncture of a vein.

PROFESSIONAL ORGANIZATIONS

Contact information for most of the professional organizations discussed in this book is listed below to assist those who require more information or who wish to join or become involved in professional activities.

Accrediting Agencies

Joint Review Committee on Education in
  Diagnostic Medical Sonography
20 North Wacker Drive, Suite 900
Chicago, IL 60606-2901
312-704-5151

Joint Review Committee on Education in
  Radiologic Technology
20 North Wacker Drive, Suite 900
Chicago, IL 60606-2901
312-704-5300
http://hudson.idt.net/~jrcert

Joint Review Committee on Education
  Programs in Nuclear Medicine
  Technology
1144 West 3300 South
Salt Lake City, UT 84119

Registries and Other Certification Agencies

American Registry of Diagnostic Medical
  Sonographers
2368 Victory Parkway, Suite 510
Cincinnati, OH 45206
800-541-9754 or 513-281-7111
http://www.ardms.org

American Registry of Radiologic
  Technologists
1255 Northland Drive
St. Paul, MN 55120-1155
612-687-0048
http://www.arrt.org

Nuclear Medicine Technology Certification
  Board
2970 Clairmont Road NE, Suite 610
Atlanta, GA 30329-1634
404-315-1739

State Licensing Agencies
  see Appendix C

Professional Societies

American Healthcare Radiology
  Administrators
111 Boston Post Road, Suite 215
P.O. Box 334
Sudbury, MA 01776
978-443-7591
http://ahra.com

American Society of Radiologic
  Technologists
15000 Central Avenue SE
Albuquerque, NM 87123-3909
505-298-4500
http://www.asrt.org

Association of Educators in Radiological
  Sciences
2021 Spring Road, Suite 600
Oak Brook, IL 60523
708-571-9183
http://www.aers.org

Association of Vascular and Interventional
  Radiographers
2021 Spring Road, Suite 600
Oak Brook, IL 60523
630-571-2266

International Society of Radiographers and
  Radiologic Technologists
ISRRT Secretary-General
52 Addison Crescent

Don Mills, Ontario M3B 1K8
Canada
http://users.aol.com/isrrt/isrrt.html

Society of Diagnostic Medical Sonographers
12770 Coit Road, Suite 508
Dallas, TX 75251
972-235-7367
http://www.sdms.org

Society of Magnetic Resonance
  Technologists/Society of Magnetic
  Resonance in Medicine/Society for
  Magnetic Resonance Imaging
2118 Milvia Street, Suite 201
Berkeley, CA 94704
510-841-1899
http://www.ismrm.org

Society of Nuclear Medicine—Technologist
  Section
1850 Samuel Morse Drive
Reston, VA 20190-5316
703-708-9000
http://www.snm.org

State and Local Radiologic Technology
  Societies
  Because many state societies do not
  maintain an executive office, we suggest
  contacting the American Society of
  Radiologic Technologists for current
  address and phone number. Local societies
  can usually be contacted through local
  radiologic technology educators or
  administrators or through the state
  society.

Radiologist Organizations

American Association of Physicists in
  Medicine
335 East 45th Street
New York, NY 10017
212-661-9404
http://www.aapm.org

American Board of Radiology
2301 West Big Beaver Road, Suite 625
Troy, MI 48084
313-643-0300

American College of Radiology
1891 Preston White Drive
Reston, VA 22091
703-648-8900
http://www.acr.org

American Institute of Ultrasound in
  Medicine
11200 Rockville Pike, Suite 205
Rockville, MD 20852-3139
301-881-2486
http://www.aium.org

The American Medical Association
515 North State Street
Chicago, IL 60610
312-464-5000
http://www.ama.org

American Roentgen Ray Society
1891 Preston White Drive
Reston, VA 22091
703-648-8992

American Society for Therapeutic Radiology
  and Oncology
1101 Market Street, Suite 1400
Philadelphia, PA 19107
215-574-3185

Radiological Society of North America
2021 Spring Road, Suite 600
Oak Brook, IL 60523
708-571-2670
http://www.rsna.org

Society of Nuclear Medicine
136 Madison Avenue
New York, NY 10016-6784
212-889-0717
http://www.snm.org

APPENDIX C

STATE LICENSING AGENCIES

Most states have licensing laws for radiographers in effect or under development (including Puerto Rico and the District of Columbia). Although the laws and regulations vary widely from state to state, all states that require licenses accept the Examination in Radiography of the American Registry of Radiologic Technologists (ARRT) to obtain a license to practice.

Students or radiographers desiring information should contact the appropriate agency for the particular state. Although addresses and phone numbers sometimes change, the most current for each are listed here.

Alabama

Radiological Health Branch
Division of Environmental Health
Department of Public Health
434 Monroe Street, Room 510
Montgomery, AL 36130-1701
334-613-5366

Alaska

Department of Health and Social Services
Division of Public Health
Radiological Health
Box H
Juneau, AK 99811-0613
907-465-3019

Arizona

State of Arizona
Medical Radiologic Technology Board of
    Examiners
4814 South 40th Street
Phoenix, AZ 85040-2940
602-255-4845

Arkansas

Licensing Accreditation and Registration
Division of Radiation Control and
    Emergency Management
4815 W. Markham, Slot 30
Little Rock, AR 72205
501-661-2301

California

State of California
Radiologic Health Branch
714 P Street, Box 942732
Sacramento, CA 95814-7320
916-445-0931

Colorado

Radiation Control Division
Colorado Department of Health
4300 Cherry Creek Drive South
Denver, CO 80222-1530
303-692-3077

Connecticut

Applications, Examinations and Licensure
Department of Public Health
Radiographer Licensure
410 Capital Avenue
MS #12 APP
Hartford, CT 06134
860-509-7568

Delaware

State of Delaware
Office of Radiation Control
Robbins Building
P.O. Box 637
Dover, DE 19903
302-736-4731

District of Columbia

Department of Consumer and Regulatory
  Affairs
Pharmaceutical Radiology and Medical
  Control Devices
Room 1016
P.O. Box 3720
Washington, DC 20013-7200
202-727-7218

Florida

State of Florida
Office of Radiation Control
1317 Winewood Boulevard
Tallahassee, FL 32399-0700
850-487-3451

Georgia

Office of Regulatory Services—X-ray Unit
Department of Human Resources
2 Peachtree Street, 19th Floor
Atlanta, GA 30303
404-657-5400

Hawaii

State of Hawaii
Radiologic Technology Board
Department of Health
Noise and Radiation Branch
Box 3378
Honolulu, HI 96801
808-586-4700

Idaho

Idaho Department of Health and Welfare
Division of Health
Radiation Control
2220 Old Penitential Road
Boise, ID 83712
208-334-2235

Illinois

State of Illinois
Division of Radiologic Technologist
  Certification
Illinois Department of Nuclear Safety
1035 Outer Park Drive
Springfield, IL 62704
217-785-9915

Indiana

State of Indiana
Department of Health
2 N. Meridian Street
Indianapolis, IN 46204
317-233-7565

Iowa

State of Iowa
Radiological Health Section
Bureau of Radiological Health
Lucas State Office Building
Des Moines, IA 50319-0075
515-281-3478

Kansas

Bureau of Radiation Control
State of Kansas
Department of Health and Environment
Bldg. #283, Forbes Field
Topeka, KS 66620
913-296-1562

Kentucky

State of Kentucky
Operator Certification Coordinator
Radiation Control Branch
275 East Main Street
Frankfort, KY 40621-0001
502-564-3700

Louisiana

Louisiana State Radiologic Technology
Board of Examiners
3108 Cleary Avenue, Suite 207
Metairie, LA 70002
504-838-5231

Maine

State of Maine
Radiologic Technology Board of Examiners
State House Station #35
Augusta, ME 04333-0035
207-624-8603

Maryland

Allied Health Programs
Department of Health and Mental Hygiene

Board of Physicians Quality Assurance
P.O. Box #2571 (4201 Patterson Avenue)
Baltimore, MD 21215-0095
410-764-4777 *or* 1-800-492-6836

Massachusetts

State of Massachusetts
Radiation Control Office
305 South Street, 7th Floor
Jamaica Plain, MA 02130
617-727-6214

Michigan

Radiation Safety Section
Department of Consumer and Industry
  Services
P.O. Box 30195
Lansing, MI 48909
517-335-8200

Minnesota

Section of Radiation Control
121 East 7th Place
P.O. Box 64975
St. Paul, MN 55164
612-215-0945

Mississippi

X-Ray Section
Division of Radiological Health
P.O. Box 1700
Jackson, MS 39215-1700
601-987-4153

Missouri

Medical Radiation Control Program
920 Wildwood Drive
P.O. Box 570
Jefferson City, MO 65102-0570
573-751-6083

Montana

State of Montana
Department of Commerce
Board of Radiologic Technologists
P.O. Box 200513
Helena, MT 59620-0513
406-444-4288

Nebraska

Nebraska Department of Health
Professional and Occupational Licensure
  Division
P.O. Box 94986
Lincoln, NE 68509-4986
402-471-4915

Nevada

Radiological Health Section
505 King Street
Carson City, NV 89710
702-687-5394

New Hampshire

Bureau of Radiological Health
Health and Welfare Building
#6 Hazen Drive
Concord, NH 03301
603-271-4588

New Jersey

State of New Jersey
Department of Environmental Protection
Radiation Protection Programs
CN 415
Trenton, NJ 08625-0415
609-984-5890

New Mexico

Radiologic Technologist Certification
  Program
New Mexico Environment Department
P.O. Box 26110
Santa Fe, NM 87502-6110
505-827-1557—Main Office

New York

Bureau of Environment Radiation
  Protection
New York State Department of Health,
  Room 325
2 University Place
Albany, NY 12203-3399
518-458-6476

North Carolina

Division of Radiation Protection
Electronic Production Radiation Section

3825 Barrett Drive
Raleigh, NC 27609-7221
919-571-4141

North Dakota

North Dakota State Department of Health
Division of Environmental Engineering
1200 Missouri Avenue, Room 304
Box 5520
Bismarck, ND 58506-5520
701-328-5188

Ohio

X-Ray Section
Ohio Department of Health
246 North High Street, P.O. Box 118
Columbus, OH 43266-0118
614-752-4319 *or* 1-800-999-1468 (Ohio
   only)

Oklahoma

Department of Environmental Quality
Radiation and Special Hazards
1000 NE 10th Street
Oklahoma City, OK 73117-1212
405-271-8118

Oregon

Board of Radiologic Technology, Suite 407
800 NE Oregon Street, #21
Portland, OR 97232
503-731-4088

Pennsylvania

Bureau of Radiation Protection
Department of Environmental Health
Health Licensing Division
P.O. Box 8469
Harrisburg, PA 17105-8469
717-787-2568

Puerto Rico

University of Puerto Rico
Medical Sciences Campus
Department of Environmental Health
G.P.O. Box 5067
San Juan, PR 00936
809-758-2525 Ext. 1424

Rhode Island

Professional Regulation
3 Capitol Hill, Room 104
Providence, RI 02908
401-277-2827

South Carolina

Division of Electronic Products
Bureau of Radiological Health
2600 Bull Street
Columbia, SC 29201
803-737-7400

South Dakota

Radiological Safety
South Dakota State Health Department
523 East Capitol
Pierre, SD 57501
605-773-3364

Tennessee

Board of Medical Examiners
Department of Health
426 5th Avenue N, 1st Floor
Nashville, TN 37247-1010
615-532-4384

Texas

Texas Department of Health
Professional Licensing and Certification
   Division
1100 West 49th Street
Austin, TX 78756-3183
512-834-6617

Utah

Division of Occupational and Professional
   Licensing
P.O. Box 45805
Salt Lake City, UT 84145-0805
801-530-6628 *or* 801-530-6551

Vermont

Vermont Board of Radiologic Technology
Office of the Secretary of State
Office of Professional Regulation
109 State Street
Montpelier, VT 05609-1106
802-828-2363

Virginia

Board of Medicine
6606 W. Broad Street, 4th Floor
Richmond, VA 23230-1717
804-662-9908 *or* 804-662-7664

Washington

Department of Licensing
1300 S.E. Quince Street
Olympia, WA 98504-7867
360-586-6100

West Virginia

West Virginia Radiologic Technology
  Board of Examiners
1715 Flat Top Road, P.O. Box 638

Cool Ridge, WV 25825
304-787-4398

Wisconsin

Section on Radiation Protection
Department of Health and Social Services
P.O. Box 309
Madison, WI 53701-0309
608-267-4784

Wyoming

Occupational Licensing Office
Wyoming Board of Radiologic Technologist
  Examiners
2020 Carey Avenue, Suite 201
Cheyenne, WY 82002
307-777-3507

PATIENT CARE LAB ACTIVITIES

STUDENT NAME: _____   DATE: _____

LAB 11–1: PATIENT TRANSFER TECHNIQUES

Objective

■ Demonstrate proper wheelchair and cart transfer techniques.

Equipment

■ Wheelchair and cart

Procedure

■ On completion of this laboratory activity, the student will be able to:

Stand-by Assist Wheelchair Transfer

	YES	NO
1 Position the wheelchair at a 45-degree angle to the table.	☐	☐
2 Move the wheelchair footrests out of the way and be sure that the wheelchair is locked.	☐	☐
3 Instruct the patient to sit on the edge of the wheelchair seat.	☐	☐
4 Instruct the patient to push down on the arms of the chair to assist in rising and then stand up slowly.	☐	☐
5 Direct the patient to reach out and hold onto the table with the hand closest to the table and then turn slowly until he or she feels the table behind him or her.	☐	☐
6 Instruct the patient to hold the table with both hands and then sit down.	☐	☐

Assisted Standing Pivot Wheelchair Transfer

	YES	NO
1 Position the wheelchair at a 45-degree angle to the table with the patient's strongest side closest to the table. If the patient has loose-fitting clothes, place a transfer belt around the patient's waist.	☐	☐
2 Move the wheelchair footrests out of the way and be sure that the wheelchair is locked.	☐	☐
3 Direct the patient to sit on the edge of the wheelchair seat, providing assistance as needed.	☐	☐
4 Instruct the patient to push down on the arms of the wheelchair to assist in rising.	☐	☐
5 Bend at the knees, keeping the back stationary, and grasp the transfer belt with both hands. Block the patient's feet and knees to provide stability, especially for paraplegic and hemiplegic patients.	☐	☐
6 Assist the patient in rising to a standing position.	☐	☐
7 Ask the patient if he or she is feeling alright. If the patient reports any feelings of dizziness or exhibits any of the other signs of orthostatic hypotension, let him or her stand for a moment until the feeling subsides.	☐	☐
8 Pivot the patient toward the table until the patient can feel the table against the back of the thighs.	☐	☐
9 Ask the patient to support himself or herself on the table with both hands and sit down, assisting as necessary.	☐	☐

STUDENT NAME: _____ DATE: _____

Two-Person Wheelchair Lift

	YES	NO
1 Plan for the lift by locating an assistant who will lift the patient's feet as you lift the patient's torso.	☐	☐
2 Lock the wheelchair, remove the arm rests, swing away or remove the leg rests, and direct the patient to cross his or her arms over the chest.	☐	☐
3 Stand behind the patient, reach under the patient's axillae, and grasp the patient's crossed forearms. Direct the assistant to squat in front of the patient and cradle the patient's thighs in one hand and the calves in the other hand.	☐	☐
4 On command, lift the patient to clear the wheelchair and move the patient as a unit to the desired place.	☐	☐

Cart Transfer With a Moving Device

	YES	NO
1 Move the cart alongside the table, preferably on the patient's strong or less affected side. Place it as close to the table as possible and then secure it by depressing the wheel locks. In addition, place sandbags or other devices on the floor to block wheels satisfactorily.	☐	☐
2 Place the patient at an oblique angle away from the table while the moving device is placed to the midpoint of the back.	☐	☐
3 Return the patient to a supine position so that he or she is halfway onto the moving device.	☐	☐
4 Grab the draw sheet and use it to slowly move the patient onto the table.	☐	☐
5 Remove the moving device, turning the patient obliquely if necessary.	☐	☐

Cart Transfer Without a Moving Device

	YES	NO
1 Move the cart alongside the table, preferably on the patient's strong or less affected side. Place it as close to the table as possible and then secure it by depressing the wheel locks. In addition, place sandbags or other devices on the floor to block wheels satisfactorily.	☐	☐
2 Begin by rolling up the draw sheet on both sides of the patient. Be sure that the draw sheet is completely under the patient and straightened before the transfer.	☐	☐
3 Support the patient's head and upper body from the far side of the radiographic table. Direct a second assistant to support the patient's pelvic girdle from the cart side and a third assistant to support the patient's legs from the table side.	☐	☐
4 Cross the patient's arms over the chest to avoid injury or interfering with a smooth transfer.	☐	☐
5 Direct the second assistant supporting the pelvic girdle to stand on the opposite side of the cart and make sure that the cart does not move away from the table during the transfer.	☐	☐
6 On command, grasp the rolled up draw sheet and slowly pull the patient to the edge of the cart. On a second command, slowly lift and pull the patient onto the table.	☐	☐

COMMENTS: _____

_____

_____

EVALUATOR'S SIGNATURE: _____

STUDENT'S SIGNATURE: _____

STUDENT NAME: _____   DATE: _____

LAB 12–1: IMMOBILIZATION DEVICES

Objective

- Demonstrate proper technique for patient immobilization.

Equipment

- Oblique sponge
- Finger sponge
- Strap
- Compression bands
- Sandbags
- Headclamp

Procedure

- On completion of this laboratory activity, the student will be able to:

		YES	NO
1	Position a patient with a sponge for an oblique lumbar spine position.	☐	☐
2	Position a patient's hand in a fan lateral position on a sponge.	☐	☐
3	Position a patient for an axial calcaneus position using a strap.	☐	☐
4	Position a patient on a table in a semi-erect position using compression bands.	☐	☐
5	Position a patient in an erect lateral cervical position using sandbags.	☐	☐
6	Position a patient for an AP skull radiograph using headclamps.	☐	☐

COMMENTS: _____

_____

_____

EVALUATOR'S SIGNATURE: _____

STUDENT'S SIGNATURE: _____

STUDENT NAME: _____   DATE: _____

LAB 12–2: PEDIATRIC IMMOBILIZATION TECHNIQUES

Objective

- Demonstrate proper techniques for pediatric immobilization.

Equipment

- Pediatric patient or doll
- Sheet
- Pigg-O-Stat
- Velcro restraint board
- Octostop

Procedure

- On completion of this laboratory activity, the student will be able to:

Mummification Technique

	YES	NO
1 Position the child in the center of a triangularly folded sheet so that the shoulders are just above the top fold.	☐	☐
2 Bring the left corner of the sheet over the left arm and under the body so that about 2 feet of the sheet extends beyond the right side of the body. Make sure the child is not lying on the left arm.	☐	☐
3 Tuck the 2 feet of sheet over the right arm and under the body. Again make sure the child is not lying on the arm.	☐	☐
4 Bring the remaining sheet over the body, tucking the sheet securely under the left side of the body. Secure the sheet in place with tape.	☐	☐

Using Specialized Pediatric Immobilization Devices

	YES	NO
1 Position a pediatric patient in a Pigg-O-Stat for an AP chest radiograph.	☐	☐
2 Position a pediatric patient on a Velcro strap restraint board.	☐	☐
3 Position a pediatric patient on an Octostop restraint board.	☐	☐

COMMENTS: _____
_____
_____

EVALUATOR'S SIGNATURE: _____

STUDENT'S SIGNATURE: _____

STUDENT NAME: _____ DATE: _____

LAB 13–1: MONITORING PATIENT VITAL SIGNS

Objective

- Measure a patient's vital signs of temperature, pulse, respiration, and blood pressure.

Equipment

- Thermometer
- Blood pressure kit

Procedure

- On completion of this laboratory activity, the student will be able to:

Temperature—Oral Method

	YES	NO
1 Place the oral thermometer under the patient's tongue.	☐	☐
2 Ensure that the thermometer is kept in place until a stable reading is obtained.	☐	☐
3 Read the oral thermometer and record the reading.	☐	☐

Respiration

	YES	NO
1 Measure a patient's respiration by observing the patient's chest or abdomen for a 60-second period.	☐	☐
2 Record the number of respirations per minute.	☐	☐

Pulse

	YES	NO
1 Measure a patient's pulse rate at the radial artery near the wrist for a 60-second period.	☐	☐
2 Record the patient's pulse rate per minute.	☐	☐

Blood Pressure

	YES	NO
1 Obtain a sphygmomanometer and stethoscope.	☐	☐
2 Place the cuff of the sphygmomanometer on the patient's upper arm midway between the elbow and shoulder.	☐	☐
3 Inflate the cuff above the systolic pressure to stop blood flow to the arm.	☐	☐
4 With the stethoscope placed over the brachial artery in the antecubital fossa of the elbow, slowly release the cuff of the sphygmomanometer.	☐	☐
5 When the first sound of blood flow is heard through the stethoscope, record the systolic pressure reading.	☐	☐
6 When the sound of blood flowing through the arm ceases, record the diastolic pressure reading.	☐	☐

COMMENTS: _____
_____
_____

EVALUATOR'S SIGNATURE: _____

STUDENT'S SIGNATURE: _____

STUDENT NAME: _____   DATE: _____

LAB 14-1: PROPER HANDWASHING TECHNIQUE

Objective

■ Demonstrate proper handwashing technique.

Equipment

■ Sink
■ Soap
■ Toweling

Procedure

■ On completion of this laboratory activity, the student will be able to:

		YES	NO
1	Approach the sink. Consider it to be contaminated. Avoid contact with clothing. Use foot or knee levels when available. If not, use toweling to handle all controls. Adjust water flow to avoid splashing. Adjust water temperature to comfort.	☐	☐
2	Wet hands thoroughly with water, keeping the hands lower than the elbows.	☐	☐
3	Apply soap. Soap should be available in liquid form and can be applied by use of foot or knee levers. Soap can also be dispensed from a pump.	☐	☐
4	Use a firm, vigorous, rotary motion, beginning at the wrist and working toward the finger tips. Rub the palms, back of the hands, between the fingers, and under the nails.	☐	☐
5	Rinse and allow water to run down over hands.	☐	☐
6	Repeat the entire process to cleanse from the elbow to the finger tips.	☐	☐
7	Turn off the water. Use toweling on handles if foot or knee levers are not available.	☐	☐
8	Dry from the elbow to the fingertips, never returning to an area.	☐	☐

COMMENTS: _____

_____

_____

EVALUATOR'S SIGNATURE: _____

STUDENT'S SIGNATURE: _____

STUDENT NAME: _____   DATE: _____

LAB 14–2: CONTACT PRECAUTIONS TECHNIQUE

Objective

- Demonstrate the proper method for performing a radiographic examination on a patient with contact precautions.

Equipment

- Cassettes and cassette bags
- Gowns, gloves, caps, masks, goggles
- Portable machine
- Lead aprons

Procedure

- On completion of this laboratory activity, the student will be able to:

		YES	NO
1	Determine the correct number of cassettes needed for the examination and place each cassette into a protective bag.	☐	☐
2	Move the portable machine to the isolated room.	☐	☐
3	Locate the isolation supplies for the room.	☐	☐
4	Remove all ornamentation, including watch, rings, earrings, and other such items, and place them in a pocket.	☐	☐
5	Put on a lead apron.	☐	☐
6	Wash hands as described previously.	☐	☐
7	Put on a clean gown, making sure it is sufficiently long to cover most of the uniform. Pick up the gown from the inside near the armhole openings and gently shake it open. Put one arm in and then the other. First tie the neck strings, then tie the waist strings.	☐	☐
8	Put on a mask, tying it securely, and then a cap. Goggles may also be worn, if available.	☐	☐
9	Put on the gloves. These should be clean but need not be sterile.	☐	☐

		YES	NO
10	Direct an assistant to put on a lead apron, gown, gloves, and a cap.	☐	☐
11	Enter the isolated area and explain to the patient who you are and what you are doing.	☐	☐
12	Position the patient and the cassette.	☐	☐
13	Direct the assistant to manipulate the machine and make the exposure.	☐	☐
14	Remove the cassette from behind the patient. Fold the edge of the protective bag back, never touching the inside.	☐	☐
15	Direct the assistant to remove the cassette, never touching the outside. Place the covering into an appropriate container. Instruct the assistant to remove the portable equipment from the room.	☐	☐
16	Untie the waist ties of the gown.	☐	☐
17	Remove the gloves. Remove the first glove with the other gloved hand, never touching the inside of the glove. Grasp the top of the glove and pull it inside out. Remove the other glove with the exposed hand, touching the inside only. Discard into an appropriate container.	☐	☐
18	Remove the cap and then untie the mask ties, touching the ties only, and remove the mask.	☐	☐
19	Untie the neck ties of the gown and pull the gown forward and down from the shoulders. Pull the gown off so that the sleeves are inside out and the front of the gown is folded inward. Avoid touching the front of the gown. Discard into an appropriate container.	☐	☐
20	Wash hands.	☐	☐
21	Direct the assistant to follow the same protocol. Clean the portable equipment with an antiseptic.	☐	☐
22	Wash hands one last time.	☐	☐

COMMENTS: _____

_____

_____

EVALUATOR'S SIGNATURE: _____

STUDENT'S SIGNATURE: _____

_____

STUDENT NAME: _____ DATE: _____

LAB 15–1: OPENING A STERILE PACKAGE

Objective

- Demonstrate the proper technique for opening a sterile package.

Equipment

- Sterile package and table

Procedure

- On completion of this laboratory activity, the student will be able to:

Open a Sterile Package on a Table

	YES	NO
1 Place the package on the center of the surface with the top flap of the wrapper set to open away from himself or herself.	☐	☐
2 Pinch the first flap on the outside of the wrapper between the thumb and index finger by reaching around (not over) the package. Pull the flap open and lay it flat on the far surface.	☐	☐

	YES	NO
3 Use the right hand to open the right flap and the left hand to open the left flap.	☐	☐
4 Grasp the turned-down corner and pull the fourth and final flap down, being sure not to touch the inner surface of any of the package with an unsterile object such as a sleeve.	☐	☐

Open a Sterile Package While Holding It

	YES	NO
1 Hold the package in one hand with the top flap opening away from himself or herself.	☐	☐
2 Pull the top flap well back and hold it away from both the contents of the package and the sterile field.	☐	☐
3 Drop the contents gently onto the sterile field from about 6 inches above the field and at a slight angle, making sure that the package wrapping does not touch the sterile field at any time.	☐	☐

COMMENTS: _____

_____

_____

EVALUATOR'S SIGNATURE: _____

STUDENT'S SIGNATURE: _____

STUDENT NAME: _____   DATE: _____

LAB 15–2: STERILE GOWNING TECHNIQUE

Objective

■ Demonstrate the proper sterile technique for self-gowning and gowning another.

Equipment

■ Surgical gown

Procedure

■ On completion of this laboratory activity, the student will be able to:

Self-Gowning

	YES	NO
1 Stand about 12 inches from the sterile area, pick up the gown by the folded edges, and lift it directly up from the package.	☐	☐
2 Step back from the table, making sure no objects are near the gown. Grasp the gown at the neck band, hold it at arm's length, unfold it, and gently shake it.	☐	☐
3 Face the inside of the gown and, holding it by the shoulder seams, raise the arms up and slip them into the sleeves.	☐	☐
4 Direct an unsterile assistant to stand behind and reach inside the sleeves, grasp the sleeves, and pull them gently to adjust the gown.	☐	☐

	YES	NO
5 For the open method of gloving, the sleeves are pulled over the hands. For the closed method of gloving, the sleeves are pulled so that only the fingertips are visible.	☐	☐
6 Direct an assistant to fasten the back and waistband of the gown.	☐	☐

Gowning Another

	YES	NO
1 After gowning and gloving using sterile technique, pick up the sterile gown by the neck band, hold it at arm's length, and allow it to unfold.	☐	☐
2 Hold the gown by the shoulder seams with the outside facing himself or herself.	☐	☐
3 Protect the sterile gloves by placing both hands under the back panel of the gown at the top shoulder seam.	☐	☐
4 Direct the person being gowned to slip the arms into the sleeves in a downward motion until the hands emerge from sleeves.	☐	☐
5 Direct the person to pull the gown over the arms and shoulders and fasten the back and waistband of the gown.	☐	☐

COMMENTS: _____

_____

_____

EVALUATOR'S SIGNATURE: _____

STUDENT'S SIGNATURE: _____

STUDENT NAME: _____ DATE: _____

LAB 15–3: STERILE GLOVING TECHNIQUE

Objective

- Demonstrate proper sterile technique for the closed and open methods of self-gloving and for gloving another.

Equipment

- Surgical gloves
- Surgical gown

Procedure

- On completion of this laboratory activity, the student will be able to:

Self-Gloving: Closed Method

		YES	NO
1	Have an assistant open the glove package so that the right glove is on his or her right side.	□	□
2	Keep the hands and fingers covered by the sterile gown when grasping the gloves.	□	□
3	Pick up the glove of the dominant hand with the nondominant hand.	□	□
4	Place the palm of the glove on the palm of the dominant hand with the fingers of the glove facing the elbow.	□	□
5	Grasp the bottom part of the cuff with the fingers of the dominant hand. With the nondominant hand, grasp the top part of the cuff and pull it over the dominant hand.	□	□
6	Pick up the other glove with the gloved hand.	□	□
7	With the ungloved hand, hold the cuff through the sterile gown.	□	□
8	Using the gloved hand, pull the other hand into the glove.	□	□
9	Adjust the fingers until comfortable.	□	□

Self-Gloving: Open Method

		YES	NO
1	With the hands pushed through the sleeves of the sterile gown, pick up the cuff of the dominant hand glove with the nondominant hand, being sure not to touch the outside surface of the glove.	□	□
2	Slip the dominant hand into the glove and pull the glove on by the nondominant hand.	□	□
3	Pick up the other glove by reaching under the cuff with the gloved (and now sterile) dominant hand, being sure to touch only the outside surface of the glove with the sterile gloved hand.	□	□
4	Pull the glove onto the nondominant hand without touching the inside surface of the glove (which is actually the outside surface of the folded cuff).	□	□

Gloving Another

		YES	NO
1	After gloving using sterile technique, open the sterile package and pick up the gloves.	□	□
2	After informing the person being gloved which hand to use, grasp the cuff and pull sideways to open the glove, with the thumb facing the hand to be gloved. Be sure to have an extremely good grasp on the cuff, as considerable force will be exerted when the hand is pushed down into the tight glove.	□	□
3	Direct the person being gloved to keep the thumb away from the glove to avoid possible contact and then put the hand in the glove using a downward motion.	□	□
4	Repeat the process for the other hand.	□	□

COMMENTS: _____

_____

_____

EVALUATOR'S SIGNATURE: _____

STUDENT'S SIGNATURE: _____

_____

STUDENT NAME: _____   DATE: _____

LAB 16–1: ASSISTING PATIENTS WITH URINAL/ BEDPAN

Objective

- Demonstrate proper technique for assisting a patient with a urinal and a bedpan.

Equipment

- Urinal
- Bedpan
- Gloves

Procedure

- On completion of this laboratory activity, the student will be able to:

Assist a Patient With a Urinal

	YES	NO
1 Put on clean, disposable gloves and raise the cover sheet sufficiently to permit adequate visibility while being careful not to expose the patient excessively.	□	□
2 Spread the patient's legs and place the urinal between them. Place the penis into the urinal far enough so that it does not slip out, and hold the urinal in place by the handle until the patient finishes voiding.	□	□
3 Remove the urinal, empty it, remove the gloves, and wash hands.	□	□

Assist a Patient With a Bedpan

	YES	NO
1 Remove the bedpan cover and place it at the end of the table.	□	□
2 If the patient is able to move, place one hand under the lower back and ask the patient to raise the hips. Place the pan under the hips, being sure the patient is covered with a sheet.	□	□
3 Direct the patient to sit up, if possible, so that the head is elevated about 60 degrees.	□	□
4 When the patient has finished using the bedpan, put on clean, disposable gloves. Direct the patient to lie back. Place one hand under the lumbar area and instruct the patient to raise up at the hips.	□	□
5 Remove the pan, cover it, and empty it in the designated area. Rinse it clean with cold water and return it to the area where used equipment is placed.	□	□
6 Offer the patient a wet paper towel or washcloth to wash hands and a paper towel to dry them. Remove the gloves and wash hands.	□	□

COMMENTS: _____
_____
_____

EVALUATOR'S SIGNATURE: _____

STUDENT'S SIGNATURE: _____

STUDENT NAME: _____ DATE: _____

LAB 17-1: THE HEIMLICH MANEUVER

Objective

- Simulate the Heimlich maneuver on a conscious adult, an unconscious adult, a pregnant victim, and an infant.

Equipment

- None

Procedure

- On completion of this laboratory activity, the student will be able to:

The Conscious Adult

	YES	NO
1 Assess the victim to determine if he or she is choking.	☐	☐
2 Stand behind the victim and wrap both arms around him or her, clutching one fist with the other hand.	☐	☐
3 Place the thumb side of the fist at the midline of the victim's abdomen, above the navel and well below the sternum.	☐	☐
4 Hold the elbows out from the victim, and exert pressure inward and upward.	☐	☐
5 Administer each thrust separately, repeating the procedure quickly six to ten times or until the obstructing object is expelled.	☐	☐

The Unconscious Adult

	YES	NO
1 Place the unconscious patient in the supine position.	☐	☐
2 Kneel astride the victim, and place the heel of one hand in the midline of the abdomen, above the navel and well below the sternum. Place the second hand directly on top of the first and apply pressure in a quick upward thrust.	☐	☐
3 Repeat the procedure until the obstructing object is expelled.	☐	☐

The Pregnant Victim

	YES	NO
1 Stand behind the pregnant victim; placing both arms under the victim's armpits and around the victim's chest. Place the thumb side of the fist in the center of the sternum and the second hand over the fist.	☐	☐
2 Apply backward thrusts until the obstructing object is expelled.	☐	☐

The Infant Victim

	YES	NO
1 Hold the infant along your arm with the head lower than the trunk and support the infant by holding the jaw.	☐	☐
2 Rest the arm holding the infant on your thigh, and, using the heel of the hand, deliver four back blows between the infant's scapulae.	☐	☐
3 Continue to support the head and neck, and turn the infant over.	☐	☐
4 Place the index finger on the sternum just below the intermammary line. Using two or three fingers, deliver four chest thrusts.	☐	☐
5 Alternately repeat back blows and chest thrusts until the obstructing object is expelled.	☐	☐

COMMENTS: _____

_____

EVALUATOR'S SIGNATURE: _____

STUDENT'S SIGNATURE: _____

STUDENT NAME: _____ DATE: _____

LAB 18–1: FILLING A SYRINGE FROM AN AMPULE AND A VIAL

Objective

- Demonstrate proper technique for filling a syringe from an ampule and a vial.

Equipment

- Glass ampule
- Vial
- Syringe
- Needle

Procedure

- On completion of this laboratory activity, the student will be able to:

Fill a Syringe From a Glass Ampule

	YES	NO
1 Direct an assistant to flick the top of the neck of the ampule until all the liquid is at the bottom of the container.	☐	☐
2 Direct the assistant to snap off the top of the ampule with a gauze pad.	☐	☐
3 Open a syringe package. Open a needle package and insert the needle on the end of the syringe without letting the end of the syringe or the end of the needle touch anything but each other.	☐	☐
4 Withdraw the contents of the ampule, being careful not to let the shaft of the needle touch the broken edge of the ampule.	☐	☐
5 After use, dispose of the ampule, syringe, and needle into an acceptable "sharps" biohazard container.	☐	☐

Fill a Syringe From a Vial

	YES	NO
1 Break the seal, expose the rubber stopper, and wipe the stopper with an alcohol swab.	☐	☐
2 Open a syringe package and pull back the syringe plunger to pull air into the syringe equal to the amount of drug that will be withdrawn from the vial.	☐	☐
3 Open a needle package and insert the needle on the end of the syringe without letting the end of the syringe or the end of the needle touch anything but each other.	☐	☐
4 Invert the vial and, with the dominant hand, insert the needle without letting the tip of the needle touch anything but the rubber stopper of the vial.	☐	☐
5 With the tip of the needle in the fluid, inject air equal to the volume of drug to be removed. Pull back on the plunger until the correct amount of drug has been drawn into the syringe.	☐	☐
6 Remove the needle and hold the syringe with the needle pointing up while tapping it with a finger to move any air bubble toward the hub where it can be expelled by gently pushing on the plunger of the syringe.	☐	☐
7 After use, dispose of entire syringe and needle into an acceptable sharps biohazard container.	☐	☐

COMMENTS: _____

_____

_____

EVALUATOR'S SIGNATURE: _____

STUDENT'S SIGNATURE: _____

STUDENT NAME: _____ DATE: _____

LAB 18–2: PREPARING A DRIP INFUSION SET-UP

Objective

- Demonstrate the proper technique for setting up a drip infusion set.

Equipment

- IV pole
- Drip infusion set
- Saline solution bag

Procedure

- On completion of this laboratory activity, the student will be able to:

	YES	NO
1 Remove the administration set from the box and straighten the tubing while checking for any cracks or holes.	☐	☐
2 Slide the clamp up to the drip chamber and close it.	☐	☐

	YES	NO
3 Place the bag on a hard surface, remove the protective cap from the tubing insertion port on the bag, and wipe it with an alcohol sponge.	☐	☐
4 Remove the protective cap from the spike on the drip chamber of the tubing and insert the spike into the port.	☐	☐
5 Check again to make certain the clamp is closed, hang the bag on the IV pole, and squeeze the drip chamber until it is half full.	☐	☐
6 Prime the IV set-up by removing the protective cap from the end of the tubing and holding it over a sink or wastebasket.	☐	☐
7 Taking care to preserve the sterility of the cap and of the end of the tubing, release the clamp and allow the solution to run freely until all air bubbles are cleared from the tubing.	☐	☐
8 Reclamp the tubing to stop the flow and replace the protective cap over the end of the tubing.	☐	☐

COMMENTS: _____
_____
_____

EVALUATOR'S SIGNATURE: _____

STUDENT'S SIGNATURE: _____

STUDENT NAME: _____ DATE: _____

LAB 18–3: VENIPUNCTURE AND INTRAVENOUS DRUG INJECTION

Objective

- Demonstrate the proper technique for venipuncture and intravenous drug injection.

Equipment

- Disposable gloves
- Butterfly needle
- Syringe
- Venipuncture Training Arm Kit

Procedure

- On completion of this laboratory activity, the student will be able to:

	YES	NO
1 Wash hands thoroughly.	☐	☐
2 Check the patient's identification.	☐	☐
3 Explain the procedure to the patient.	☐	☐
4 Assemble all needed supplies and prepare the drug for administration.	☐	☐
5 Put on disposable gloves.	☐	☐
6 Once an appropriate site for venipuncture has been selected, cleanse it with an alcohol swab, using a circular motion while moving from the center to the outside.	☐	☐
7 Apply a tourniquet above the site, using sufficient tension to impede the flow of blood in the vein. Ask the patient to open and close the fist to distend the vein fully. When the vein has been identified, ask the patient to hold the fist in a clenched position.	☐	☐
8 To stabilize the vein, place the thumb on the tissue just below the site and gently pull the skin and vein toward the hand.	☐	☐
9 Hold the needle with the bevel facing upward. Pinch the wings of the butterfly needle together tightly.	☐	☐
10 Insert the needle next to the vein at a 15-degree angle and gently advance it into the vein. Blood will flow back into the tubing when the needle is correctly positioned.	☐	☐
11 If the tubing of the butterfly needle has not previously been filled with solution, allow the blood to flow from the hub before attaching the syringe to ensure that no air bubbles are contained in the system.	☐	☐
12 Remove the tourniquet and inject the drug.	☐	☐
13 Unless otherwise instructed, remove the needle and apply gentle pressure to the site with an alcohol swab.	☐	☐
14 Dispose of the syringe and needle properly.	☐	☐
15 Chart all relevant information.	☐	☐

COMMENTS: _____

_____

_____

EVALUATOR'S SIGNATURE: _____

STUDENT'S SIGNATURE: _____

THE AMERICAN REGISTRY OF RADIOLOGIC TECHNOLOGISTS' CODE OF ETHICS

The Code of Ethics forms the first part of the *Standards of Ethics*. The Code of Ethics shall serve as a guide by which Registered Technologists and Applicants may evaluate their professional conduct as it relates to patients, health care consumers, employers, colleagues, and other members of the health care team. The Code of Ethics is intended to assist Registered Technologists and Applicants in maintaining a high level of ethical conduct and in providing for the protection, safety, and comfort of patients. The Code of Ethics is aspirational.

1 The Radiologic Technologist conducts himself or herself in a professional manner, responds to patient needs, and supports colleagues and associates in providing quality patient care.

2 The Radiologic Technologist acts to advance the principal objective of the profession to provide services to humanity with full respect for the dignity of mankind.

3 The Radiologic Technologist delivers patient care and service unrestricted by the concerns of personal attributes or the nature of the disease or illness, and without discrimination, regardless of sex, race, creed, religion, or socioeconomic status.

4 The Radiologic Technologist practices technology founded on theoretical knowledge and concepts, utilizes equipment and accessories consistent with the purposes for which they have been designed, and employs procedures and techniques appropriately.

5 The Radiologic Technologist assesses situations, exercises care, discretion, and judgment, assumes responsibility for professional decisions, and acts in the best interest of the patient.

6 The Radiologic Technologist acts as an agent through observation and communication to obtain pertinent information for the physician to aid in the diagnosis and treatment management of the patient, and recognizes that interpretation and diagnosis are outside the scope of practice for the profession.

7 The Radiologic Technologist utilizes equipment and accessories, employs techniques and procedures, performs services in accordance with an accepted standard of practice, and demonstrates expertise in limiting the radiation exposure to the patient, self, and other members of the health care team.

8 The Radiologic Technologist practices ethical conduct appropriate to the profession and protects the patient's right to quality radiologic technology care.

9 The Radiologic Technologist respects confidences entrusted in the course of professional practice, respects the patient's right to privacy, and reveals confidential information only as required by law or to protect the welfare of the individual or the community.

10 The Radiologic Technologist continually strives to improve knowledge and skills by participating in educational and professional activities, sharing knowledge with colleagues, and investigating new and innovative aspects of professional practice. One means available to improve knowledge and skill is through professional continuing education.

YOUR RIGHTS AS A HOSPITAL PATIENT*

We consider you a partner in your hospital care. When you are well informed, participate in treatment decisions, and communicate openly with your doctor and other health professionals, you help make your care as effective as possible. This hospital encourages respect for the personal preferences and values of each individual.

While you are a patient in the hospital, your rights include the following:

- You have the right to considerate and respectful care.
- You have the right to be well informed about your illness, possible treatments, and likely outcome and to discuss this information with your doctor. You have the right to know the names and roles of people treating you.
- You have the right to consent to or refuse a treatment, as permitted by law, throughout your hospital stay. If you refuse a recommended treatment, you will receive other needed and available care.
- You have the right to have an advance directive, such as a living will or health care proxy. These documents express your choices about your future care or name someone to decide if you cannot speak for yourself. If you have a written advance directive, you should provide a copy to the hospital, your family, and your doctor.
- You have the right to privacy. The hospital, your doctor, and others caring for you will protect your privacy as much as possible.
- You have the right to expect that treatment records are confidential unless you have given permission to release information or reporting is required or permitted by law. When the hospital releases records to others, such as insurers, it emphasizes that the records are confidential.
- You have the right to review your medical records and to have the information explained, except when restricted by law.
- You have the right to expect that the hospital will give you necessary health services to the best of its ability. Treatment, referral, or transfer may be recommended. If transfer is recommended or requested, you will be informed of risks, benefits, and alternatives. You will not be transferred until the other institution agrees to accept you.
- You have the right to know if this hospital has relationships with outside parties that may influence your treatment and care. These relationships may be with educational institutions, other health care providers, or insurers.
- You have the right to consent or decline to take part in research affecting your care. If you choose not to take part, you will receive the most effective care the hospital otherwise provides.
- You have the right to be told of realistic care alternatives when hospital care is no longer appropriate.
- You have the right to know about hospital rules that affect you and your treatment and about charges and payment methods. You have the right to know about hospital resources, such as patient representatives or ethics committees, that can help you resolve problems and questions about your hospital stay and care.

---

*Reprinted by permission of the American Hospital Association, © Copyright 1992.

You have responsibilities as a patient. You are responsible for providing information about your health, including past illnesses, hospital stays, and use of medicine. You are responsible for asking questions when you do not understand information or instructions. If you believe you can't follow through with your treatment, you are responsible for telling your doctor.

This hospital works to provide care efficiently and fairly to all patients and the community. You and your visitors are responsible for being considerate of the needs of other patients, staff, and the hospital. You are responsible for providing information for insurance and for working with the hospital to arrange payment, when needed.

Your health depends not just on your hospital care but, in the long term, on the decisions you make in your daily life. You are responsible for recognizing the effect of life-style on your personal health.

A hospital serves many purposes. Hospitals work to improve people's health; treat people with injury and disease; educate doctors, health professionals, patients, and community members; and improve understanding of health and disease. In carrying out these activities, this institution works to respect your values and dignity.

ANSWERS TO REVIEW QUESTIONS

CHAPTER 1	CHAPTER 2	CHAPTER 3	CHAPTER 4
1 C	1 B	1 D	1 B
2 C	2 D	2 D	2 D
3 D	3 B	3 B	3 E
4 C	4 B	4 C	4 B
5 C	5 D	5 B	5 C
6 B	6 C	6 A	6 E
7 A	7 D	7 C	7 E
8 D	8 B	8 D	8 D
9 B	9 A	9 A	9 E
10 D	10 D	10 B	10 B

CHAPTER 5	CHAPTER 6	CHAPTER 7	CHAPTER 8
1 C	1 B	1 C	1 C
2 D	2 A	2 A	2 D
3 B	3 D	3 B	3 A
4 A	4 C	4 D	4 B
5 B	5 A	5 B	5 C
6 C	6 D	6 A	6 C
7 A	7 D	7 C	7 C
8 A	8 D	8 A	8 A
9 A	9 A	9 D	9 D
10 D	10 C	10 A	10 B

CHAPTER 9	CHAPTER 10	CHAPTER 11	CHAPTER 12
1 A	1 C	1 B	1 B
2 D	2 C	2 C	2 B
3 B	3 A	3 D	3 A
4 A	4 D	4 D	4 C
5 D	5 A	5 D	5 B
6 D	6 A	6 B	6 D
7 D	7 D	7 A	7 C
8 A	8 D	8 A	8 C
9 C	9 D	9 C	9 D
10 C	10 B	10 C	10 A

CHAPTER 13	CHAPTER 14	CHAPTER 15	CHAPTER 16
1 B	1 C	1 D	1 A
2 C	2 A	2 A	2 C
3 A	3 D	3 B	3 B
4 A	4 B	4 B	4 C
5 D	5 D	5 C	5 B
6 C	6 A	6 B	6 D
7 D	7 B	7 B	7 B
8 A	8 D	8 A	8 B
9 B	9 C	9 A	9 A
10 D	10 D	10 B	10 A

CHAPTER 17	CHAPTER 18	CHAPTER 19	CHAPTER 20
1 A	1 D	1 C	1 D
2 C	2 A	2 C	2 D
3 D	3 B	3 D	3 D
4 D	4 D	4 A	4 D
5 C	5 D	5 B	5 C
6 B	6 A	6 A	6 D
7 B	7 B	7 B	7 C
8 C	8 C	8 D	8 E
9 D	9 C	9 A	9 A
10 C	10 B	10 C	10 B

CHAPTER 21	CHAPTER 22
1 B	**1** A
2 A	**2** C
3 C	**3** B
4 B	**4** D
5 A	**5** B
6 C	**6** C
7 B	**7** D
8 A	**8** B
9 A	**9** D
10 D	**10** C

Index

Page numbers in *italics* denote illustrations; page numbers followed by t refer to tables.

409